ANTIANXIETY AGENTS

Drugs in psychiatry

Volume 2

1984

ELSEVIER
AMSTERDAM · NEW YORK · OXFORD

Antianxiety agents

Edited by

GRAHAM D. BURROWS
TREVOR R. NORMAN
and
BRIAN DAVIES

Department of Psychiatry,
University of Melbourne,
Australia

1984

ELSEVIER
AMSTERDAM · NEW YORK · OXFORD

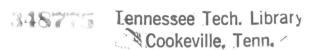

ISBN Vol. 2: 0-444-80555-9
ISBN Series: 0-444-80490-0

Vol. 1: Antidepressants, Burrows/Norman/Davies (eds) 1983.

PUBLISHED BY:

Elsevier Science Publishers B.V.
P.O. Box 211
1000 AE Amsterdam
The Netherlands

SOLE DISTRIBUTORS FOR THE U.S.A. AND CANADA:

Elsevier Science Publishing Company, Inc.
52 Vanderbilt Avenue,
New York, N.Y. 10017
U.S.A.

Library of Congress Cataloging in Publication Data
Main entry under title:

Antianixiety agents.

  (Drugs in psychiatry ; v. 2)
  Includes index.
  1. Antidepressants. I. Burrows, Graham D. II. Norman, Trevor R., 1946-   . III. Davies, Brian, 1928-   . IV. Series. [DNLM: 1. Anxiety disorders–Drug therapy. 2. Tranquilizing agents, Minor. Wl DR893T v.2. / QV 77.9 A629]
RM332.A56 1984   616.85'27061   84-1477
ISBN 0-444-80555-9

Printed in the Netherlands

Preface

This volume on antianxiety agents is the second of a series on drugs used in psychiatry. It was decided to attempt to cover the area from basic pharmacology to clinical applications. Frequently, volumes on this subject highlight one aspect only. We hope this volume will be suitable for the researcher, the specialist and the general practitioner. The third volume to follow will be on *Antipsychotics*.

We are extremely grateful for the exceptional editorial assistance of Mrs. Gertrude Rubinstein.

GRAHAM D. BURROWS
TREVOR R. NORMAN
BRIAN DAVIES

List of contributors

Darrell R. Abernethy   79
  Tufts University School of Medicine, Boston, U.S.A.

Thomas A. Ban   143
  *Tennessee Neuropsychiatric Institute and Vanderbilt
  University, Nashville, Tennessee, U.S.A.*

Graham D. Burrows   1, 33, 93
  *Department of Psychiatry, University of Melbourne, Austin
  Hospital, Heidelberg, Victoria, Australia*

Brian Davies   1
  *Department of Psychiatry, University of Melbourne, Royal
  Melbourne Hospital, Victoria, Australia*

Marcia Divoll   79
  *Tufts University School of Medicine and New England
  Medical Center, Boston, Massachusetts, U.S.A.*

Sandra E. File   13
  *Department of Pharmacology, The School of Pharmacy,
  University of London, U.K.*

Ann Fulton   33, 71
  *Department of Biochemistry, The Blood Bank, South
  Melbourne, Victoria, Australia*

Silvio Garattini 43
Istituto di Ricerche Farmacologiche 'Mario Negri', Milan,
Italy

Louis A. Gottschalk 157, 177
Department of Psychiatry and Human Behavior, University
of California, Irvine Medical Center, Orange, California,
U.S.A.

David J. Greenblatt 79
Division of Clinical Pharmacology, New England Medical
Center Hospital, Boston, Massachusetts, U.S.A.

Ian Hindmarch 217
Human Psychopharmacology Research Unit, University of
Leeds, Leeds, U.K.

Leo E. Hollister 107
Department of Psychiatry and Pharmacology, Stanford
University School of Medicine, Stanford, California, U.S.A.

Malcolm Lader 127
Department of Pharmacology, Institute of Psychiatry,
University of London, Decrespigny Park, London, U.K.

Kay P. Maguire 71
Department of Psychiatry, University of Melbourne, Royal
Melbourne Hospital, Victoria, Australia

Richard J. Moldawsky 177
Department of Psychiatry and Human Behavior, University
of California, Irvine Medical Center, Orange, California,
U.S.A.

Trevor R. Norman 33, 93, 199
Department of Psychiatry, University of Melbourne, Austin
Hospital, Heidelberg, Victoria, Australia

Hermann R. Ochs 79
Medizinische Universitätsklinik, University of Bonn,
Bonn-Bad Godesberg, F.R.G.

Contents

Burrows/Norman/Davies (eds) Antianxiety agents
© *Elsevier Science Publishers B.V., 1984*

Chapter 1

Recognition and management of anxiety

GRAHAM D. BURROWS

University of Melbourne, Austin Hospital, Heidelberg, Australia

and

BRIAN DAVIES

University of Melbourne, Royal Melbourne Hospital, Australia

Anxiety symptoms are among the most common that are presented to family doctors and specialists. For efficient management correct diagnosis is required, so that the appropriate drug can be chosen and combined with nonpharmacological therapy. It is important to recognize and distinguish anxiety states from related disorders such as depression which responds to antidepressants rather than antianxiety drugs. These issues have aroused increasing interest with the development of new drugs which combine antianxiety and antidepressant properties (see Chapter 13).

Everyone experiences a certain degree of anxiety, which serves a useful function by inducing arousal, and enables us to 'rise to the occasion'. However, a prolonged state of anxiety will result in a state of continuing stress. The stress response, 'fight or flight', was evolved for short-term emergency needs, with a built-in homoeostatic control for return to normal physiological conditions. The anxious person, who shows exaggerated responses to the ordinary stresses of everyday life, cannot reduce his state of arousal, and maintains a prolonged alarm reaction which results in diminished coping and reduced functioning.

DEFINITION

The term anxiety involves two distinct components, a subjective experience and a pattern of behaviour observed by others of the anxious person. An 'operational' definition of anxiety used by neurophysiologists, psychologists and psychobiologists has been derived from the subjective definition. Anxiety is a characteristic, unpleasant emotion induced by the anticipation of danger or frustration which threatens the security or homoeostasis of the individual or the group to which he or she belongs. Pathological or morbid anxiety refers to the occurrence of anxiety of a severity, frequency or duration which interferes with well-being or efficiency.

The term 'anxiety state' refers to a disorder in which anxiety is the primary and dominant part of the clinical picture, with the mood being relatively fixed and persistent. The state may be acute or chronic, and may vary in intensity and severity. State anxiety is a 'here and now' phenomenon, it is anxiety experienced at a given moment of time; trait anxiety refers to an habitual tendency to be anxious. A high proportion of patients will have suffered from anxiety of prolonged duration, with remissions and relapses, in general the aim with these patients is to help them over difficult periods. Restoring them to a completely normal baseline may be difficult or impossible. Acute or state anxiety may be much easier to manage.

Occurrence of anxiety

The prevalence of anxiety states has been given as 2–5% of the total population and 7–16% of psychiatric patients. Of the 15% who suffer some form of mental disorder through the year (U.S. figures) more than half will be treated by their general practitioner (Brown et al., 1979). Half of all these disorders are neuroses, mild to moderate depressions or anxiety states. In addition, anxiety states are often associated with organic disorders, either as causative factors or as secondary consequences. In either case they are exacerbating conditions. Balter (1974) found that an antianxiety drug was prescribed on 12% of all office visits. Since patients with mental disorders have a higher rate of organic illness, they must visit their doctor more often and receive more prescriptions (Eastwood and Trevelyan, 1972). This means that the general practitioner sees the majority of patients suffering from anxiety, whether as presenting complaint or associated disorder. All age groups are subject to anxiety, from the child with separation anxiety to the elderly patient who is anxious about his failing health. The doctor needs to be able to recognize it in all its manifestations and possess the basic skills for its management.

Causes of anxiety

There are at least two forms of anxiety, differing in causation from each other. The patient may be suffering from primary or 'free-floating' anxiety, a feeling of impending disaster, of fearful anticipation, or a worry that he is 'going mad'. This usually represents a maladaptive response to an anxiety-provoking situation, but one in which the intensity of emotion provoked is out of all proportion to the stimulus. In contrast, anxiety may be secondary to organic disease, due to concern about the course and outcome of the disease. This is more properly termed fear or apprehension, and is an appropriate response to a threat of danger. Obviously these two classes of patients require different treatments. Not all anxious patients will admit to their anxiety and the doctor may have to elicit the true cause of their problem. The alert doctor will recognize the signs of anxiety, but will not be distracted by bodily symptoms or the co-existence of physical illness, and will offer the kind of treatment that is appropriate.

Recognition of anxiety

The prevalence of anxiety seems to be fairly constant through all age groups, but the young report psychological complaints more frequently, whereas the older patient tends to do so through physical complaints.

Somatic symptoms. Anxiety symptoms are both somatic and psychological, but it is usually the somatic complaints that are first presented to the doctor. The patient with an anxiety state may have a tense, apprehensive attitude, with the increased muscle tension being shown in the facial expression and posture. The patient may have difficulty in relaxing, and may sit on the edge of the chair during the interview, jumping at sudden noise. Tremors may be visible if muscle tension is marked. The palpebral fissures tend to be wide and the pupils dilated. The patient may lick his lips as the mouth tends to be dry. Other bodily concomitants include aches and pains, sweating – particularly the palms, axillae and forehead. Tachycardia, palpitations, increased blood pressure and peripheral vasoconstriction of the hands and feet give rise to the typical pallor and cold extremities, whereas the arterioles of the blushing area of the neck and upper chest are usually dilated. Anxiety patients tend to have shallow breathing, sometimes with sighing respiration. Occasionally appetite is impaired but usually over-eating occurs.

Some patients do not present overt symptoms of anxiety, but complain of bodily symptoms like tension headaches, inability to take a deep breath, constriction or pain in the chest, muscle aches and pains, muscle stiffness, palpitations or gastrointestinal symptoms. The patient may actually be convinced that he is suffering from some dreaded disease.

Anxiety may be present to a high degree in painful conditions. Pain is a subjective experience involving autonomic and defense reactions, but emotional elements may become associated through neuronal elements of the hypothalamus, limbic system and cortical association areas. In their bodily manifestations the various forms of anxiety and fear demonstrate the same autonomic stress symptoms as intense pain. Although benzodiazepines are useful for the relief of muscle spasm (see Chapter 8), antidepressants rather than antianxiety agents are indicated for the relief of severe chronic pain (see Volume 4).

Psychological symptoms.   Most patients will, if asked, describe the anxious, uptight feeling that usually accompanies the somatic symptoms, or the unpleasant feeling may be present without any somatic complaints. The patient may develop worrying thoughts about his somatic symptoms, with intercurrent personal problems acquiring disproportionate dimensions. All of these keep him awake at night when he tries to sleep. He may feel more secure in familiar company than when alone, but uncomfortable with strangers or authority figures. His fears may be specific, or phobic anxiety such as fear of fainting in a large crowd, crossing an open space, having difficulty with speech, and so forth. The patient may also be suffering from 'free-floating' anxiety, experiencing feelings of impending disaster. He is over-alert, with no relaxation of his alertness. He develops irritability with those around him, and with himself for being unreasonable.

Physical examination.   It is important not to ignore the need for a physical examination. With both organic and psychological illnesses, anxiety is commonly present. The diagnosis of anxiety and evaluation of its severity require recognition of the signs of anxiety and any other disease, and the relative importance of each (See Fig. 1). A physical examination will not only detect the occasional physical problem such as thyrotoxicosis or hypoglycaemia which give rise to a classical anxiety reaction, but will reassure the patient in the absence of these conditions. In addition, it helps to establish a rapport with the patient, which will play a large part in successful management.

DIFFERENTIAL DIAGNOSIS AND CLASSIFICATION

The basis of good treatment is a proper diagnosis. Recent trends in the nosology of psychiatric disorders have grouped anxiety states under the headings – *Panic Disorder, Generalized Anxiety Disorder* and *Obsessive Compulsive Disorder*. In addition, there are the related *Simple Phobias*.

Diagnostic criteria for *panic attacks* are that discrete periods of apprehension and fear are accompanied by at least four of the following: choking or smothering sensations; feelings of unreality; dizziness; vertigo or unsteady feelings; paraesthesias; hot and cold flushes; sweating; faintness; trembling or shaking; and fear of dying, going crazy, or doing something uncontrolled during an attack. If panic attacks occur at least once a week during 3 weeks and they appear in situations other than during physical exertion or life-threatening situations, the clinical picture will be diagnosed as panic disorder (DSM III).

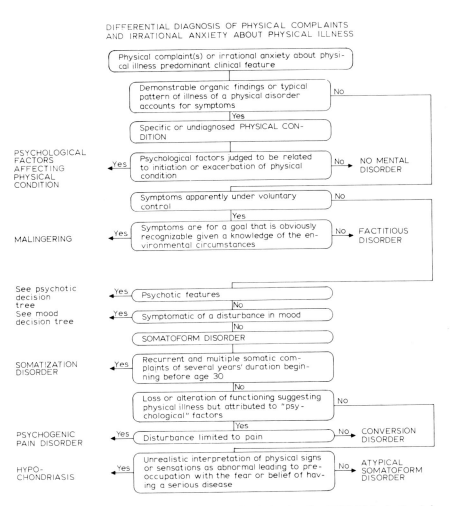

DIFFERENTIAL DIAGNOSIS OF PHYSICAL COMPLAINTS
AND IRRATIONAL ANXIETY ABOUT PHYSICAL ILLNESS

Fig. 1. Decision tree for anxiety/physical illness discrimination. See DSM III for further information. From DSM III (Mini-D) pp. 206–207. American Psychiatric Association, Washington D.C.

In *Generalized Anxiety Disorder*, the essential feature is generalized and persistent anxiety of at least one month's duration and without any of the specific symptoms which characterize *Phobic Disorders*, *Panic Disorders* or *Obsessive Compulsive Disorder* or any other physical or mental disorder. Symptoms are manifest from three of the following categories: motor tension; autonomic hyperactivity; apprehensive expectation; vigilance and scanning. In *Panic Disorder*, there is often chronic generalized anxiety between panic attacks; if these are overlooked an incorrect diagnosis of *Generalized Anxiety Disorder* may be made.

The essential feature of *Obsessive Compulsive Disorder* is the presence of persistent, recurrent ideas, thoughts or impulses that invade consciousness and are experienced as senseless and repugnant (obsessions), or repetitive, stereotyped behaviours (compulsions). Compulsive behaviour may provide a release of tension, without any pleasurable feelings. Depression and anxiety frequently accompany obsessive compulsive disorder.

In *Agoraphobia* with panic attacks, the patient avoids being outside alone, being in public places such as crowds, tunnels or bridges, and utilizing public transportation. Both panic attacks and agoraphobia result in considerable impairment.

The above diagnoses should not be made if due to a physical disorder or another mental disorder such as major depression, somatization disorder or schizophrenia (DSM III).

Anxiety or depression

Anxiety appearing for the first time in middle-aged or elderly patients must make the doctor consider whether the anxiety symptoms are the presenting features of a depressive illness. This is important since specific antidepressant treatment is likely to be helpful in the latter. Important depressive symptoms to ask about are: 1) loss of interest in work and recreation; 2) inability to concentrate; 3) guilty, self-depreciatory thoughts; 4) tiredness; 5) loss of appetite and weight; 6) waking at night and being unable to fall asleep again. Suicidal thoughts should also be asked about. The actual depressive feeling is described by different patients in different ways, e.g. 'the spark is gone'; or 'it's as if a cloud comes over me'. In all instances, depressive symptoms vary in severity from day-to-day and within the day, with periods of being back to normal. Any problem of diagnosis can then be solved by seeing the patient's spouse or children. A description of a change in the patient – irritability, moodiness with loss of appetite and loss of interest together with sleep disturbance – is characteristic of a depressive illness and should be treated accordingly.

MANAGEMENT OF ANXIETY

The doctor having recognized that the patient is suffering from anxiety has to decide on the appropriate treatment. Unfortunately most research studies reporting on the treatment of anxiety come from psychiatrists who see patients long after the appearance of symptoms, which have already become well established and more or less severely disabling. These cases are obviously the 'failed to respond' at a family practice level, and are in the minority. Although no specifically effective treatment exists, there are a number of measures that will bring symptomatic relief. These may be broadly grouped as psychological and physical therapies. The psychological measures include psychotherapy of the supportive kind, with direct counselling, as well as behavioural modification techniques, autogenic relaxation and medical hypnosis principles. Controlled studies of antianxiety drugs have indicated that they are more effective than placebo in alleviating the symptoms of anxiety. Several studies have compared interpersonal therapy and medication; the consensus is that the combination of psychological and physical intervention surpasses either treatment alone.

Introductory treatment

Supportive care. Interested listening, explanation and reassurance are the basic ingredients of supportive care. They imply an interest in the patient as a person with his own unique development, experiences and response to current life situations.

Explanation. Patients with unpleasant somatic symptoms should be told how bodily symptoms can be caused by emotions. Usually an example helps, e.g. 'you remember how you get palpitations after a near accident in the car?'

Reassurance. The physical examination and explanation of how symptoms occur should reassure the patient about his health. Some patients *will* need investigation and specialist referral, since the occurrence of physical complaints together with anxiety symptoms is not uncommon. The doctor's experience will help him decide the relative importance of these two factors in the particular patient; in some cases this also may need specialist opinion.

Symptomatic treatment – the pharmacological approach

Many drugs relieve anxiety, and alcohol is the one with the longest history. These drugs however all produce sedation, i.e. drowsiness and sleepiness; antianxiety drugs should reduce anxiety without producing undue sedation. The barbiturates, used for many years for anxiety symptoms, should not be used today. The benzodiazepines have considerable advantages over the barbiturates. They are safe on overdosage and have been shown in many trials to produce significant antianxiety effects. Beta-adrenergic blocking agents effectively counter some of the bodily symptoms of anxiety such as palpitations, diarrhoea and sweating, but irritability and worry may not be helped.

The antianxiety drugs are more effective in the treatment of the patient with severe symptoms of anxiety, than when they are moderate or mild. For the patient with milder symptoms, a non-drug therapy is usually more successful. Since anxiety fluctuates in severity over a period, flexible dosage schedules are appropriate, and lower drug consumption is encouraged if the drug is taken only when needed. The patient may learn to tolerate short intervals of anxiety, knowing medication is at hand if needed.

8

The long-term use of benzodiazepines carries with it many problems. Their effectiveness frequently diminishes as tolerance develops. It is highly desirable to make attempts every few months to take the patient off these drugs for as long as possible to diminish dependency problems. There is no convincing evidence that any of the benzodiazepines are therapeutically more effective than the others, but clinical experience shows that individual patients sometimes prefer one particular drug. Despite the accumulation of extensive laboratory data, in particular their half-lives, the precise nature of their mode of action remains unclear. Chapter 8 offers a more detailed account of the clinical use of antianxiety drugs.

Some guidelines that have been found useful for benzodiazepine prescribing in a *Family Medicine Centre* are as follows:

1) Benzodiazepines should be used less frequently with increasing age;
2) short-acting benzodiazepines are preferable to long-acting benzodiazepines in all age groups;
3) patients 65 years of age and over should be given half the daily dosage of benzodiazepines prescribed for under 65;
4) long-term use of benzodiazepines for more than one month, is of minimal or no pharmacological benefit, and should be discouraged (Rosser et al., 1980, Rosser, 1984).

This study uncovered a 'trap' for the unwary physician in that contrary to physicians' perception, the older age group were receiving the highest rate of prescription. This was due to the more frequent visits of the older, chronically ill patient to his doctor.

Response to antianxiety drugs

The effectiveness of antianxiety drugs is well documented in patients suffering from certain forms of anxiety, but they are not effective in all conditions which the DSM III has classified under anxiety disorders. They afford relief in what Freud called actual neuroses (neurasthenia, hypochondriasis and anxiety neuroses), but are not always effective in what he termed transference neuroses (phobias, hysteria and obsessive neuroses) (Grunhaus et al., 1981).

Following the use of iproniazid by West and Dally (1959) in 'atypical depression', Sargant and Dally (1962) found phenelzine efficacious in the treatment of anxiety states. Recent studies have established the value of monoamine oxidase inhibitors in the treatment of phobic and agoraphobic patients, avoidance anxiety and panic attacks, and also hysteroid dysphoria (regarded as a form of separation anxiety in young women following a bereavement). Monoamine oxidase inhibitors, tricyclic antidepressants and beta-blocking agents have all been used for the management of panic attacks, but some recently developed drugs (Chapter 13) show promising results in the treatment of these anxiety-related disorders. See Nies (Volume 1) for clinical applications of MAOIs. Volume 4 will contain a chapter on current advances in the pharmacotherapy of panic attacks, and also a chapter on the management of chronic pain, a condition with which anxiety is frequently associated. Both of these conditions respond better to antidepressant-type drugs than to simple antianxiety compounds.

Symptomatic treatment – the psychological approach

All too frequently the easy shortcut appears to be to prescribe an antianxiety agent rather than to help the patient understand and cope with his anxiety, but it is well known that medication alone is not a complete answer. All patients should receive time to discuss their stress problems and their feelings with an understanding, tolerant doctor who at least attempts to empathize with the patient. Psychotherapy can be described as either 'uncovering' or 'covering'; in general the 'covering', or supportive or directive psychotherapy is the more usual approach for the family doctor. In Chapter 8, Hollister gives some admirably simple but effective hints for 'psychotherapeutic' adjuncts to pharmacotherapy.

In the acute stage of anxiety, the simplest and most effective therapy is to remove the patient from the disturbing factors, sedate with medication, and ensure sleep. Psychological help at this stage should be confined to support, reassurance and simple explanation. In longer-standing anxiety, the treatment aims are twofold. The more severe manifestations of anxiety and associated depression, phobic symptoms, feelings of unreality (depersonalization), and panic attacks need to be brought under control by measures aimed directly at the disabling symptoms. Some attempt should be made to help the patient acquire an understanding of the vulnerable facets in his personality that have contributed, and the manner in which they have arisen.

In general practice, unless the doctor has special training and experience in one or more behavioural/psychotherapeutic approaches, the treatment should be restricted to supportive care and symptomatic treatment with drugs.

Referral to a psychiatrist

No matter how well a doctor usually manages anxious patients, there are times when nothing seems to work, and then referral for psychiatric advice or even a period of hospitalization may be necessary. Patients who fail to improve after a few weeks of active treatment, patients with severe phobic anxiety, or those with symptoms that affect the patient's sexual life are best referred to a psychiatrist. Some patients may benefit from referral for family therapy, marriage counselling, or individual or group therapy; marital stresses have been shown to be very significant in the anxious patient. Patients with long-standing personality problems or

10

difficulties in personal relationships may benefit from the non-pharmacological approach.

CONCLUSION

This introductory chapter has dealt briefly with the recognition and management of anxiety. Chapter 2–7 of this volume deals with research studies aimed at an eventual understanding of the mode of action of antianxiety drugs, which will possibly also help to an understanding of the condition of anxiety. The other seven chapters present clinical aspects of the drug treatment of anxiety; the use of antianxiety drugs and a number of specific problems associated with their usage.

Anxiety disorders are notoriously chronic or recurrent. Two recent advances which may improve management are the changes in the DSM III in an attempt to delineate more accurately their diagnosis and classification, and the development of new drugs with both antianxiety and antidepressant properties.

Medical practitioners must be able to recognize and treat anxiety symptoms. It is also important to recognize that the patient who presents anxiety, but is also suffering from depression, phobia or chronic pain, needs fundamentally different treatment. The benzodiazepines are safe and effective drugs for the relief of anxiety; they should be prescribed on an individual basis. Few experts would recommend drugs as the sole therapy for the management of anxiety. The doctor who has good interaction with a patient who wants to get well, can include drugs as adjunctive therapy. At the same time the doctor should not underestimate the effect of seeing the patient regularly. It is vital to remember, and to help the patient realize, that no drug in itself will solve the problem of anxiety.

REFERENCES

American Psychiatric Association (1980) Diagnostic and Statistical Manual for Mental Disorders (DSM III). American Psychiatric Association, Washington D.C.

Balter, M. B., Levine, J. and Manheimer, D. I. (1974) Cross-national study of the extent ot antianxiety/sedative drug use. N. Engl. J. Med. 290, 769–774.

Brown, B. S., Regier, D. A. and Balter, M. B. (1979) Key interactions among psychiatric disorders, primary care and the use of psychotropic drugs. In: B. S. Brown (Ed.), Clinical Anxiety-Tension in Primary Medicine. Proceedings of a Colloquium, Washington, D.C., 1977. Excerpta Medica, Amsterdam, ICS 448, pp. 3–13.

Burrows, G. D., Norman, T. R. and Davies B. (Eds) (1984) Antimanics, anticonvulsants and other drugs in psychiatry. In: Drugs in Psychiatry, Vol. 4, Elsevier Science Publ., Amsterdam/New York (in preparation).

Eastwood, M. R. and Trevelyan, M. H. (1972) Relationship between physical and psychiatric disorder. Psychol. Med. 2, 363–372.

Grunhaus, L., Gloger, S. and Weisstub, E. (1981) Panic attacks. A review of treatments and pathogenesis. J. Nerv. Ment. Dis. 169, 608–613.

Nies, A. (1983) Clinical applications of MAOIs. In: G. D. Burrows, T. R. Norman and B. Davies (Eds), Drugs in Psychiatry, Vol. 1, Antidepressants. Elsevier Science Publ., Amsterdam/New York, pp. 290–247.

Rosser, W. W. (1984) Physician education in the use of tranquillizers. In: G. D. Burrows and J. S. Werry (Eds), Advances in Human Psychopharmacology, Vol. 3. JAI Press. Greenwich, Conn., pp. 165–186.

Sargant, W. and Dally, P. J. (1962) Treatment of anxiety states by antidepressant drugs. Br. Med. J. 1, 509.

West, E. D. and Dally, P. J. (1959) Effects of iproniazed in depressive illness. Br. Med. J. 1, 1491–1494.

Burrows/Norman/Davies (eds) Antianxiety agents
© *Elsevier Science Publishers B.V., 1984*

Chapter 2

The neurochemistry of anxiety

SANDRA E. FILE

Department of Pharmacology, The School of Pharmacy, University of London, 29/39 Brunswick
Square, London WC1N 1AX, U.K.

INTRODUCTION

There is a contrast between the clinical efficacy of the drugs available to treat anxiety and our knowledge of the underlying neural mechanisms. The benzodiazepines have been in use for 20 years and an understanding of how these drugs work should have revealed the neurochemical basis of anxiety. The discovery of stereospecific benzodiazepine binding sites in the brain (Braestrup and Squires, 1977; Mohler and Okada, 1977) tells us at which receptors the benzodiazepines act, but we still know little of the subsequent neurotransmitter pathways mediating anxiolysis. Since the benzodiazepines have many behavioural effects other than their anxiolytic ones, e.g. amnesic, sedative, anticonvulsive, muscle relaxant, care must be taken that any neurochemical changes that are detected do relate to anxiety reduction rather than to some other behavioural effect of the drugs.

There is evidence that the benzodiazepines enhance GABA-ergic transmission and this has led to a study of the possible role of GABA in anxiety, either directly or indirectly by inhibiting transmission in serotonergic pathways. Hormones have modulatory roles in anxiety and since the discovery of benzodiazepine receptors there has been a search for endogenous anxiolytic or anxiogenic substances. Diverse central and peripheral changes contribute to the biochemistry of anxiety and it is unlikely that a change in any one neurotransmitter will have sole and crucial importance. Even the same neurochemical change, e.g. an enhancement of GABA, may have different consequences in different anatomical areas. The recent introduction of several novel anxiolytics that do not share all the other behavioural effects of the benzodiazepines should aid research into which neuro-chemical changes are crucial to anxiety reduction.

BENZODIAZEPINE RECEPTORS

In 1977 Braestrup and Squires and Mohler and Okada demonstrated the presence of high-affinity binding sites for ^{3}H-diazepam in the rat brain. Since then similar stereospecific binding sites have been found in the CNS of several species, including man. There are good correlations between the affinities of different benzodiazepine derivatives for these sites and their average therapeutic doses in man or their potencies in various pharmacological tests (Braestrup and Squires, 1978; Mohler and Okada, 1978). The benzodiazepine binding sites are widely distributed in the CNS, but there is marked regional variation in their density. To some extent this corresponds to the anatomical regions implicated in the various behavioural actions of benzodiazepines, e.g. frontal cortex and amygdala with anxiolytic effects and cerebellum with ataxia; but some high density areas, e.g. retina and occipital cortex are not yet associated with any marked benzodiazepine action.

The high correlation between the affinities for these sites of various benzodiazepines and their efficacy in a range of behavioural tests suggests that all actions of the benzodiazepines are mediated initially through these receptors. How then is this initial step translated into an anxiolytic action? What other transmitters and modulators are involved and what specific anatomical pathways are concerned?

BENZODIAZEPINES AND GABA

In 1974 Polc et al. provided electrophysiological evidence that diazepam enhanced presynaptic inhibition in the spinal cord, which could be blocked by GABA antagonists and synthesis inhibitors. In the cuneate nucleus both pre- and postsynaptic inhibitions are GABA mediated and both are enhanced by benzodiazepines (Polc and Haefely, 1976). Haefely et al. (1975) proposed that benzodiazepines facilitated GABA inhibition at all sites in the CNS, and Haefely (1978) suggested that the behavioural actions of the benzodiazepines could result from a GABA inhibition of other neurotransmitters.

Support for a functional link between GABA and benzodiazepines came from studies of ^{3}H-diazepam binding. GABA and its analog muscimol enhanced the binding of ^{3}H-diazepam by increasing the affinity of the receptor; this enhanced binding was blocked by the GABA antagonist bicuculline, which acts at the GABA recognition site; but not by picrotoxin, which acts at a different site, the GABA-receptor dependent chloride channel (Tallman et al., 1978). There are regional differences in the magnitude of the GABA potentiation of benzodiazepine binding (Karobath et al., 1979), but it is not clear whether this is due to heterogeneity of benzodiazepine receptors, of GABA receptors or to the extent that the two receptors are coupled. At present there is evidence for a supramole-cular complex with GABA and benzodiazepine receptors, a picrotoxin binding site and a chloride ionophore (Costa et al., 1979; Gallager et al., 1980), with GABA and benzodiazepines acting to open the chloride channel.

Thus both electrophysiological and biochemical evidence supports a functional link between benzodiazepines and GABA. However, not all neurones have shown a benzodiazepine enhancement of GABA inhibition (Curtis et al., 1976; Dray and Straughan, 1976), and in some regions even antagonism has been reported (Gah-wiler, 1976; Steiner and Felix, 1976). Furthermore, the phylogenetic, ontogenet-ic and regional distributions of GABA receptors and benzodiazepine receptors are poorly correlated (Braestrup and Nielsen, 1980), and certainly some GABA receptors are not associated with a benzodiazepine site (Candy and Martin, 1979; Young and Kuhar, 1979). This indicates that whereas some of the behavioural actions of the benzodiazepines might be GABA mediated (e.g. muscle-relaxant effects, Schmidt et al., 1967, and anticonvulsant effects, Haefely, 1980), others may be independent of GABA. What then is the behavioural evidence for the role of GABA in anxiety?

GABA AND ANXIETY

Raising brain GABA levels by preventing its breakdown has no effects in animal tests of anxiety (Cook and Sepinwall, 1975; File and Hyde, 1977; Tye et al., 1979). The GABA agonist muscimol does not produce a reliable anxiolytic profile, although it has a clearly synergistic action with diazepam's depressant effects (Sepinwall and Cook, 1980).

Although the evidence for GABA agonists as anxiolytics is not strong there is a growing body of data implicating the picrotoxin site as one that can mediate anx-iogenic actions. Picrotoxin (2 mg/kg) antagonised the anticonflict effects of oxa-zepam, reflected in a reduction in the number of punished lever presses, whereas unpunished responding was reduced only at 4 mg/kg (Stein et al., 1977). Howev-er, Sepinwall and Cook (1978) found that picrotoxin (2 mg/kg) reduced both punished and unpunished responding. Because picrotoxin reduces spontaneous motor behaviour (Soubrie and Simon, 1978; File, 1982a) there will always be problems distinguishing specific effects on anxiety from non-specific behavioural changes resulting from sedation. However, in three different animal tests picro-toxin and pentylenetetrazole have been shown to have intrinsic anxiogenic effects (Lal and Shearman, 1982; Lal et al., 1982; File and Lister, 1983a; Prado de Carvalho et al., 1983) and the latter, in subconvulsant doses, causes anxiety in man (Rodin et al., 1979).

It has been suggested that benzodiazepines reduce anxiety via a GABA-mediated inhibition of 5-HT (Stein et al., 1975). There is an inhibitory GABA input to the 5-HT cells of the dorsal raphe nucleus (Gallager, 1978), and although benzodiazepines do not alter spontaneous activity of raphe neurones they enhance the GABA-mediated inhibition (Gallager et al., 1980). Injections of high concentrations of chlordiazepoxide ($5 \times 10^{-5}M$) into the dorsal raphe resulted in an anxiolytic profile in a conflict test, as did equi-molar injections of GABA (Thiebot et al., 1980a). However, lower concentrations ($5 \times 10^{-7}M$) of GABA failed to enhance the disinhibitory effects of 5×10^{-9} or $5 \times 10^{-7}M$ chlordiazepoxide, which makes it improbable that a GABA-ergic mechanism is inhibiting 5-HT to reduce anxiety (Thiebot et al., 1980b); there is no evidence that when given systemically the benzodiazepines exert their anxiolytic action by this mechanism.

SEROTONIN (5-HT) AND ANXIETY

There is good evidence that serotonin pathways are involved in some way in anxiety. Parachlorophenylalanine (PCPA), an inhibitor of 5-HT synthesis, produces an anxiolytic profile in several animal tests (Tenen, 1967; Robichaud and Sledge, 1969; Stevens and Fechter, 1969; Geller and Blum, 1970; File and Hyde, 1977; File and Deakin, 1980). Wise et al. (1973) reversed the effects of PCPA by injections of the 5-HT precursor 5-hydroxytryptophan. Injections of the serotonin neurotoxins 5,6 or 5,7-dihydroxytryptamine into the cerebral ventricles or the medial forebrain bundle resulted in anxiolytic profiles (Pelham et al., 1975; Tye et al., 1979).

The effects of intraventricular serotonin in the conflict test were complex and triphasic (Stein et al., 1973), possibly reflecting differing roles of forebrain and spinal 5-HT, but in general were anxiogenic. Likewise, a 5-HT uptake inhibitor had an anxiogenic action in the social interaction test (File, 1981). The effects of 5-HT antagonists depend on the behavioural test. They have an anxiolytic action in conflict tests (Stein et al., 1973; Geller et al., 1974; Cook and Sepinwall, 1975), no effect in the social interaction test (File, 1981) and an anxiogenic action in rats lever-pressing to avoid periaqueductal grey stimulation (Schenberg and Graeff, 1978). The poor pharmacological specificity of the currently available 5-HT antagonists, together with doubts that some of them penetrate the blood-brain barrier, preclude firm conclusions from the effects of these drugs.

Several lines of evidence indicate a particular importance of the dorsal raphe ascending serotonergic system. Stimulation of the dorsal raphe by carbachol has an anxiogenic action that can be reversed by benzodiazepines (Stein et al., 1973), and inhibition of the dorsal raphe by high concentrations of GABA results in an anxiolytic profile (Thiebot et al., 1980b). The application of chlordiazepoxide directly into the dorsal raphe nucleus produces an anxiolytic profile (Thiebot et al., 1980a), as do small 5,7-dihydroxytryptamine lesions of the nucleus (File et al., 1979b). This latter effect was specific to 5-HT since the concentrations of seven amino acids were unchanged (Collins et al., 1979, and Table 1), and injections of the catecholamine neurotoxin, 6-hydroxydopamine, into the dorsal raphe did not

TABLE 1

Cortical amino acid concentrations (μmole/g wet weight) in control (vehicle injected) animals and in those with 5,7-dihydroxytryptamine lesions of the dorsal raphe nucleus (yielding an anxiolytic profile).

	Controls	Lesioned
Taurine	2.7	2.2
Aspartate	3.35	3.88
Glutamate	4.55	4.02
Glutamine	1.46	1.44
Glycine	0.69	0.68
Alanine	0.47	0.67
GABA	2.32	2.48

produce an anxiolytic profile. However, efforts to pursue this role of 5-HT further, by making larger raphe lesions or by lesioning the 5-HT input from the dorsal raphe into the amygdala, failed to produce an anxiolytic profile and resulted in general hypoactivity (File and Deakin, 1980; File et al., 1981).

An additional way in which the role of 5-HT in anxiety has been explored is by measuring the effects of benzodiazepines on brain serotonergic function. Chase et al. (1970) found benzodiazepines increased 5-HT concentrations in the brain, probably due to a decrease in 5-HT turnover (Lidbrink et al., 1973; Pratt et al., 1979). Wise et al. (1972) compared the effects on serotonin turnover of a single dose of oxazepam with those after 6 daily doses. Both acute and chronic treatments reduced 5-HT turnover. Cook and Sepinwall (1975) did not find reduced serotonin turnover after a single dose of chlordiazepoxide (10 mg/kg) when there is only a weak anti-conflict effect, but did after repeated injections, when there were good anti-conflict effects. However, the maximum anti-conflict effect was not accompanied by the maximum reduction in 5-HT turnover. File and Vellucci (1978) found no changes in 5-HT turnover after a single dose of chlordiazepoxide (5 mg/kg), which had a sedative, but not an anxiolytic, action, but did find reduced turnover after 5 days of daily injections when there was a clear anxiolytic effect. Rastogi et al. (1978) found that chronic, but not acute, administration of diazepam enhanced 5-HT synthesis and synaptosomal tryptophan levels and ^{3}H-5-HT uptake. Both acute and chronic diazepam administration raised the levels of synaptosomal 5-HT, but the effect was much greater with chronic treatment. Relatively high doses of benzodiazepines, or long-term administration of low doses raise 5-HIAA levels (Chase et al., 1970; Rastogi et al., 1978; Vellucci and File, 1979).

In summary, although a reduction in 5-HT turnover cannot account totally for anxiolytic effects it does seem to have an important role, with the ascending pathways from the dorsal raphe nucleus being of particular relevance. What we do not yet know is which other neurotransmitter changes are necessary to act together with these 5-HT changes to produce anxiolysis.

CATECHOLAMINES AND ANXIETY

Benzodiazepines reduce the turnover of dopamine (Fuxe et al., 1975; Keller et al., 1976), and it has been suggested (Haefely, 1978) that the reduction in the striatum is mediated by inhibitory GABA neurones. The changes in dopamine turnover produced by diazepam and the potentiation by diazepam of catalepsy induced by neuroleptics can both be reversed by picrotoxin (Haefely et al., 1975), supporting a link with GABA. Beer et al. (1972) found neuroleptics to have an anxiolytic action in the thirsty rat conflict test, but in general they do not have anxiolytic effects in animal tests (Margules and Stein, 1967; Cook and Davidson, 1973; Lippa et al., 1979a; and Fig. 1). However, buspirone, a drug that binds only to dopamine receptors (Taylor et al., 1980), is as clinically effective as diazepam at reducing anxiety (Goldberg and Finnerty, 1979). In some respects buspirone resembles apomorphine and piribedil in its actions (Riblet et al., 1980), and at low doses it may act as an agonist at presynaptic dopamine receptors. In the social interaction test of anxiety the effects of low doses of buspirone resembled those of low doses of piribedil (Fig. 2 and File, 1981), but these are not identical with those of the benzodiazepines (Fig. 2 and File, 1980). Presynaptic inhibitory dopamine receptors located on synaptic endings of non-dopaminergic neurones could alter transmission in other transmitter pathways to mediate the anxiolytic action of buspirone. Much more evidence is needed before it can be concluded that dopamine has an important role in the biochemistry of anxiety.

It has been suggested (Redmond, 1977; Redmond and Huang, 1979) that the locus coeruleus noradrenergic system is essential to the behavioural and electrophysiological expression of anxiety. The evidence for this is that stimulation of the locus electrically or by administration of piperoxane produces the same behavioural changes in monkeys as do threatening stimuli. These can be diminished by various classes of drugs: tricyclic antidepressants, clonidine, morphine, propranolol, acute administration of diazepam and electrolytic lesions of the locus coeruleus. All these treatments are sedative and no attempt has been made to distinguish between sedative and anxiolytic actions; certainly the rate of firing in locus coeruleus neurones relates to the animal's general state of alertness (Jones et al., 1978). There is little experimental evidence from other laboratories to support Redmond's hypothesis. Central depletion of dopamine and noradrenaline by intraventricular injection of 6-hydroxydopamine failed to produce an anti-conflict effect or to modify the effect of diazepam (Lippa et al., 1979a). Specific lesions of the locus coeruleus ascending noradrenergic pathways do not produce an anxiolytic profile in any animal test (Crow et al., 1978; File et al., 1979a; Mason and

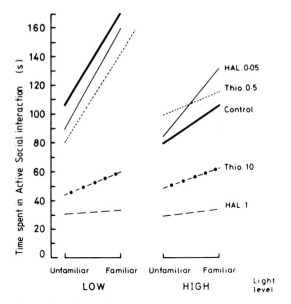

Fig. 1. Mean time (s) spent in active social interaction during a 7.5-min test by pairs of male rats tested under low or high light in an arena which was familiar or unfamiliar to them. Six pairs of rats were tested in each drug and test condition: vehicle controls, haloperidol (0.05 and 1 mg/kg), thioridazine (0.5 and 10 mg/kg).

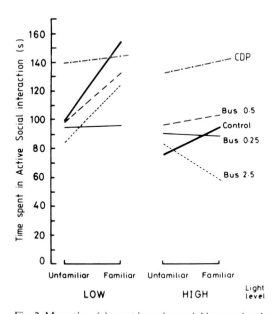

Fig. 2. Mean time (s) spent in active social interaction during a 7.5-min test by pairs of male rats tested under low or high light in an arena which was familiar or unfamiliar to them. Six pairs of rats were tested in each condition: water-injected controls, buspirone (0.25, 0.5 and 2.5 mg/kg) and chlordiazepoxide (5 mg/kg daily for 5 days).

er, 1979a,b; Tye, cited in Iversen, 1979), and in one case even resulted in an xiogenic action (Mason et al., 1978). The effects of noradrenaline when injected into the ventricles or into the amygdala have been reported to be anxiolytic, i.e. the opposite effect to that predicted from Redmond's theory (Margules, 1971; Stein et al., 1973). Neither α- nor β-receptor antagonists have anxiolytic effects in animal tests (Wise et al., 1972, 1973; Stein et al., 1973; File, 1980).

It is more likely that changes in central noradrenaline are responsible for modifying overall levels of activity. Since intraventricular injections of noradrenaline increased unpunished as well as punished responding in rats it is perhaps more accurate to describe its effects as stimulant, rather than anxiolytic. This suggests that a reduction in noradrenaline function may have a general sedative or depressant action. This is supported by the finding that acute treatment with benzodiazepines reduces noradrenaline turnover and causes sedation, whereas after a few days of treatment there is tolerance to both of these effects (Stein et al., 1975). However, even this finding is controversial, as Cook and Sepinwall (1978) did not find reduced noradrenergic turnover until after the second injection, whereas the behavioural effects of sedation are greatest after the first dose. Rastogi et al. (1978) found that both acute and chronic diazepam treatment raised synaptosomal levels of noradrenaline and dopamine and decreased the levels of their metabolites, indicating reduced turnover. Neither acute nor chronic treatment altered the synthesis of catecholamines.

Although there is little evidence for a role of central catecholamines in anxiety, these amines may play an important part in withdrawal. Rats withdrawn from chronic diazepam treatment showed a rebound hyperactivity, accompained by an increased rate of catecholamine synthesis, decreased synaptosomal levels of dopamine and noradrenaline, and raised concentrations of homovanillic acid (a metabolite of dopamine) and of 4-hydroxy-3-methoxyphenylglycol (MOPEG, a major metabolite of noradrenaline) (Rastogi et al., 1978). Raised MOPEG levels have also been found in patients withdrawn from benzodiazepines (Lader, personal communication). Inhibition of the locus coeruleus reduces ethanol and morphine withdrawal symptoms (Gold et al., 1978; Kostowski and Trzaskowska, 1980). The role of catecholamines in general, and perhaps the locus coeruleus noradrenergic system in particular, in withdrawal seems worthy of further investigation.

The clinical efficacy of β-blockers in alleviating at least the autonomic symptoms of anxiety (Granville-Grossman and Turner, 1966; Tyrer and Lader, 1974) suggests a role for peripheral noradrenaline in the somatic expression of anxiety (Darwin, 1872; Lader, 1974), especially as even those that penetrate the brain only poorly (e.g. practolol) are effective in reducing somatic symptoms. But a central action of these drugs cannot be excluded. Several of the β-blockers penetrate the central nervous system and a main side-effect is drowsiness; the sedative effects in mice and rats may therefore be due to central actions (Haydee et al.,

1972; Speizer and Weinstock, 1973). Intravenous administration of DL-oxprenolol and DL-propranolol reduce the EEG-arousal response evoked by electrical stimulation of the mesencephalic reticular formation or of the locus coeruleus (Koella, 1978). However, even if the sedation is caused by a central action of β-blockers, it cannot necessarily be assumed that the relevant action is the blockade of β-receptors, since many of these drugs also have a non-specific membrane-stabilising action. For example, D-propranolol (which has little β-blocking action) is as potent a sedative (Speizer and Weinstock, 1973) and is as good at counteracting amphetamine-hyperactivity (Weinstock and Speizer, 1974) as the racemic mixture.

The major central action of the β-blockers seems to relate to sedation and to central nervous system depression, but peripheral β-receptors have an important role in the expression of anxiety. Feedback from the periphery to the central nervous system can then provide an interaction between autonomic arousal and cognitive factors in anxiety (Schacter, 1966; Lader, 1974).

MODULATION OF ANXIETY BY CORTICOSTERONE AND ACTH

The hypothalamo-pituitary-adrenal system is triggered by several stressors and seems to have a role in anxiety. It is a complex system involving the release from the hypothalamus of corticotrophin-releasing-factor (CRF), that acts on the pituitary to release ACTH (corticotrophin) that in turn acts on the adrenal cortex to stimulate synthesis and release of glucocorticoids. The neural pathways controlling CRF release are complex, but the bulk of experimental evidence suggests that α-adrenergic pathways inhibit secretion, 5-HT pathways stimulate secretion in stress and mediate the diurnal rhythm, acetylcholine stimulates and GABA tonically inhibits secretion (Buckingham, 1981). Benzodiazepines could reduce CRF secretion by inhibiting the 5-HT stimulatory pathway, but it has recently been suggested that they might act through an indole system other than 5-HT (Lahti and Barsuhn, 1980).

The effect of the benzodiazepines on the hypothalamo-pituitary-adrenal system has usually been assessed by measuring the endpoint of plasma corticosteroid concentrations. Benzodiazepines block the stress-induced rise in corticosterone (Krulik and Cerny, 1971; Lahti and Barsuhn, 1975, 1980; Keim and Sigg, 1977; LeFur et al., 1979; File and Peet, 1980). This action is not at the adrenal since benzodiazepines do not affect corticosterone secretion stimulated by injection of ACTH (Lahti and Barsuhn, 1974) and are without effect when the release of ACTH is blocked by betamethasone (Marc and Morselli, 1969). A central site of action is supported by the finding that benzodiazepines reduce ACTH concentrations (Bruni et al., 1980).

ACTH is also secreted by central cells other than those in the pituitary and persists in the brain after hypophysectomy (Krieger et al., 1977). During stress both ACTH and β-endorphin are released from central neurones and benzodiaze-pines may also inhibit release of ACTH from these sites. The dipeptide trypto-phanglycine inhibits ^{3}H-diazepam binding and occurs along with other active amino acids in $ACTH_{1-12}$. It has therefore been speculated that the endogenous ligand for the benzodiazepine receptor is a peptide with a sequence homologous to $ACTH/\beta$-lipotropin (Squires et al., 1979).

Benzodiazepines block the rise in plasma corticosterone induced by the test conditions in two animal tests of anxiety (Lippa et al., 1977; File, 1980). Rats show less social interaction when the test apparatus is unfamiliar or brightly lit and this is accompanied by elevations of plasma corticosterone (File, 1980; File and Peet, 1980). Table 2 shows a time course for the response to a 10-min exposure to a low light, familiar or a high light, unfamiliar arena. Both raise the levels above that found in the home cage, but the elevation in the latter condition is higher and continues to rise longer. In another animal test where an infant monkey is sepa-rated from its mother (Coe and Levine, 1981), plasma cortisol concentrations closely parallel behavioural indices of anxiety.

Lippa et al. (1977) found that while neither adrenalectomy nor hypophysecto-my alone influenced responding in a conflict test they each enhanced the anxiolyt-ic action of diazepam. This suggests that both ACTH and corticosterone have modulatory anxiogenic actions. Certainly ACTH increases arousal and attention to environmental cues (Beckwith et al., 1976; Sandman et al., 1980) and if these cues are aversive its action is anxiogenic (Weiss et al., 1970; File and Vellucci, 1978; Clarke, 1981). This is compatible with the suggestion that a similar amino-acid sequence could be an endogenous ligand for the benzodiazepine receptors (Squires et al., 1979). The situation for corticosterone is less clear. In the social interaction test, adrenalectomised rats maintained the same level of responding in all the test conditions, but the overall level of social interaction was reduced com-pared with the controls, marking interpretation difficult. Low doses of corticoste-rone had an anxiolytic effect and even at high doses no anxiogenic action could be detected (File et al., 1979c). Low doses of corticosterone have opposite central nervous system effects to ACTH (Steiner et al., 1969; Pfaff et al., 1971) and, like benzodiazepines, low doses of corticosterone raise 5-HT concentrations (Telegdy et al., 1976), whereas ACTH raises the concentration of its metabolite 5-hydroxy-indole acetic acid (File and Vellucci, 1978). ACTH and corticosterone have oppo-site behavioural effects in avoidance responding (Weiss et al., 1970) and on extinction of active avoidance (Bohus et al., 1968; Van Wimersma Greidanus, 1970; de Wied, 1974). However, they do not always have opposite effects, espe-cially at high doses of corticosterone. To further complicate interpretation there are feedback loops within the hypothalamo-pituitary-adrenal system and, for example, high levels of corticosterone will inhibit the release of pituitary ACTH (Jones et al., 1972).

Thus, although the release of ACTH and corticosterone contribute to the bio-

TABLE 2

Mean (± SEM) Plasma corticosterone concentrations (μg/100 ml) in rats placed in pairs for 12 mins in a low light, familiar arena, or a high light, unfamiliar arena. Plasma was sampled immediately (0 mins), 10 or 30 mins after the test.

Time since test (mins)	0	10	30
Low light familiar arena	35.8± 11.35	41.6± 5.84	46.2± 7.35
High light unfamiliar arena	36.2± 4.29	66.6± 4.57	92 ± 4.55

chemical changes in anxiety, their roles are complex. Plasma corticosteroid concentration may be a useful measure of anxiety, but this does not necessarily mean that it enhances anxiety, its action could be compensatory.

ENDOGENOUS LIGANDS AND ANXIOGENIC AGENTS

The discovery of benzodiazepine binding sites triggered a search for endogenous substances that might act as transmitters at these receptors. The possibility of a peptide ligand has already been discussed. Two purines were isolated from brain fractions (Skolnick et al., 1978) with low affinity for the benzodiazepine receptor. But they are more potent at inhibiting GABA-enhanced benzodiazepine binding (Paul et al., 1981), possibly by acting at the chloride ionophore (Olsen and Leeb-Lundberg, 1980). There is no evidence yet that the purines influence anxiety and behaviourally they produce sedation (Marley and Nistico, 1972; Hanlika et al., 1973; Crawley et al., 1981) and counteract pentylenetetrazol-induced seizures (Paul et al., 1981). Nicotinamide has also been isolated from extracts of rat brain (Mohler et al., 1979) and has an anxiolytic action in a conflict test. However, the affinity of nicotinamide for the benzodiazepine receptor is 4 – 5 times lower than those for purines, so it must be questioned whether it would naturally be present in sufficient concentration to have an anxiolytic effect.

Braestrup et al. (1980) extracted β-carboline 3-carboxylic acid ethyl ester from human urine, and found it to have high affinity for the benzodiazepine receptor, and a low affinity for 5-HT receptors. However, this particular compound was a product of the extraction procedure and does not normally occur in vivo. The presence of a methoxy group in position 6 or 7 of the β-carbolines, necessary to produce the hallucinations associated with these compounds, prevents good binding to benzodiazepine receptors (Braestrup and Nielsen, 1980).

There is good evidence that the β-carbolines that act at the benzodiazepine receptors have anxiogenic actions in animal tests (File et al., 1982b; Ninan et al., 1982; Corda et al., 1983; Prado de Carvalho et al., 1983). One β-carboline, FG 7142, has been shown to be anxiogenic in man (Dorow et al., 1983). In general, the β-carbolines have behavioural effects opposite to those of the benzodiazepines, for example, they promote seizures (see File, 1983). Two other compounds, the imidazodiazepine Ro 15-1788 (Hunkeler et al., 1981) and a triazoloquinoline CGS 8216 (Czernik et al., 1982) that displace benzodiazepines from their binding sites also have opposite behavioural effects, i.e. they are anxiogenic (File et al., 1982b; File and Lister, 1983b; Hoffman and Britton, 1983; Petersen et al., 1983). Thus the benzodiazepine receptor seems clearly able to mediate anxiogenic as well as anxiolytic effects. The compounds with anxiogenic actions do not show GABA-stimulation of their binding to the benzodiazepine receptors, whereas those with anxiolytic actions do show such enhancement (Braestrup et al., 1982).

Interest has recently focussed on the antagonist actions of the methylxanthines. Caffeine and theophylline inhibit GABA-stimulated benzodiazepine binding (Paul et al., 1981), although they have no direct effect on benzodiazepine binding in vivo (Polc et al., 1981). An alternative site of interaction of these compounds is with adenosine. Benzodiazepines inhibit adenosine uptake (Traversa and Newman, 1979; Bender et al., 1980) and their potency in this correlates well with clinical efficacy (Wu et al., 1981). Benzodiazepines also increase the release of ^{3}H-adenosine from rat cerebral cortex and this is antagonised by theophylline (Phillis et al., 1980). The methylxanthines bind to adenosine receptors and their affinities correlate well with central stimulant actions (Snyder et al., 1981). There is thus the possibility of an antagonistic interaction between the methylxanthines and the benzodiazepines and this has been found in several animal tests (Polc et al., 1981) and in tests on normal volunteers (File et al., 1982a). Is there any evidence that caffeine antagonises the anxiolytic actions of benzodiazepines?

Low doses of caffeine abolished the anti-conflict effect of diazepam in rats (Polc et al., 1981) and in student volunteers caffeine (500 mg) reversed the anxiolytic action of lorazepam (File et al., 1981). It is too early to conclude that these interactions are based on purinergic mechanisms and it may be that caffeine and benzodiazepines are acting at different sites to achieve their opposite effects.

NOVEL ANXIOLYTICS

Recently, several drugs have been synthesised that reduce anxiety, without having all of the other behavioural properties of the benzodiazepines. One of these, SQ-65396, is a pyrazolopyridine with anxiolytic effects in the thirsty rat conflict (Beer et al., 1972) and in man, but without sedative effects and with only weak anticonvulsant activity. SQ-65396 does not affect GABA-receptor binding (Williams and Risley, 1979), but does enhance the binding of ^{3}H-diazepam, by increasing the affinity of the receptor (Beer et al., 1978). This effect is dependent on the presence of chloride ions and is inhibited by picrotoxin (Supavilai and Karobath, 1979). Another pyrazolopyridine, SQ-20009, has recently been shown to have two modulatory effects on benzodiazepine binding: a direct and chloride ion dependent stimulatory effect, which is in turn modulated by the state of the GABA receptor; and an indirect effect of enhancing the GABA-stimulated benzodiazepine binding (Supavilai and Karobath, 1980).

Another group of novel anxiolytics is the triazolopyridazines, e.g. CL-218872. This drug inhibits ^{3}H-diazepam binding with a potency approximating that of the benzodiazepines and has anxiolytic and sedative actions (Lippa et al., 1979b; File 1982b; McElroy and Feldman, 1982; Straughan et al., 1982; Melchior et al., 1983). This drug has structural similarities with the indole portion of some peptides and with the purines. Further experiments on the biochemical effects of this drug should elucidate whether neurotransmitters such as GABA and 5-HT have any essential role in anxiety.

Recently, a third class of drugs that inhibit ^{3}H-diazepam binding, phenylquinoline derivatives, e.g. PK-8165 and PK-9084, have been proposed as potential anxiolytics (LeFur et al., 1981). These drugs are active in a drink conflict test, but have proved weak in the social interaction test (File and Lister, 1983b). Interestingly, these compounds are proconvulsant (File and Simmonds, 1984).

SUMMARY

As mentioned in the Introduction no firm conclusions on the biochemical basis of anxiety can be offered. The advent of several new classes of anxiolytics that do not share all the other behavioural properties of the benzodiazepines provides the opportunity of distinguishing the changes relevant to anxiety from those associated with sedation and anticonvulsant actions. So far the evidence is pointing to the possibility of multiple benzodiazepine binding sites, but the functional relevance of these is unknown. Some of the benzodiazepine sites are not linked to GABA and it is these that we know least about. The most recent evidence has come from the anxiogenic, rather than the anxiolytic, effect of drugs. Both the benzodiazepine and the picrotoxin binding sites can mediate anxiogenic effects.

REFERENCES

Beckwith, B. E., Sandman, C. A., and Kastin, A. J. (1976) Influences of three short-chain peptides (α-MSM, MSH/ACTH$_{4-10}$, MIF) on dimensional attention. Pharmacol. Biochem. Behav. 5, 11–16.

Beer, B., Chasin, M., Clody, D. E., Vogel, J. R. and Horovitz, Z. P. (1972) Cyclic adenosine monophosphate phosphodiesterase in brain: effect on anxiety. Science 176, 428–430.

Beer, B., Klepner, C. A., Lippa, A. S. and Squires, R. F., (1978) Enhancement of ^{3}H-diazepam binding by SQ 65396: a novel anti-anxiety agent. Pharmacol. Biochem. Behav. 9, 849–851.

Bender, A. S., Phillis, J. W. and Wu, P. H. (1980) Diazepam and flurazepam inhibit adenosine uptake by rat brain synaptosomes. J. Pharm. Pharmacol. 32, 293–294.

Bohus, B., Nyakas, C. and Endroczi, E. (1968) Effects of adrenocorticotropic hormone on avoidance behavior of intact and adrenalectomised rats. Int. J. Neuropharmacol. 7, 307–314.

Braestrup, C. and Nielsen, M. (1980) Searching for endogenous benzodiazepine receptor ligands. Trends Pharmacol. Sci. 1, 424–427.

Braestrup, C. and Squires, R. F. (1977) Specific benzodiazepine receptors in rat brain characterised by high-affinity ^{3}H-diazepam binding. Proc. Natl. Acad. Sci. USA 74, 3805–3809.

Braestrup, C. and Squires, R. F. (1978) Brain specific benzodiazepine receptors. Br. J. Psychiatry 133, 249–260.

Braestrup, C., Nielsen, M. and Olsen, C. E. (1980) Urinary and brain β-carboline-3-carboxylates as potent inhibitors of brain benzodiazepine receptors. Proc. Natl. Acad. Sci. USA 77, 2288–2292.

Braestrup, C., Schmiechen, R., Neef, G., Nielsen, M. and Petersen, E. N. (1982) Interaction of convulsive ligands with benzodiazepine receptors. Science 216, 1241–1243.

Bruni, G., Dalpra, P., Dotti, M. T. and Segre, G. (1980) Plasma ACTH and cortisol in benzodiazepine treated rats. Pharmacol. Res. Commun. 12, 163–175.

Buckingham, J. C. (1981) Neural mechanisms controlling the secretion of corticotrophin releasing factor. Br. J. Clin. Pharmacol. 11, 216–218.

Candy, J. M. and Martin, I. L. (1979) The postnatal development of the benzodiazepine receptor in the cerebral cortex and cerebellum of the rat. J. Neurochem. 32, 655-658.

Chase T. N., Katz, R. I. and Kopin, I. J. (1970) Effect of diazepam on fate of intracisternally injected serotonin-C^{14}. Neuropharmacology 9, 103–108.

Clarke, A. (1981) The effects of ACTH-related peptides in animal test of anxiety. Unpublished University of London Ph. D. Thesis.

Coe, C. L. and Levine, S. (1981) Normal responses to mother-infant separation in nonhuman primates. In: D. F. Klein and J. G. Rabkin (Eds.), Anxiety: New Research and Changing Concepts. Raven Press, New York, pp. 155–178.

Collins, G. G. S., File, S. E., Hyde, J. R. G. and Macleod, N. K. (1979) The effects of 5,7-dihydroxytryptamine lesions of the median and of the dorsal raphe nuclei on social interaction in the rat. Br. J. Pharmacol. 66, 114–115P.

Cook, L. and Davidson, A. B. (1973) Effects of behaviorally active drugs in a conflict-punishment procedure in rats. In: S. Garattini, E. Mussini and L. O. Randall (Eds.), The Benzodiazepines. Raven Press, New York, pp. 327–345.

Cook, L., and Sepinwall, J. (1975) Behavioral analysis of the effects and mechanisms of action of benzodiazepines. In: E. Costa and P. Greengard (Eds), Mechanism of Action of Benzodiazepines. Raven Press, New York, pp. 1–28.

Corda, M., Blaker, W. D., Mendelson, W. B., Guidotti, A. and Costa, E. (1983) β-carbolines enhance shock-induced suppression of drinking in rats. Proc. Natl. Acad. Sci. USA 80, 2072–2076.

Costa, T., Rodbard, D. and Pert, C. B. (1979) Is the benzodiazepine receptor coupled to a chloride anion channel? Nature 277, 315–317.

Crawley, J., Marangos, P. J., Paul, S. M., Skolnick, P. and Goodwin, F. K. (1981) Purine-benzodiazepine interaction: inosine reverses diazepam-induced stimulation of mouse exploratory behavior. Science 211, 725–727.

Crow, T. J., Deakin, J. F. W., File, S. E., Longden, A. and Wendlandt, S. (1978) The locus coeruleus noradrenergic system – evidence against a role in attention, habituation, anxiety and motor activity. Brain Res. 155, 249–261.

Curtis, D. R., Lodge, D., Johnston, G. A. R. and Brand, S. J. (1976) Central actions of benzodiazepines. Brain Res. 118, 344–347.

Czernik, A. J., Petrack, B., Kalinsky, H. J., Psychoyos, S., Cash, W. D., Tsai, C., Rinehart, R. K., Granat, F. R., Lovell, R. A., Brundish, D. E. and Wade, R. (1982) CGS 8216: receptor binding characteristics of a potent benzodiazepine antagonist. Life Sci. 30, 363–372.

Darwin, C. (1872) The Expression of Emotion in Man and Animals. Murray, London.

De Wied, D. (1974) Pituitary-adrenal system hormones and behavior. In: The Neurosciences, 3rd Study Program. F. O. Schmitt and F. G. Worden (Eds), MIT Press, Cambridge pp. 653–666.

Dray, A. and Straughan, D. W. (1976) Benzodiazepines: GABA and glycine receptors on single neurones in the rat medulla. J. Pharm. Pharmacol. 28, 314–315.

Dorow, R., Horowski, R., Paschelke, G., Amin, M. and Braestrup, C. (1983) Severe anxiety induced by FG 7142. A β-carboline ligand for benzodiazepine receptors. Lancet (July), 98–99.

File, S. E. (1980) The use of social interaction as a method for detecting anxiolytic activity of chlordiazepoxide-like drugs. J. Neurosci. Methods 2, 219–238.

File, S. E. (1981) Behavioural effects of serotonin depletion. In: E. Clifford Rose (Ed.), Metabolic Disorders of the Nervous System. Pitmans, London, pp. 429–445.

File, S. E. (1982a) Chlordiazepoxide-induced ataxia, muscle relaxation and sedation in the rat: effects of muscimol, picrotoxin and naloxone. Pharmac. Biochem. Behav. 17, 1165–1170.

File, S. E. (1982b) Animal anxiety and the effects of benzodiazepines. In: E. Usdin, P. Skolnick, J. Tallman, D. Greenblatt and S. Paul (Eds), Pharmacology of Benzodiazepines. MacMillan Press, London, pp. 355–364.

File, S. E. (1983) Behavioural actions of benzodiazepine antagonists. In: M.R. Trimble (Ed.), Benzodiazepines Divided. John Wiley & Sons Ltd., London, pp. 129–138.

File, S. E. and Deakin, J. F. W. (1980) Chemical lesions of both dorsal and median raphe nuclei and changes in social and aggressive behaviour in rats. Pharmacol. Biochem. Behav. 12, 855-859.

File, S. E. and Hyde, J. R. G. (1977) The effects of p-chlorophenylalanine and ethanolamine-O-sulphate in an animal test of anxiety. J. Pharm. Pharmacol. 29, 735–738.

File, S. E. and Lister, R. G. (1983a) Anxiogenic actions of picrotoxin and pentylenetetrazole: reversal by chlordiazepoxide. Br. J. Pharmacol. 79, 286 p.

File, S. E. and Lister, R. G. (1983b) Quinolines and anxiety: anxiogenic effects of CGS 8216 and partial anxiolytic profile of PK 9084. Pharmac. Biochem. Behav. 18, 185–188.

File, S. E. and Peet, L. A. (1980) The sensitivity of the rat corticosterone response to environmental manipulations and to chronic chlordiazepoxide treatment. Physiol. Behav. 25, 753–758.

File, S. E. and Simmonds, M. A. (1984) Interactions of two phenylquinolines with picrotoxin and benzodiazepines in vivo and in vitro. Eur. J. Pharmacol. (in press).

File, S. E. and Vellucci, S. V. (1978) Studies on the role of ACTH and of 5-HT in anxiety, using an animal model. J. Pharm. Pharmacol. 30, 105–110.

File, S. E., Deakin, J. F. W., Longden, A. and Crow, T. J. (1979a) An investigation of the role of the locus coeruleus in anxiety and agonistic behaviour. Brain Res. 169, 411–420.

File, S. E., Hyde, J. R. G. and Macleod, N. K. (1979b) 5,7-dihydroxytryptamine lesions of dorsal and median raphe nuclei and performance in the social interaction test of anxiety and in a home-cage aggression test. J. Affect. Dis. 1, 115–122.

File, S. E., Vellucci, S. V. and Wendlandt, S. (1979c) Corticosterone – an anxiogenic or an anxiolytic agent? J. Pharm. Pharmacol. 31, 300–305.

File, S. E., James, T. A. and Macleod, N. K. (1981) Depletion in amygdaloid 5-hydroxytryptamine concentration and changes in social and aggressive behaviour. J. Neural Trans. 50, 1–12.

File, S. E., Bond, A. J. and Lister, R. G. (1982a) Interaction between effects of caffeine and lorazepam in performance tests and self-ratings. J. Clin. Psychopharmacol. 2, 102–106.

File, S. E., Lister, R. G. and Nutt, D. A. (1982b) The anxiogenic action of benzodiazepine antagonists. Neuropharmacology 21, 1033–1037.

Fuxe, K., Agnati, L. F., Bolme, P., Hokfelt, T., Lidbrink, P., Ljungdahl, A., Perez de la Mora, M. and Ogren, S. O. (1975) The possible involvement of GABA mechanisms in the action of benzodiazepines on catecholamine neurons. In: E. Costa and P. Greengard (Eds), Mechanism of Action of Benzodiazepines. Raven Press, New York, pp. 45–61.

Gahwiler, B. H. (1976) Diazepam and chlordiazepoxide: powerful GABA antagonists in explants of rat cerebellum. Brain Res. 107, 176–179.

Gallager, D. W. (1978) Benzodiazepines: Potentiation of a GABA inhibitory response in the dorsal raphe nucleus. Eur. J. Pharmacol. 49, 133–143.

Gallager, D. W., Mallorga, P., Thomas, J. W. and Tallman, J. F. (1980) GABA-benzodiazepine interactions: physiological, pharmacological and development aspects. Fed. Proc. 39, 3043–3049.

Geller, I. and Blum, K. (1970) The effects of 5-HT on parachlorophenylalanine (p-CPA) attenuation of 'conflict' behavior. Eur. J. Pharmacol. 9, 319–324.

Geller, I., Hartmann, R. J. and Croy, D. J. (1974) Attenuation of conflict behavior with cinanserin, a serotonin antagonist: reversal of the effect with 5-hydroxytryptophan and α-methyltryptamine. Res. Commun. Chem. Pathol. Pharmacol. 7, 165–174.

Gold, M. E., Redmond, D. E. and Kleber, H. D. (1978) Clonidine blocks acute opiate-withdrawal symptoms. Lancet 2, 599-602.

Goldberg, H. L. and Finnerty, R. J. (1979) The comparative efficacy of buspirone and diazepam in the treatment of anxiety. Am. J. Psychiatry 136, 1184–1187.

Granville-Grossman, K. L. and Turner, P. (1966) The effect of propranolol on anxiety. Lancet i, 788–790.

Haefely, W. E. (1978) Behavioral and neuropharmacological aspects of drugs used in anxiety and related states. In: M. A. Lipton, A. Di Mascio and K. F. Killam (Eds), Psychopharmacology: A Generation of Progress. Raven Press, New York, pp. 1359–1374.

Haefely, W. E. (1980) GABA and the anticonvulsant action of benzodiazepines and barbiturates. Brain Res. Bull. 5, (Suppl. 2), 873–878.

Haefely, W. E., Kullsar, A., Mohler, H., Pieri, L., Polc, P. and Schaffner, R. (1975) Possible involvement of GABA in the central actions of benzodiazepines. Adv. Biochem. Psychopharmacol. 14, 131–151.

Hanlika, I., Ababei, L., Branisteanu, D. and Topoliceanu, F. (1973) Preliminary data on the possible hypnogenic role of adenosine. J. Neurochem. 21, 1019–1020.

Haydee, E. M., Fabian, H. E. M. and Izquierdo, J. A. (1972) Effect of β-adrenergic blocking agents on the spontaneous motility of mice. Arzneim. Forsch. 22, 1375–1376.

Hoffman, D. K. and Britton, D.R. (1983) Anxiogenic-like properties of benzodiazepine antagonists. Soc. Neurosci. Abstr., 9, 129.

Hunkeler, W., Mohler, H., Pieri, L., Polc, P., Bonetti, E. P., Cumin, R., Schaffner, R. and Haefely, W. (1981) Selective antagonists of benzodiazepines. Nature 290, 514–516.

Iversen, S. D. (1979) Animal models of relevance to biological psychiatry. In: H. M. van Praag, M. H. Lader, O. J. Rafaelson and E. J. Sachar (Eds), Handbook of Biological Psychiatry, Part I. Disciplines Relevant to Biological Psychiatry. Marcel Dekker Inc., New York, pp. 303–335.

Jones, G., Foote, S. L., Segal, M. and Bloom, F. (1978) Locus coeruleus neurones in freely behaving rats exhibit pronounced alterations of firing rate during sensory stimulation and stages of the sleep-wake cycle. Soc. Neurosci. Abstr. 4, 856.

Jones, M. T., Brush, F. R. and Neame, R. L. B. (1972) Characteristics of fast feedback control of corticotrophin release by corticosteroids. J. Endocrinol. 55, 489–497.

Karobath, H., Placheta, P., Lippitsch, M and Krogsgaard-Larsen, P. (1979) Is stimulation of benzodiazepine a novel GABA receptor? Nature, (London) 278, 748–749.

Keim, K. L. and Sigg, E.B. (1977) Plasma corticosterone and brain catecholamines in stress: effect of psychotropic drugs. Pharmacol. Biochem. Behav. 6, 79–85.

Keller, H. H., Schaffner, R. and Haefely, W. (1976) Interaction of benzodiazepines with neuroleptics at central dopamine neurons. Naunyn-Schmiedebergs Arch. Pharmacol. 294, 1–7.

Koella, W. P. (1978) Central effects of β-adrenergic-blocking agents: mode and mechanisms of action. In: P. Keilholz (Ed), A Therapeutics Approach to the Psychic via the β-adrenergic system. Baltimore University Park Press, pp. 11–29.

Kostowski, W. and Trzaskowsa, E. (1980) Effect of lesion of the locus coeruleus and clonidine treatment on ethanol withdrawal symptom in rats. Pol. J. Pharmacol. Pharm. 32, 617–623.

Krieger, D. T., Liotta, A. and Brownstein, M. J. (1977) Presence of corticotrophin in brain of normal and hypophysectomised rats. Proc. Natl. Acad. Sci. USA 74, 648–652.

Krulik, R. and Cerny, M. (1971) Effect of chlordiazepoxide on stress in rats. Life Sci. 10, 145–151.

Lader, M. H. (1974) The peripheral and central role of the catecholamines in the mechanisms of anxiety. Int. Pharmacopsychiatry 9, 125–137.

Lahti, R. A. and Barsuhn, C. (1974) The effect of minor tranquillizers on stress-induced increases in plasma corticosteroids. Psychopharmacologia 35, 215–220.

Lahti, R. A. and Barsuhn, C. (1975) The effect of various doses of minor tranquillisers on plasma corticosteroids in stressed rats. Res. Commun. Chem. Pathol. Pharmac. 11, 595–602.

Lahti, R. A. and Barsuhn, C. (1980) Benzodiazepines, stress and rat plasma corticosteroids: the role of indoleamines. Res. Commun. Psychol. Psychiatr. Behav. 5, 369–383.

Lal, H., and Shearman, G. (1982) Attenuation of chemically induced anxiogenic stimuli as a novel method for evaluating anxiolytic drugs: a comparison of clobazam with other benzodiazepines. Drug Develop. Res. Supp. 1, 127–134.

Lal, H., Bennett, D., Elmesallamy, F. and Gherezghiher, T. (1982) Anxiogenic potential of β-carboline compounds as bioassayed by generalization to interoceptive discriminable stimuli produced by pentylenetetrazol. Abstr. Soc. Neurosci. 8, 571.

Le Fur, G., Guillova, F., Mitrani, N., Mizoule, J. and Uzan, A. (1979) Relationships between plasma corticosteroids and benzodiazepines in stress. J. Pharmacol. Exp. Ther. 211, 305–308.

Le Fur, G., Mizoule, J., Burgeuin, M. C., Ferris, O., Heaulme, M., Gauthier, A., Gueremy, C. and Uzan, A. (1981) Multiple benzodiazepine receptors: evidence of a dissociation between anticonflict and anticonvulsant properties by PK 8165 and PK 9084 (two quinoline derivatives). Life Sci. 28, 1439–1448.

Lidbrink, P., Corrodi, H., Fuxe, K. and Olson, L. (1973) The effects of benzodiazepines meprobamate and barbiturates on central monoamine neurons. In: S. Garattini, E. Mussini and L. O. Randall (Eds), The Benzodiazepines. Raven Press, New York, pp. 203–224.

Lippa, A. S., Greenblatt, E. N. and Pelham, R. W. (1977) The use of animal models for delineating the mechanisms of action of anxiolytic agents. In: I. Hanin and E. Usdin (Eds), Animal Models in Psychiatry and Neurology. Pergamon Press, Oxford, pp. 279–291.

Lippa, A. S., Nash, P. A. and Greenblatt, E. N. (1979a) Preclinical neuropsychopharmacological testing procedures for anxiolytic drugs. In: S. Fielding and H. Lal (Eds), Anxiolytics. Futura Pub. Co. Inc., Mount Kisco, New York, pp. 41–81.

Lippa, A. S., Critchett, D. J., Sano, M. C., Klepner, C. A., Greenblatt, E. N., Coupet, J. and Beer, B. (1979b) Benzodiazepine receptors: cellular and behavioral characteristics. Pharmacol. Biochem. Behav. 10, 831–843.

Marc, V. and Morselli, P. L. (1969) Effect of diazepam on plasma corticosterone levels in the rat. J. Pharm. Pharmacol. 21, 784–785.

Margules, D. L. (1971) Alpha and beta-adrenergic receptors in amygdala: reciprocal inhibitors and facilitators of punished operant behavior. Eur. J. Pharmacol. 16, 21–26.

Margules, D. L. and Stein, L. (1967) Neuroleptics vs. tranquillizers: evidence from animal studies of mode and site of action. In: H. Brill, J. O. Cole, P. Deniker, H. Hippius and P. B. Bradley (Eds), Neuropsychopharmacology. Excerpta Medica, Amsterdam, pp. 108–120.

Marley, E. and Nistico, A. (1972) Effects of catecholamines and adenosine derivatives given into the brain of fowls. Br. J. Pharmacol. 46, 619–636.

Mason, S. T. and Fibiger, H. C.   (1979a)   Anxiety: the locus coeruleus disconnection. Life Sci. 25, 2141–2147.

Mason, S. T. and Fibiger, H. C.   (1979b)   Noradrenaline, fear and extinction. Brain Res. 165, 47–56.

Mason, S. T., Roberts, D. C. S. and Fibiger, H. C.   (1978)   Noradrenaline and neophobia. Physiol. Behav. 21, 353–361.

McElroy, J. F. and Feldman, R. S.   (1982)   Generalization between benzodiazepine-and triazolo-pyridazine-elicited discriminative cues. Pharmac. Biochem. Behav. 17, 709–713.

Melchior, C. L., Garrett, K. and Tabakoff, B.   (1983)   Proconvulsant effects of the benzodiazepine agonist, CL 218, 872. Abstr. Soc. Neurosci. 9, 129.

Mohler H. and Okada, T.   (1977)   Benzodiazepine-receptor: demonstration in the central nervous system. Science 198, 849–851.

Mohler, H. and Okada, T.   (1978)   The benzodiazepine-receptor in normal and pathological human brain. Br. J. Psychiatry 133, 261–268.

Mohler, H., Polc, P., Cumin, R., Pieri, L. and Kettler, R.   (1979)   Nicotinamide is a brain constituent with benzodiazepine-like actions. Nature 278, 563–565.

Ninan, P. T., Insel, T. M., Cohen, R. M., Cook, J. M., Skolnick, P. and Paul, S. M.   (1982)   Benzodiazepine receptor-mediated experimental 'anxiety' in primates. Science 218, 1332–1334.

Olsen, R. W. and Leeb-Lundberg, R.   (1980)   Endogenous inhibitors of picrotoxinin-convulsant binding sites in rat brain. Eur. J. Pharmacol. 65, 101–104.

Paul, S. M., Marangos, P. J. and Skolnick, P.   (1981)   The benzodiazepine-GABA-chloride iono-phore receptor complex: common site of minor tranquillizer action. Biol. Psychiatry 16, 213–229.

Pelham, R. W., Osterberg, A. C., Thibault, L. and Tanikella, T.   (1975)   Interactions between plasma corticosterone and anxiolytic drugs on conflict behavior in rats. Presented at 4th Int. Cong. Soc. Psychoneuroendocrinol., Aspen, Colorado.

Petersen, E. N., Jensen, L. H., Honore, T. and Braestrup, C.   (1983)   Differential pharmacological effects of BZ receptor inverse agonists. In: G. Biggio and E. Costa (Eds), Benzodiazepine Recognition Site Ligands: Biochemistry and Pharmacology. Raven Press, New York, pp. 57–64.

Pfaff, D. W., Silva, M. T. A. and Weiss, J. M.   (1971)   Telemetered recording of hormone effects on hippocampal neurons. Science 172, 394–395.

Phillis, J. W., Bender, A. S. and Wu, P. H.   (1980)   Benzodiazepines inhibit adenosine uptake into rat brain synaptosomes. Brain Res. 195, 494–498.

Polc, P. and Haefely, W.   (1976)   Effects of two benzodiazepines, phenobarbitone and baclofen on synaptic transmission in the cat cuneate nucleus. Naunyn-Schmiedebergs Arch. Pharmacol. 294, 121–131.

Polc, P., Mohler, H. and Haefely, W.   (1974)   The effect of diazepam on spinal cord activities: possible sites and mechanisms of action. Naunyn-Schmiedebergs Arch. Pharmacol. 284, 319–337.

Polc, P., Bonetti, E. P., Pieri, L., Cumin, R., Angioi, R. M., Mohler, H. and Haefely, W. E.   (1981)   Caffeine antagonizes several central effects of diazepam. Life Sci. 28, 2265–2275.

Prado de Carvalho, L., Venault, P., Rossier, J. and Chapouthier, G.   (1983)   Anxiogenic properties of convulsive agents. Abstr. Soc. Neurosci. 9, 128.

Pratt, J., Jenner, P., Reynolds, E. H. and Marsden, C. D.   (1979)   Clonazepam induces decreased serotonergic activity in the mouse brain. Neuropharmacology 18, 791–799.

Rastogi, R. B., Lapierre, Y. D. and Singhal, R. L.   (1978)   Synaptosomal uptake of norepinephrine and 5-hydroxytryptamine and synthesis of catecholamines during benzodiazepine treatment. Can. J. Physiol. Pharmacol. 56, 777–784.

Redmond, D. E.   (1977)   Alterations in the function of the nucleus locus coeruleus: a possible model for studies of anxiety. In: I. Hanin and E. Usdin (Eds), Animal Models in Psychiatry and Neurology. Pergamon Press, Oxford, pp. 293–304.

Redmond, D. E. and Huang, Y. H. (1979) New evidence for a locus coeruleus-norepinephrine connection with anxiety. Life Sci. 25, 2149–2162.

Riblet, L. A., Allen, L. E., Hyslop, D. K., Taylor, D. P. and Wilderman, R. C.(1980) Pharmacologic activity of buspirone, a novel non-benzodiazepine antianxiety agent. Fed. Proc. 39, 752.

Robichaud, R. C. and Sledge, K. L. (1969) The effects of p-chlorophenylalanine on experimentally induced conflict in the rat. Life Sci. 8, 965–969.

Rodin, E., Rodin, M. and Lavine, L. (1979) Electroclinical and ultrastructural changes associated with subconvulsant doses of pentylenetetrazol. Exp. Neurol. 64, 386–400.

Sandman, C. A., Beckwith, B. E. and Kastin, A. J., (1980) Are learning and attention related to the sequence of amino acids in ACTH/MSH peptides? Peptides 1, 277-280.

Schacter, S. (1966) The interaction of cognitive and physiological determinants of emotional state. In: C. D. Spielberger (Ed.), Anxiety and Behaviour. Academic Press, New York pp. 193–224.

Schenberg, L. C. and Graeff, F. G. (1978) Role of the periaqueductal gray substance in the antianxiety action of benzodiazepines. Pharmacol. Biochem. Behav. 9, 287–295.

Schmidt, R. F., Vogel, M. E. and Zimmermann. M. (1967) Die wirkung von Diazepam auf die präsynaptische Hemmung und andere Rückenmarksreflexe. Naunyn-Schmiedebergs Arch. Exp. Pathol. Pharmakol. 258, 69–82.

Sepinwall, J. and Cook, L. (1978) Behavioral pharmacology of antianxiety drugs. In: L. L. Iversen, S. D. Iversen and S. H. Snyder (Eds), Handbook of Psychopharmacology, Vol. 13. Plenum Press, New York, pp. 345–393.

Sepinwall, J. and Cook, L. (1980) Relationship of γ-aminobutyric acid (GABA) to antianxiety effects of benzodiazepines. Brain Res. Bull. 5 (Suppl. 2), 839–848.

Skolnick, P., Marangos, P. J., Goodwin, F. K., Edwards, M. and Paul, S. M. (1978) Identification of inosine and hypoxanthine as endogenous inhibitors of ^{3}H-diazepam binding in the central nervous system. Life Sci. 23, 1473–1480.

Snyder, S. H., Katims, J. J., Annau, Z., Bruns, R. F. and Daly, J. W. (1981) Adenosine receptors and behavioral actions of methylxanthines. Proc. Natl. Acad. Sci. USA 78, 3260–3264.

Soubrie, P. and Simon, P. (1978) Comparative study of the antagonism of bemegride and picrotoxin on behavioural depressant effects of diazepam in rats and mice. Neuropharmacology 17, 121–125.

Speizer, Z. and Weinstock, M. (1973) The influence of propranolol on abnormal behaviour induced in rats by prolonged isolation – an animal model for mania? Br. J. Pharmacol. 48, 348P.

Squires, R. F., Benson, D. I., Braestrup, C., Coupet, J., Klepner, C. A., Myers, V. and Beer, B. (1979) Some properties of brain specific benzodiazepine receptors: new evidence for multiple receptors. Pharmacol. Biochem. Beh. 10, 825–830.

Stein, L., Wise, C. D. and Berger, B. D., (1973) Antianxiety action of benzodiazepines: decrease in activity of serotonin neurons in the punishment system. In: S. Garattini, E. Mussini and L. O. Randall (Eds), The Benzodiazepines. Raven Press, New York, pp. 299–326.

Stein, L., Wise, C. D. and Belluzzi, J. D. (1975) Effects of benzodiazepines on central serotonergic mechanisms. In: E. Costa and P. Greengard (Eds), Mechanism of Action of Benzodiazepines. Raven Press, New York, pp. 299–326.

Stein, L., Belluzzi, J. D. and Wise, C. D. (1977) Benzodiazepines: behavioral and neurochemical mechanisms. Am. J. Psychiatry 134, 665–668.

Steiner, F. A. and Felix, D. (1976) Antagonistic effects of GABA and benzodiazepines on vestibular and cerebellar neurons. Nature (London) 260, 346–347.

Steiner, F. A., Ruf, K. and Akert, K. (1969) Steroid-sensitive neurones in rat brain: anatomical localization and responses to neurohumours and ACTH. Brain Res. 12, 74–85.

Stevens, D. A. and Fechter, L. D., (1969) The effects of p-chlorophenylalanine, a depletor of brain serotonin, on behavior. II. Retardation of passive avoidance learning. Life Sci. 8, 379–385.

Straughan, D. W., Oakley, N. R. and Jones, B. J.   (1982)   Is the BZ_1 selective agent CL 218,872 a non-sedative anxiolytic? Abstr. Soc. Neurosci. 8, 468.

Supavilai, P. and Karobath, M.   (1979)   Stimulation of benzodiazepine receptor binding by SQ 20009 is chloride-dependent and picrotoxin-sensitive. Eur. J. Pharmacol. 60, 111–113.

Supavilai, P. and Karobath, M.   (1980)   Interaction of SQ 20009 and GABA-like drugs as modulators of benzodiazepine receptor binding. Eur. J. Pharmacol. 62, 229–233.

Tallman, J. F., Thomas, J. W. and Gallager, D. W.   (1978)   GABA-ergic modulation of benzodiazepine binding site sensitivity. Nature 274, 383–385.

Tallman, J. F., Paul, S. M., Skolnick, P. and Gallager, D. W.   (1980)   Receptors for the age of anxiety: pharmacology of the benzodiazepines. Science 207, 274–281.

Taylor, D. P., Hyslop, D. K. and Riblet, L. A.   (1980)   Buspirone: a model for anxioselective drug action. Soc. Neurosci. Abstr. 6, 791.

Telegdy, G., Kovacs, G. L. and Vermes, I.   (1976)   Action of corticosteroids on brain serotonin metabolism in correlation with avoidance behaviour in rats. Acta Physiol. Acad. Sci. Hung. 48, 417–419.

Tenen, S. S.   (1967)   The effects of p-chlorophenylalanine, a serotonin depletor, on avoidance acquisition, pain sensitivity, and related behavior in the rat. Psychopharmacologia 10, 204–219.

Thiebot, M., Jobert, A. and Soubrie, P.   (1980a)   Conditioned suppression of behavior: its reversal by intraraphe microinjection of chlordiazepoxide and GABA. Neurosci. Lett. 16, 213–217.

Thiebot, M., Jobert, A. and Soubrie, P.   (1980b)   Effects of intraraphe chlordiazepoxide and GABA microinjections on behavioral inhibition in rats. Abstracts of 12th CINP Congress, Goteborg, 340.

Traversa, U. and Newman, M.   (1979)   Stereospecific influence of oxazepam hemisuccinate on cyclic AMP accumulation elicited by adenosine in cerebral cortical slices. Biochem. Pharmacol. 28, 2363–2365.

Tye, N. C., Iversen, S. D. and Green, A. R.   (1979)   The effects of benzodiazepines and serotonergic manipulations on punished responding. Neuropharmacology 18, 689–695.

Tyrer, P. J. and Lader, M. H.   (1974)   Response to propranolol and diazepam in somatic anxiety. Br. Med. J. 2, 14–16.

Van Wimersma Greidanus, T.   (1970)   Effects of steroids on extinction of an avoidance response in rats. A structure-activity relationship study. Prog. Brain Res. 32, 185–191.

Vellucci, S. V. and File, S. E.   (1979)   Chlordiazepoxide loses its anxiolytic action with long-term treatment. Psychopharmacology 62, 61–65.

Weinstock, M. and Speizer, Z.   (1974)   Modification by propranolol and related compounds of motor activity and stereotype behaviour induced in the rat by amphetamine. Eur. J. Pharmacol. 25, 29–35.

Weiss, J. M., McEwen, B. S., Silva, M. T. and Kalkut, M.   (1970)   Pituitary-adrenal alterations and fear responding. Am. J. Physiol. 218, 864–868.

Williams, M. and Risley, E. A.   (1979)   Enhancement of the binding of ^{3}H-diazepam to rat brain membranes in vitro by SQ 20009, a novel anxiolytic, γ-amino-butyric acid (GABA) and muscimol. Life Sci. 24, 833–842.

Wise, C. D., Berger, B. D. and Stein, L.   (1972)   Benzodiazepines: anxiety-reducing activity by reduction of serotonin turnover in the brain. Science 177, 180–183.

Wise, C. D., Berger, B. D. and Stein, L.   (1973)   Evidence of α-noradrenergic reward receptors and serotonergic punishment receptors in the rat brain. Biol. Psychiatry 6, 3–21.

Wu, P. H., Phillis, J. W. and Bender, A. S.   (1981)   Do benzodiazepines bind at adenosine uptake sites in CNS? Life Sci. 28, 1023–1031.

Young, W. S. and Kuhar, M. J.   (1979)   Autoradiographic localization of benzodiazepine receptor in the brains of humans and animals. Nature 280, 393–395.

Young, W. S. and Kuhar, M. J.   (1980)   Radiohistochemical localization of benzodiazepine receptors in rat brain. J. Pharmacol. Exp. Ther. 212, 337–346.

Burrows/Norman/Davies (eds) Antianxiety agents
© *Elsevier Science Publishers B.V., 1984*

Chapter 3

Benzodiazepines: Receptors and clinical implications of molecular mechanisms

ANN FULTON, TREVOR R. NORMAN

and

GRAHAM D. BURROWS

*Department of Psychiatry, University of Melbourne, Austin and Larundel Hospitals, Heidelberg
3084, Victoria, Australia*

INTRODUCTION

Benzodiazepines have been available to the clinician since 1960 when chlordiazepoxide (Librium) was first introduced. Many other benzodiazepines have subsequently been introduced into clinical usage since that time. Of the psychotropic medications, the benzodiazepines are the most widely prescribed drugs, with as many as 1 in 10 of the population receiving a prescription for them in some countries (Ban et al., 1981).

Benzodiazepines have a characteristic pharmacological profile (Greenblatt and Shader, 1974). Their most distinctive feature is their antianxiety effect and the disinhibition of certain behavioural responses. They are also the most potent anticonvulsant agents known, being effective against chemically and electrically induced seizures. The sedative properties of the benzodiazepines are well recognized, with two aspects being apparent – the clinically desirable effect of damping excessive response to normal stimuli and the undesirable property of reducing the normal response to excessive stimuli. Facilitation of sleep by the benzodiazepines can be useful clinically and several short-acting drugs have been marketed specifically as hypnotics. The muscle-relaxant properties of these agents usually appears at sedative doses and is difficult to distinguish from sedation. Benzodiazepines exert their effects centrally and are virtually devoid of activity outside the central nervous system. In addition they have a very low toxicity and overdosage of a benzodiazepine alone is rarely fatal. They have few adverse effects on fertility and teratogenic, mutagenic and carcinogenic effects occur at doses far in excess of those used clinically. A detailed review of these properties has recently been published (Haefely, 1983). Any attempts to explain the mechanism of action of these drugs must account for all of the physiological and biochemical properties of the benzodiazepines.

Haefely (1978) has suggested that the psychotropic effects of a drug can be explained by the chain of events initiated when that drug binds to its specific receptor. Binding may either activate or inactivate the receptor thereby inducing or preventing changes in subcellular elements of the target cell respectively, which leads to the characteristic effects of the drug (see Fig. 1). Such a conceptualization has been helpful for the understanding of the biological actions of the benzodiazepines.

MECHANISM OF ACTION

Early efforts to understand the mechanism of action of the benzodiazepines focussed on their effects on the turnover of the biogenic amines (Haefely, 1978). Catecholamine turnover was found to be unaffected or slightly reduced; the effect on serotonin turnover remains controversial. Reduced acetylcholine turnover has been found. The high doses of benzodiazepines required to produce these effects make it unlikely that their specific actions can be explained in terms of reduced biogenic amine turnover. Data from electrophysiological investigations have shown that the limbic system, the thalamus and spinal cord are particularly sensitive to the action of the benzodiazepines. However, studies at this level have not been able to provide much insight into the mechanism of action since nearly all brain regions so far investigated have been shown to be affected by the benzodiazepines.

Other studies have focussed on the inhibitory neurotransmitter γ-aminobutyric acid (GABA), which constitutes up to 30% of all the synapses in the brain (Iversen and Bloom, 1972). GABA binds specifically to receptors in the synaptic membrane which are coupled to chloride ion channels. Activation of these receptors results in the opening of the channels, permitting the flow of chloride ions through the membrane. Usually this is an inward flow causing a hyperpolarization. The effect of a depolarizing excitatory transmitter will be attenuated.

The effects of benzodiazepines in various parts of the central nervous system have been explained by their actions on GABA transmission. The evidence supporting this hypothesis includes the specific ability of the benzodiazepines to

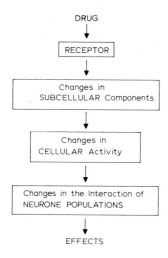

Fig. 1. Events caused by the binding of a drug to its receptor. (Modified from Haefely, 1978.)

relieve convulsions associated with a partial inhibition of brain GABA-ergic transmission. Secondly, the benzodiazepines have an agonistic action on post-synaptic GABA-ergic mechanisms in a number of brain nuclei where GABA-ergic transmission is operative. Thirdly, the benzodiazepines have a capacity to enhance GABA-mediated presynaptic inhibition or to mimic the effects of GABA presynaptically on preganglionic terminals. Finally, when GABA-ergic transmission between postsynaptic neurons of certain cells is decreased, benzodiazepines have the capacity to reduce the amount of cGMP that would have been produced. Clearly the benzodiazepines have important effects on GABA-ergic transmission but the molecular mechanisms involved in their action are still unclear. It is almost certain however that the benzodiazepines act postsynaptically. They could act by increasing GABA release, by inhibiting GABA reuptake or by facilitating GABA actions at the postsynaptic receptor. It is important to note that the benzodiazepines do not have a direct GABA-mimetic effect. They exert their GABA-mimetic actions only when GABA transmission is functional; GABA-mimetic compounds in contrast exert their effects even when GABA transmission is not functional.

The benzodiazepines given in anxiolytic doses fail to change GABA metabolism or to increase or decrease GABA content. The benzodiazepines do not cause a release of GABA from storage sites in nerve terminals. Since the benzodiazepines are not GABA-mimetic, do not act presynaptically by modifying synthesis, release or uptake of GABA, it must be concluded that they act postsynaptically by facilitating the action of GABA on receptors. The mechanism should depend on specific high-affinity binding of the benzodiazepines to a regulatory site near the

36

GABA receptor. Perhaps this site, by an allosteric mechanism, facilitates the interaction between GABA and its receptor. Consistent with this hypothesis is the discovery of high-affinity binding sites for the benzodiazepines distinct from those for GABA.

CLINICAL IMPLICATIONS OF HIGH-AFFINITY SPECIFIC BENZO-DIAZEPINE BINDING SITES

Specific benzodiazepine binding sites have been characterized in several vertebrate species (Braestrup and Squires, 1977, 1978; Möhler and Okada, 1977 a,b; Robertson et al., 1978; Speth et al., 1978). Most clinically and pharmacologically active benzodiazepines displace ^{3}H-diazepam or ^{3}H-flunitrazepam from the binding site(s) with inhibitory constants that correlate well with ED_{50} values for pharmacological tests predictive of anxiolytic activity (Braestrup and Squires, 1978). This suggests that the binding sites have relevance to the in vivo effects of the benzodiazepines.

The benzodiazepine receptors are characterized by four pricipal properties: a) their location; b) their specificity; c) their ability to be modulated; and d) their multiplicity.

a) *Location.* Specific high-affinity binding sites for the benzodiazepines have been found in cortical and limbic areas of the CNS and in the spinal cord (Möhler and Okada, 1977; Squires and Braestrup, 1977). Low-affinity binding sites were reported in mammalian platelets (Wang et al., 1980). The absence of high-affinity binding sites in such major organs as the heart, kidneys, lungs, effectively confines benzodiazepine actions to the CNS. The lack of secondary effects on these organs following benzodiazepine administration (and therefore the safety) is likely to be due to the limited distribution of the receptors in the body and also to their specificity of binding.

b) *Specificity.* Binding studies have demonstrated that the benzodiazepines and their receptors have a mutual specificity. The benzodiazepine drugs are weak displacers of tritiated spiperone, clonidine, WB-4101 (Fulton and Burrows, 1983) and haloperidol (Burt et al., 1976) from serotonin, α-adrenergic and dopamine receptor sites. Conversely, non-benzodiazepine compounds do not readily displace bound diazepam (Braestrup and Squires, 1978; Müller et al., 1978). This selectiveness in binding results in an absence of side effects which can originate from interactions with other neurotransmitter systems. For example, the anticholinergic effects (dry mouth, blurred vision, cardiac irregularities, etc.) quite frequently accompany the administration of the tricyclic antidepressants, which have potent effects on muscarinic-cholinergic receptors (Snyder and Yamamura, 1977; Golds et al., 1980).

c) *Modulation*. Several groups of neurotransmitter receptors have the property of responding to exposure to agonists and antagonists (Bonnet, 1979). Chronic blockade by antagonist drugs can result in receptors with heightened sensitivity to their agonists and in an increase of binding site population (Ezrin-Waters and Seeman, 1977). The opposite effect has also been recorded: chronic dosage with agonists may result in the development of subsensitive responses to agonistic challenge (Martres et al., 1977) due sometimes to a reduction in the number of functional receptors (Quik and Iverson, 1978). Recent animal studies have shown that benzodiazepine binding sites are also liable to such alterations. The clinical phenomenon of tolerance might be explained by these changes.

The time course of the development of subjective side effects following single and multiple dose administration of benzodiazepines to man supports the idea of receptor site adaptation. Following the initiation of drug therapy drowsiness is commonly experienced, but usually abates with continued administration of the same dose, even though plasma and tissue concentrations of the drug are higher (Greenblatt and Shader, 1978). It appears that tolerance to the therapeutic actions of the drug develop more slowly, so that the anxiolytic and sedative effects become dissociated on chronic dosing.

Acute benzodiazepine administration to rats had been reported to increase binding site density within 15 min (Speth et al., 1979). Chronic administration reduced ^{3}H-diazepam in rat cortex (Chiu and Rosenberg, 1978). Decreased binding was specific to prolonged receptor occupation and not an adaptation to chronic depression of the central nervous system as barbital administration did not affect diazepam binding characteristics (Rosenberg and Chiu, 1979). The receptor number returned to pretreatment values within 24 hours of cessation of drug treatment (Rosenberg and Chiu, 1981).

Extrapolation from the animal model suggests that tolerance to the benzodiazepines may correspond with the development of receptor subsensitivity. Development of subsensitivity may explain tolerance to the sedative effects of the benzodiazepines as described above. Further, the lack of evidence for the efficacy of continuous long-term treatment of anxiety with benzodiazepines (Committee on the Review of Medicines, 1980) might be explained by the development of receptor subsensitivity. The same committee noted the lack of evidence for efficacy of the long-term use of benzodiazepines in the treatment of insomnia, or justification for the preferential use of short-acting agents as hypnotics. This is in agreement with experimental evidence that subsensitivity develops as rapidly with short-acting as with long-acting drugs.

d) *Multiplicity*. Evidence for multiple benzodiazepine binding sites has been described (Squires et al., 1979; Sieghart and Karobath, 1980; Supavilai and Karobath, 1980) and extensively reviewed (Braestrup and Nielsen, 1980; Lippa et al., 1982). Based on studies with a new class of agents, the triazolopyridazines (see

Fig. 2), Squires and coworkers (1979) demonstrated the presence of at least two distinct benzodiazepine binding sites. Consistent with possibly different physiological roles for the binding sites was the demonstration that some members of the triazolopyridazines exhibited activity in animal behavioural tests predictive of antianxiety effects in man, and had anticonvulsant properties, but did not produce sedation or ataxia. Klepner et al. (1979) suggest that the two types of receptors may be classified as GABA and chloride-independent (type I) or GABA and chloride-dependent (type II). Further, interaction with type I receptors produces the antianxiety effects of a drug and interaction with type II the sedation and ataxia. An uneven regional distribution of these two types of receptors in brain was demonstrated in this study.

Further evidence for multiple benzodiazepine receptors was obtained in photoaffinity labelling experiments using ^{3}H-flunitrazepam binding with subsequent gel electrophoresis (Sieghart and Karobath, 1980). In the cerebellum, the radioligand bound predominantly to a single protein band of molecular weight 51,000 (P_{51}). In other brain areas the major part of radioactivity was localized in this band but two other bands of molecular weights 55,000 (P_{55}) and 59,000 (P_{59}) were also shown to be present. The triazolopyridazine CL-218872 bound preferentially to the P_{51} protein (Sieghart and Karobath, 1980). Perhaps the antianxiety activity of drugs is related to this GABA/benzodiazepine-P_{51} receptor complex and the other protein complexes may perhaps regulate anticonvulsant and sedative effects.

Le Fur et al. (1981) studied the effects of two quinoline derivatives PK-8165 and PK-9084 (see Fig. 2) on ^{3}H-diazepam binding and found that they readily displaced this ligand from its binding site. Both compounds in animal studies produced anticonflict behaviour (anxiolysis) without sedation or ataxia and did not have anticonvulsive properties. It was proposed that they acted on – and therefore the anticonflict behaviour was due to an interaction with – a GABA-independent benzodiazepine receptor associated with a chloride ionophore. Other compounds, such as the pyrazolopyridines, which act as modulators of the GABA/benzodiazepine receptor complex, have been described (Karobath et al., 1981; Supavilai and Karobath, 1981). These compounds, which are also structurally unrelated to GABA and the benzodiazepines, exhibit antianxiety activity in animal tests (Beer et al., 1972). Pyrazolopyridine stimulation of benzodiazepine receptor binding appears to be a preferential effect on the P_{51}-containing receptor type (Supavilai and Karobath, 1980), which again supports the notion of this being the 'anxiolytic' receptor site.

ENDOGENOUS LIGAND FOR THE BENZODIAZEPINE RECEPTOR

The existence of the benzodiazepine receptor implies the presence of an endogenous ligand for the binding of which the receptors have evolved. Such a substance

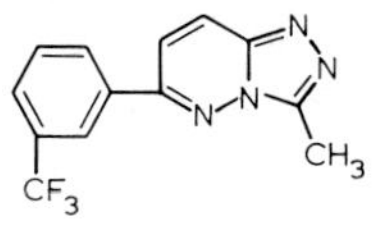

Fig. 2.

could be the body's own antianxiety, anticonvulsant or hypnotic agent. Its identification is a problem which is presently receiving the attention of various groups of workers. A number of purinergic compounds (Asano and Spector, 1979; Skolnick et al., 1979) have been proposed as the endogenous factor, and a substance, β-carboline-3-carboxylic acid (β-CCE), was isolated from human urine by Braestrup's group (Braestrup et al., 1980). Beta-CCE readily displaced bound ^{3}H-diazepam (Braestrup et al., 1980) and while the endogenous ligand may prove to be a molecule of a similar structure, its identity is as yet unknown.

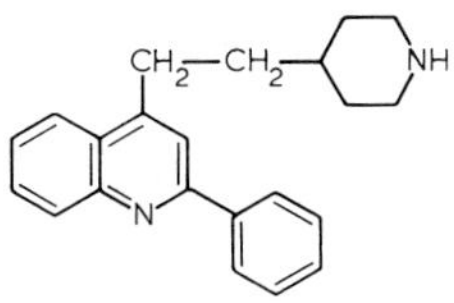

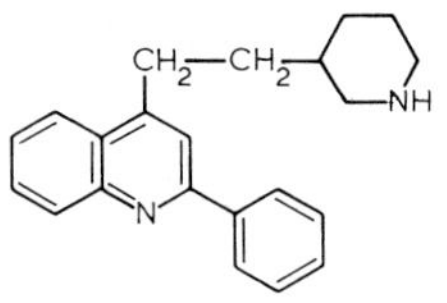

BENZODIAZEPINE ANTAGONISTS

Modification of the basic benzodiazepine structure has led to the production of antagonists to their actions. For example, Ro 15-1788 (Fig. 3) is one such compound which has a high affinity for the benzodiazepine receptor (Hunkeler et al., 1981) and reverses the effects of benzodiazepines in man (Darragh et al., 1981). It is assumed that antagonists act at the level of the central benzodiazepine receptor to inhibit the binding of the typical benzodiazepines.

Another compound CGS-8216 (Fig. 3) has a high affinity for the benzodiazepine receptor (Czernik et al., 1982) but is inactive in pharmacological screens for benzodiazepine-like drugs. Instead it prevents the effects of diazepam in animal models. Clinical studies are not yet available, but like Ro 15-1788 it may have desirable effects, e.g. on mental alertness, in the management of benzodiazepine overdose, or reversal of the unwanted side effects of benzodiazepines given for surgical or diagnostic procedures.

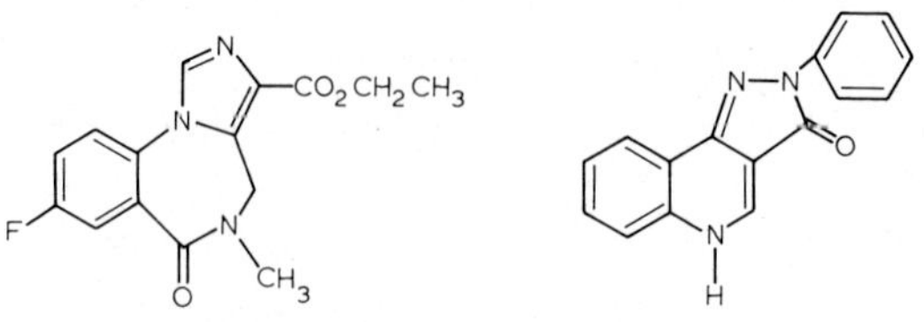

Ro 15-1788   CGS 8216

Fig. 3.

CONCLUSIONS

It now seems clear that benzodiazepines exert their clinical effects by binding to specific receptors in brain. Pharmacological, biochemical and other evidence indicates that rather than a single homogeneous population of receptors there are at least two (probably three) types of benzodiazepine receptor. Recent evidence suggests that the actions of the benzodiazepines could be due to their effects on the receptor subtypes. Non-benzodiazepinoid compounds with specific antianxiety properties have been developed but their efficacy in man awaits detailed clinical evaluation. They hold the hope of effective treatment of anxiety without the unwanted side effects. Further development of benzodiazepine antagonists should lead to a clinically useful group of compounds. Further research on the molecular mechanism of action of the benzodiazepines should lead to an understanding of the relationship between receptor heterogeneity and the various clinical manifestations of these drugs.

More pessimistically, this receptor model cannot account for all clinically effective antianxiety agents. For example, the azaspirodecadione, buspirone, which is anxioselective in animals and man (Hartman and Geller, 1981; Rickels et al., 1982), does not interact with the benzodiazepine/GABA receptor system (Taylor et al., 1982). It is believed to exert its anxiolytic effect through the dopaminergic system. Clearly this group of compounds presents a challenge to the recently developed ideas on the biochemical aetiology of anxiety and its alleviation by benzodiazepines. They may also provide important new clues to the nature of anxiety and its treatment.

REFERENCES

Asano, T. and Spector, S. (1979) Identification of inosine and hypoxanthine as endogenous ligands for the brain benzodiazepine binding sites. Proc. Natl. Acad. Sci. U.S.A. 74, 3805–3809.

Ban, T. A., Brown, W. T., DaSilva, T., Gagnon, M. A., Lamont, H. E., Lehmann, H. E., Lowy, F. W., Ruedy, J. and Sellers, E. M. (1981) Therapeutic monograph on anxiolytic-sedative drugs. Can. Pharm. J. 114, 301–308.

Beer, B., Chasin, M., Clody, D. E., Vogel, J. R. and Horovitz, Z. P. (1972) Cyclic adenosine monophosphate phosphodiesterase in brain: effect on anxiety. Science 176, 428–430.

Bonnet, K. A. (1979) Adaptive alterations in receptor mediated processes and their implications for some mental disorders. Adv. Exper. Med. Biol. 116, 247–259.

Braestrup, C. and Nielsen, M. (1980) Multiple benzodiazepine receptors. Trends in Neuroscience 3, 301–303.

Braestrup, C. and Squires, R. F. (1977) Specific benzodiazepine receptors in rat brain characterized by high affinity ^{3}H-diazepam binding. Proc. Natl. Acad. Sci. U.S.A. 74, 3805–3809.

Braestrup, C. and Squires, R. F. (1978) Pharmacological characterization of benzodiazepine receptors in the brain. Eur. J. Pharmacol. 48, 263–270.

Braestrup, C., Nielsen, M. and Olsen, C. E. (1980) Urinary and brain beta-carboline-3-carboxylates as potent inhibitors of brain benzodiazepine receptors. Proc. Natl. Acad. Sci. U.S.A. 77, 2288–2292.

Burt, D., Creese, I. and Snyder, S. H. (1976) Properties of ^{3}H-haloperidol and ^{3}H-dopamine binding associated with dopamine receptor in calf brain membranes. Mol. Pharmacol. 12, 800–812.

Chiu, T. H. and Rosenberg, H. (1978) Reduced diazepam binding following chronic benzodiazepine treatment. Life Sci. 23, 1153–1157.

Committee on the Review of Medicines (1980) Systematic review of the benzodiazepines. Br. Med. J. 1, 910–912.

Czernik, A. J., Petrack, B., Kalinsky, H. J., Psychoyos, S., Cash, W. D., Tsai, C., Rinehart, R. K., Granat, F. R., Lovell, R. A., Brundish, D. E. and Wade, R. (1982) CGS–8216: Receptor binding characteristics of a potent benzodiazepine antagonist. Life Sci. 30, 363–372.

Darragh, A., Lambe, R., Scully, M. and Brick, I. (1981) Investigation in man of a benzodiazepine antagonist, Ro 15–1788. Lancet 2, 8–10.

Ezrin-Waters, C. and Seeman, P. (1977) L-DOPA reversal of hyperdopaminergic behaviour. Life Sci. 22, 1027–1032.

Fulton, A. and Burrows, G. D. (1983) Benzodiazepine action and affinities for serotonergic and adrenergic receptors. Prog. Neuropsychopharmacol. (in press).

Golds, P. R., Przyslo, F. R. and Strange, P. G. (1980) The binding of some antidepressant drugs to brain muscarinic acetylcholine receptors. Br. J. Pharmacol. 68, 541–549.

Greenblatt, D. J. and Shader, R. I. (1974) Benzodiazepines in Clinical Practice. Raven Press, New York.

Greenblatt, D. J. and Shader, R. I. (1978) Dependence, tolerance and addiction to benzodiazepines: clinical and pharmacokinetic considerations. Drug Metab. Rev. 8, 13–28.

Haefely, W. E. (1978) Central actions of benzodiazepines: general introduction. Br. J. Psychiatry 133, 231–238.

Haefely, W. E. (1983) Tranquillizers. In: D. G. Grahame-Smith and P. J. Cowen (Eds), Psychopharmacology 1: Preclinical Psychopharmacology. Excerpta Medica, Amsterdam. pp. 107–151.

Hartman, R. J. and Geller, I. (1981) Effects of buspirone on conflict behaviour of laboratory rats and monkeys. Proc. West. Pharmacol. Soc. 24, 179–181.

Hunkeler, W., Möhler, H., Pieri, L., Polc, P., Bonetti, E., Cumin, R., Schattner, R. and Haefely, W. (1981) Selective antagonists of benzodiazepines. Nature 290, 514–516.

Iversen, L. L. and Bloom, F. E. (1972) Studies on the uptake of ^{3}H-GABA and ^{3}H-glycine in slices and homogenates of rat brain and spinal cord by electron microscopic autoradiography. Brain Res. 41, 131–143.

Karobath, M., Supavilai, P., Placheta, P. and Sieghart, W. (1981) Interactions of anxiolytic drugs with benzodiazepine receptors. In: B. Angrist, G. Burrows, M. Lader, O. Lingjaerde, G. Sedvall and D. Wheatley (Eds), Recent Advances in Neuropsychopharmacology. Pergamon Press, Oxford, pp. 229–238.

Klepner, C. A., Lippa, A. S., Benson, D. I., Sano, M. C. and Beer, B. (1979) Resolution of two biochemically and pharmacologically distinct benzodiazepine receptors. Pharmacol. Biochem. Behav. 11, 457–462.

Le Fur, G., Mizoule, J., Burgevin, M. C., Ferris, O., Heaulme, M., Gauthier, A., Gueremy, C. and Uzan, A. (1981) Multiple benzodiazepine receptors and evidence of a dissociation between anti-conflict and anticonvulsant properties by PK8165 and PK9084. Life Sci. 28, 1439–1448.

Lippa, A. S., Meyerson, L. R. and Beer, B. (1982) Molecular substrates of anxiety: clues from the heterogeneity of benzodiazepine receptors. Life Sci. 31, 1409–1417.

Martres, M. P., Costentin, J., Baudry, M., Marcais, H., Protais, P. and Schwartz, J. C. (1977) Long term changes in the sensitivity of pre- and post-synaptic dopamine receptors in mouse striatum evidenced by behavioural and biochemical studies. Brain Res. 136, 319–337.

Möhler, H. and Okada, T. (1977a) Properties of ^{3}H-diazepam binding to benzodiazepine receptors in rat cerebral cortex. Life Sci. 20, 2101–2110.

Möhler, H. and Okada, T. (1977b) Benzodiazepine receptor demonstration in the central nervous system. Science 198, 849–851.

Müller, W., Schläfer, U. and Wollert, U. (1978) Benzodiazepine receptor binding: the interactions of some non-benzodiazepine drugs with specific ^{3}H-diazepam binding to rat brain synaptosomal membranes. Naunyn-Schmiedebergs Arch. Pharmacol. 305, 23–26.

Quik, M. and Iversen, L. L. (1978) Subsensitivity of the rat striatal dopaminergic system after treatment with bromocriptine. Naunyn-Schmiedebergs Arch. Pharmacol. 304, 141–145.

Rickels, K., Weisman, K., Norstad, N., Singer, M., Stoltz, D., Brown, A. and Danton, J. (1982) Buspirone and diazepam in anxiety: a controlled study. J. Clin. Psychiatry 43, 81–86.

Robertson, H. A., Martin, I. L. and Candy, J. M. (1978) Differences in benzodiazepine receptor binding in Maudsley reactive and Maudsley non-reactive rats. Eur. J. Pharmacol. 50, 455–457.

Rosenberg, H. C. and Chiu, T. H. (1979) Decreased ^{3}H-diazepam binding as a specific response to chronic benzodiazepine treatment. Life Sci. 24, 803–808.

Rosenberg, H. C. and Chiu, T. H. (1981) Tolerance during chronic benzodiazepine treatment associated with decreased receptor binding. Eur. J. Pharmacol. 70, 453–460.

Sieghart, W. and Karobath, M. (1980) Molecular heterogeneity of benzodiazepine receptors. Nature 286, 285–287.

Skolnick, P., Syapin, P. J., Paugh, B. H., Moneada, V., Marangos, P. J. and Paul, S. M. (1979) Inosine, an endogenous ligand of the brain benzodiazepine receptor antagonizes pentylenetetrazole-evoked seizures. Proc. Natl. Acad. Sci. U.S.A. 76, 1515–1518.

Snyder, S. H. and Yamamura, H. I. (1977) Antidepressants and the muscarinic acetylcholine receptor. Arch. Gen. Psychiatry 34, 236–239.

Speth, R. C., Wastek, G. J., Johnson, P. G. and Yamamura, H. I. (1978) Benzodiazepine binding in human brain: characterization using ^{3}H-flunitrazepam binding. Life Sci. 22, 859–866.

Speth, R. C., Bresolin, N. and Yamamura, H. I. (1979) Acute diazepam administration produces rapid increases in brain benzodiazepine receptor density. Eur. J. Pharmacol. 59, 159–160.

Squires, R. F. and Braestrup, C. (1977) Benzodiazepine receptors in rat brain. Nature 266, 732–734.

Squires, R. F., Benson, D., Braestrup, C., Coupet, J., Klepner, C., Myers, V. and Beer, B. (1979) Some properties of brain specific benzodiazepine receptors: new evidence for multiple receptors. Pharmacol. Biochem. Behav. 10, 825–830.

Supavilai, P. and Karobath, M. (1980) Heterogeneity of benzodiazepine receptors in rat cerebellum and hippocampus. Eur. J. Pharmacol. 64, 91–93.

Supavilai, P. and Karobath, M. (1981) Action of pyrazolopyridines as modulators of ^{3}H-flunitrazepam binding to the GABA/benzodiazepine receptor complex of the cerebellum. Eur. J. Pharmacol. 70, 183–193.

Taylor, D. P., Riblet, L. A., Stanton, H. C., Eison, A. S., Eison, M. S. and Temple, D. S. (1982) Dopamine and antianxiety activity. Pharmacol. Biochem. Behav. 17 (Suppl. 1), 25–35.

Wang, J. K., Taniguchi, T. and Spector, S. (1980) Properties of ^{3}H-diazepam binding sites on rat blood platelets. Life Sci. 27, 1881–1888.

Burrows/Norman/Davies (eds) Antianxiety agents
© *Elsevier Science Publishers B.V., 1984*

Chapter 4

Metabolism of some benzodiazepines

SILVIO GARATTINI

and

VALERIO REGGI

Istituto di Ricerche Farmacologiche 'Mario Negri', Via Eritrea 62, 20157 Milan, Italy.

INTRODUCTION

More than 20 different benzodiazepines (BDZ) are currently marketed through-out the world although it is well known that the pharmacological effects of these various compounds are similar, differing more in quantitative than qualitative aspects. Thus most if not all the claims for selective effects should be taken as based on a very skilful marketing policy rather than on knowledge drawn from scientifically sound studies (Greenblatt and Shader, 1974; Lader, 1976; Garattini et al., 1977; Sellers, 1978; Bellantuono et al., 1980).

Many BDZ undergo metabolic transformation resulting in molecules that account for or prolong the activity of the parent compound. The study of BDZ metabolism is therefore important in understanding the pharmacology of this class of drugs. Information from this type of study is particularly relevant for the rational use of these drugs in clinical situations where diseases or particular phys-iological conditions may affect the rate at which active metabolites are formed and/or inactivated. A by-product of such study is the observation that two of the three main active metabolites of the first BDZ marketed, chlordiazepoxide, joined the parent compound on the market about 10 years later as 'new' antianxiety agents.

44

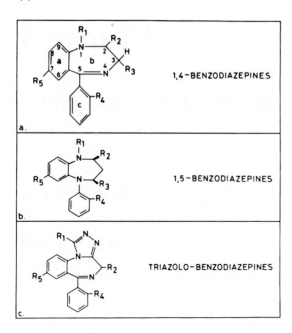

Fig. 1. General chemical structures of the benzodiazepines.

CHEMISTRY AND STRUCTURE-ACTIVITY RELATIONSHIP

The general structures of 1,4-, 1,5-, and triazolo-BDZ are shown in Fig. 1. The chemical differences between the single compounds are specified in Fig. 2.

The BDZ can be classified according to different criteria, but the one proposed here is based on the metabolic fate in man of the different compounds (see later), grouping them according to the main steps of their biotransformation towards inactivation. Following this criterion we have grouped the compounds shown in Fig. 2 in: 1) pro-nordiazepam-like compounds. They are usually formed by a process of N-dealkylation and they are metabolized by a hydroxylation at position 3; 2) oxazepam-like compounds, molecules whose main metabolic transformation is conjugation; 3) NO_2-BDZ, and 4) triazolo-BDZ, which undergo specific metabolic pathways.

Studies on structure-activity relationships (Sternbach, 1973) have shown that substitutions can fruitfully be operated at position 1 of ring b (see Fig. 1a), position 7 of ring a and ortho-position in ring c. It has been observed that activity is particularly enhanced:

a) when an electron-withdrawing group is introduced at position 7 of ring a (e.g. halogen, CF_3, NO_2, CN);

b) when an atom of F or Cl is substituted at one or both orthopositions of ring c;

1- PRO-NORDIAZEPAM COMPOUNDS	R₁ (•)	R₂ (•)	R₃ (•)	R₄(•)	R₅(•)
BROMAZEPAM (see above) (•)					
CHLORDESMETHYLDIAZEPAM	-H	=O	-H	-Cl	-Cl
CHLORDIAZEPOXIDE (see above)					
CLOBAZAM (••)	-CH₃	=O	=O	-H	-Cl
CLORAZEPATE	-H	$=O \leftrightarrow <^{OH}_{OK}$	-COOK	-H	-Cl
DESMETHYLDIAZEPAM	-H	=O	-H	-H	-Cl
DIAZEPAM	-CH₃	=O	-H	-H	-Cl
FLURAZEPAM	$-CH_2-CH_2-N<^{C_2H_5}_{C_2H_5}$	=O	-H	-F	-Cl
FOSAZEPAM	$-CH_2-P^{\nearrow O}_{\searrow (CH_3)_2}$	=O	-H	-H	-Cl
HALAZEPAM	-CH₂-CF₃	=O	-H	-H	-Cl
MEDAZEPAM	-CH₃	$<^H_H$	-H	-H	-Cl
PHENAZEPAM	-H	=O	-H	-Cl	-Br
PINAZEPAM	-CH₂-C≡CH	=O	-H	-H	-Cl
PRAZEPAM	-CH₂-◁	=O	-H	-H	-Cl
TRIFLUBAZAM (••)	-CH₃	=O	=O	-H	-CF₃
2- OXAZEPAM-LIKE COMPOUNDS					
CAMAZEPAM	-CH₃	=O	$-OOCN<^{CH_3}_{CH_3}$	-H	-Cl
LORAZEPAM	-H	=O	-OH	-Cl	-Cl
LORMETAZEPAM	-CH₃	=O	-OH	-Cl	-Cl
OXAZEPAM	-H	=O	-OH	-H	-Cl
TEMAZEPAM	-CH₃	=O	-OH	-H	-Cl
3- NITRO-BENZODIAZEPINES					
CLONAZEPAM	-H	=O	-H	-Cl	-NO₂
FLUNITRAZEPAM	-CH₃	=O	-H	-F	-NO₂
NITRAZEPAM	-H	=O	-H	-H	-NO₂
4- TRIAZOLO-BENZODIAZEPINES					
TRIAZOLAM (fig 1c)	-CH₃	-H		-Cl	-Cl
ESTAZOLAM	-H	-H		-H	-Cl

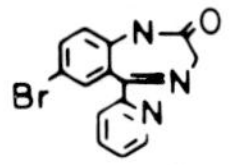

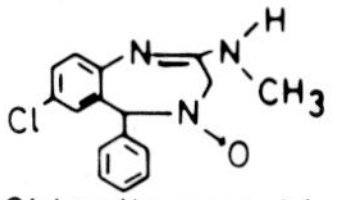

(•) = see general structure in Fig. 1a   (••) = see general structure in Fig. 1b
(•) = see text , section 6.1.2.

Fig. 2. Chemical differences between selected benzodiazepines.

c) when a CH₃ group is substituted at position 1 of ring *b*.
Substituents at meta- or para-positions of ring *c*, at positions 8 and 9 of ring *a* and electron-releasing substituents at position 7 of ring *a* all result in loss of activity.

MEASUREMENT OF THE BENZODIAZEPINES IN BIOLOGICAL SAMPLES

Given at therapeutic dosages, BDZ reach levels lower than 100 ng/ml in human plasma. In addition, BDZ are biotransformed to pharmacologically active metabolites. This process results in low plasma concentrations of different but chemically similar compounds. Thus the determination of BDZ in biological samples requires highly sensitive, specific methods. The discussion of analytical methods is beyond the scope of this paper, but it is worth recalling that gas-chromatography is at present the most suitable method for determination of BDZ in biological samples. Details can be found in Table 1 (See also Chapter 5).

TABLE 1

Analytical methods for the measurement of some benzodiazepines in biological samples.

Drug	Method*	Reference
Bromazepam	EC-GLC	Klotz, 1981
	EC-GLC+DPP	Kaplan et al., 1976
Chlordesmethyldiazepam	EC-GLC	Lanzoni et al., 1979
Chlordiazepoxide	EC-GLC	Garattini et al., 1969
Clobazam	EC-GLC	Caccia et al., 1979
Desmethyldiazepam	EC-GLC	Arnold, 1975; Garattini et al., 1969
Diazepam	EC-GLC	Arnold, 1975; Garattini et al., 1969
Flurazepam	TLC+SPF+SP	de Silva and Strojny, 1971
Medazepam	EC-GLC	de Silva and Puglisi, 1970
Phenazepam	EC-GLC	Zherdev et al., 1981
Pinazepam	GLC-MS	Trebbi et al., 1975
Camazepam	EC-GLC	Marcucci et al., 1978
Lorazepam	EC-GLC	Greenblatt et al., 1978b
Lormetazepam	TLC	Hümpel et al., 1979
Oxazepam	EC-GLC	Arnold, 1975; Garattini et al., 1969
Temazepam	EC-GLC	Belvedere et al., 1972
Clonazepam	EC-GLC	de Silva et al., 1974b
Flunitrazepam	EC-GLC	de Silva et al., 1974b
Nitrazepam	EC-GLC	Kangas, 1977

* Preference is given to GLC methods whenever available.
Abbreviations:
EC-GLC = electron-capture gas-liquid chromatography; DPP = differential pulse polarography; TLC = thin layer chromatography; SPF+SP = spectrophotofluorometry + spectrophotometry; MS = mass spectrometry.

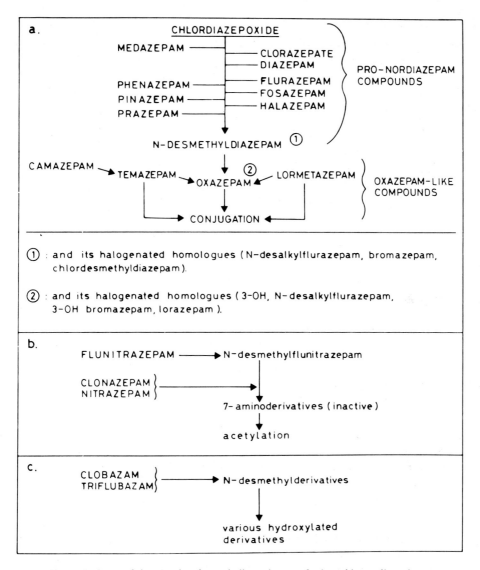

Fig. 3. General scheme of the postulated metabolic pathways of selected benzodiazepines.

GENERAL SCHEME OF METABOLIC PATHWAYS

Figure 3 shows the general metabolic pathways postulated for the BDZ considered in this paper; the scheme is mainly intended to stress similarities and relationships between the different compounds. Since details are given in a later section, here we make the following points of general clinical interest:

a) As shown in Fig. 3a, a number of BDZ undergo biotransformations resulting in

the same (or similar) compound, N-desmethyldiazepam (nordiazepam). The formation of this active metabolite is particularly important because its further biotransformation towards elimination proceeds much more slowly than for the parent compound so that N-desmethyldiazepam (or its homologues) is the compound that actually accumulates in the body after a few days of treatment (Garattini et al., 1973; Greenblatt et al., 1975; Mandelli et al., 1978). This is why we refer to this group of BDZ as pro-nordiazepam-like compounds. The limiting step in the metabolism of pro-nordiazepam BDZ is hydroxylation at position 3 (see Fig. 4) to give oxazepam (or oxazepam-like structures). This process is prolonged in premature and at term newborn infants, elderly patients, and those with severe liver diseases (Mandelli et al., 1978; Bellantuono et al., 1980).
b) Oxazepam-like compounds share the characteristic of having a -OH group at position 3 (see Fig. 4). These BDZ are thus ready for conjugation with no major previous biotransformation. The process of conjugation does not seem to be influenced by age or by liver disease (Greenblatt, 1981). This observation supports the indication of oxazepam-like compounds as BDZ of choice in elderly and seriously hepatopathic patients.

In vitro metabolism

Discussion of in vitro metabolic studies does not fall within the scope of the present paper on account of the scarce clinical relevance of the topic. For those interested we suggest reviews by Garattini et al. (1977) and Nau et al. (1979).

Single compounds

All BDZ for which information is available will be discussed here as regards their in vivo metabolism in man and the clinical relevance of metabolite formation and elimination. Drugs are discussed in the order set on page 45.

PRO-NORDIAZEPAM-LIKE COMPOUNDS

Discussed here are all BDZ which a) undergo dealkylation at position 1 of ring *b*

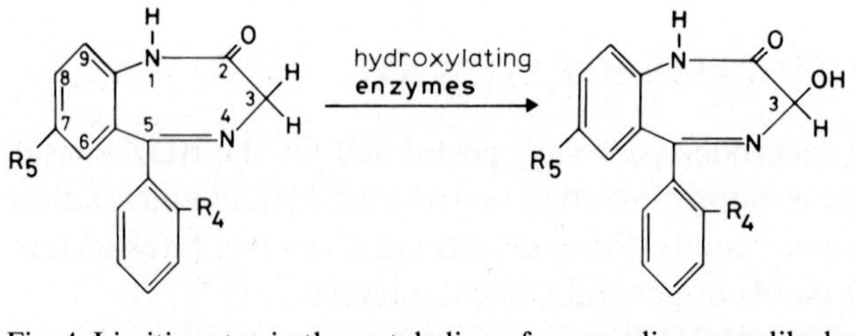

Fig. 4. Limiting step in the metabolism of pro-nordiazepam-like benzodiazepines.

and are then hydroxylated to be eliminated or b) do not have any substituent at position 1 of ring *b* but need to be hydroxylated for elimination.

These compounds have been classified as pro-nordiazepam-like BDZ even if they are transformed to structures chemically different from nordiazepam, as is the case of bromazepam, chlordesmethyldiazepam, clobazam, flurazepam and phenazepam. The chemical differences between nordiazepam and the latter four BDZ must be very slight since pharmacological activity, site of metabolic attack and/or elimination half-life are substantially comparable. The fact worth stressing here is that all BDZ of this group (with the exception of bromazepam) are biotransformed into – or start out as – metabolites sharing the pharmacological activity of the parent compound but with a much longer elimination half-life.

This means that a patient for whom a BDZ of this group is prescribed will after a few days of treatment have in his body a large amount of an active compound. The clinical consequences of this accumulation are not yet clarified, but interaction with other sedative substances (e.g. alcohol) and/or higher probability of experiencing unwanted effects are likely. Furthermore, as stated before, this accumulation is greater in elderly patients or in those with severe liver diseases.

For brevity's sake and easier reading, subject matter here is set out as 1) a description of the main steps of metabolic transformation in humans with 2) stress on the clinically relevant aspects of metabolite formation.

N-desmethyldiazepam

Metabolism in man: N-desmethyldiazepam (NDZ), also called nordiazepam, was shown to be an active metabolite of both chlordiazepoxide and diazepam (Marcucci et al., 1968; Schwartz, 1973). Its metabolic transformation is shown in Fig. 5. NDZ is hydroxylated to oxazepam which is then conjugated with glucuronic acid, the latter process resulting in inactivation.

Clinically relevant remarks: the elimination half-life of NDZ from human plasma ranges from 51 to 120 hours (Mandelli et al., 1978). This very long process is

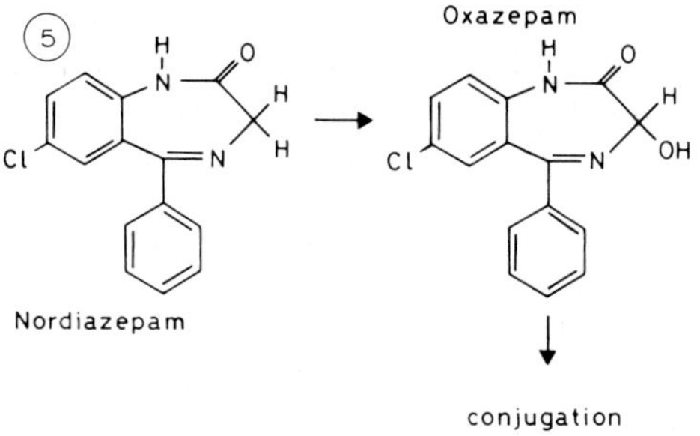

Fig. 5. Metabolic pathways of *N*-desmethyldiazepam.

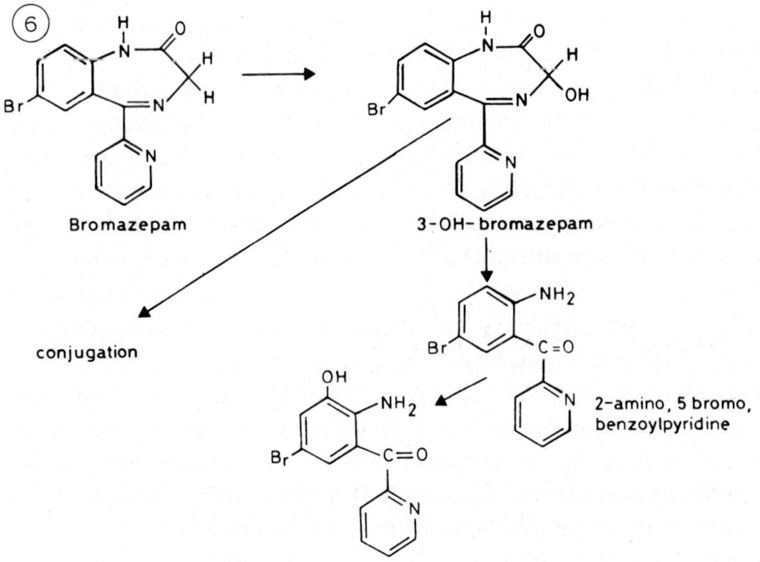

50

Fig. 6. Metabolic pathways of bromazepam (after Kaplan et al., 1976).

due to the slow hydroxylation at position 3. As mentioned above (see p. 48) the rate of hydroxylation depends on age and liver function, older age and severe liver disease slowing it. NDZ is always the compound that accumulates during chronic treatment with pro-nordiazepam BDZ (Mandelli et al., 1978).

Bromazepam

Metabolism in man: as shown in Fig. 6, bromazepam (BRZ) undergoes hydroxylation at position 3 and is then inactivated partly by conjugation with glucuronic acid and partly by breaking of the 7-atom ring to give 2-amino, 5-bromo-benzoylpyridine; the latter is promptly hydroxylated to the 3-hydroxyderivative.

Clinically relevant remarks: BRZ can be considered an exception within the group of pronordiazepam compounds since it has been reported (Kaplan et al., 1976) that hydroxylation at position 3 occurs with a half-life of only 11.9 hours (range 7.9–19.3). This value is very low compared with all the other pro-nordiazepam compounds whose hydroxylation involves a half-life of 51–120 hours. Inclusion of BRZ in the pro-nordiazepam BDZ group is therefore arbitrary, and is based more on analogies in the metabolic transformation pathway (hydroxylation at position 3) than on consideration of the fast elimination rate. Whether the hydroxylation of BRZ is affected by age or liver disease is not known.

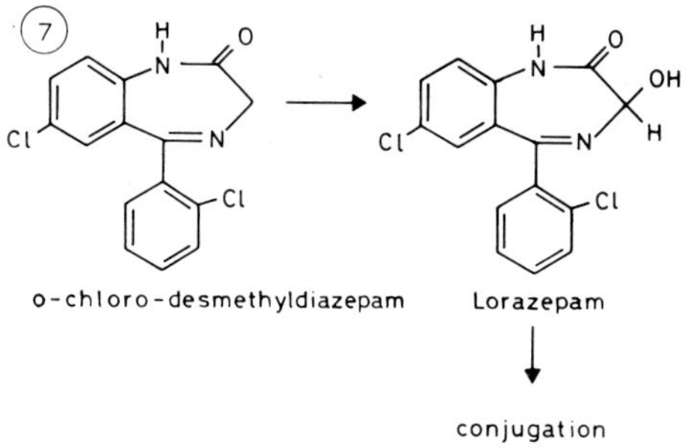

Fig. 7. Metabolic pathways of *o*-chloro-desmethyldiazepam.

Chlordesmethyldiazepam

Metabolism in man: metabolic biotransformation of *o*-chloro-*N*-desmethyldiazepam (CDDZ) is shown in Fig. 7. The main metabolite of CDDZ is lorazepam which is its 3-OH derivative (de Silva et al., 1974a; Garattini et al., 1977).

Clinically relevant remarks: CDDZ has been grouped with the pronordiazepam compounds because 1) it is chemically a halogenated homologue of NDZ and 2) it follows the same metabolic fate as NDZ with a comparable elimination half-life (Dal Bo et al., 1980). Although no specific studies have been performed and hence no data are available, it can be assumed that hydroxylation at position 3 is dependent on age and liver function as for NDZ because of the similarities in the elimination kinetic parameters for the two compounds.

Chlordiazepoxide

Metabolism in man: Figure 8 shows the main steps of chlordiazepoxide (CDX) biotransformation. CDX is hydrolyzed to demoxepam through desmethyl-CDX; demoxepam is then partly inactivated via opening of the lactam and further conjugation, and partly converted to desmethyldiazepam which, in turn, follows the metabolic pathway described in section on *N*-desmethyldiazepam.

Clinically relevant remarks: the conversion of demoxepam into desmethyldiazepam is clinically relevant because it results in the formation of pharmacologically active metabolites: 1) whose elimination is slower than that of the parent compound; 2) which accumulate in the human body during chronic treatment and 3) whose elimination is very much slower in elderly patients or those with severe liver disease (Greenblatt et al., 1978a).

52

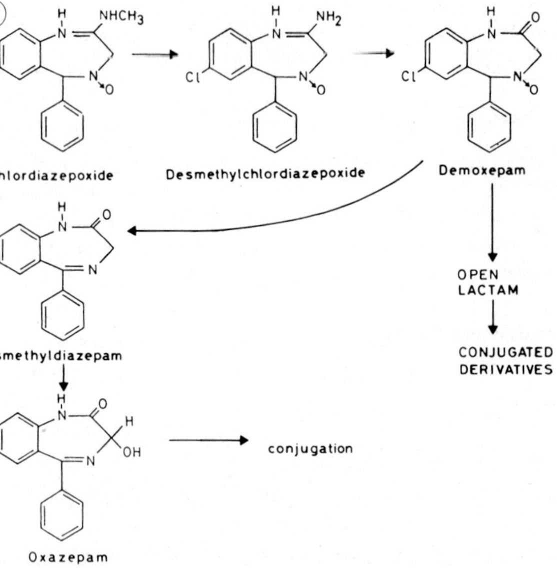

Fig. 8. Metabolic pathways of chlordiazepoxide (after Greenblatt et al., 1978a).

Clobazam

Metabolism in man: clobazam (CBZ) is a 1.5-BDZ and its metabolism is shown in Fig. 9. CBZ undergoes 1) demethylation resulting in *N*-desmethyl-CBZ, and 2) hydroxylation at position 4′ or at positions 3′ and 4′. Desmethyl-CBZ is then hydroxylated at position 4′ or at positions 4′ and 3′. 4′ hydroxy-CBZ is partly desmethylated and partly eliminated directly. All the metabolites mentioned are found in human urine, partially in the conjugated form. An important difference between 1.4 and 1.5-BDZ is that none of the hydroxylated metabolites of the latter are active (Volz et al., 1979). Another important difference is that no hydroxylation occurs at position 3 of 1.5 BDZ.

Clinically relevant remarks: the rationale for grouping CBZ with the pro-nordiazepam compounds lies in the fact that the *N*-demethylated derivative is pharmacologically active (Caccia et al., 1980) and has an elimination half-life longer than the parent compound. It therefore accumulates in the human body during chronic treatment. In this sense CBZ is, conceptually if not chemically, a pro-nordiazepam compound.

Whether and what step(s) of CBZ metabolism are affected by age or disease is not known.

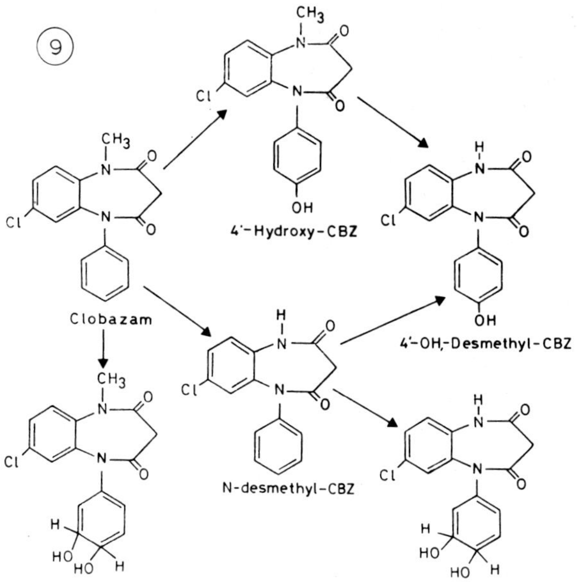

53

Fig. 9. Metabolic pathways of clobazam (CBZ) (after Volz et al., 1979).

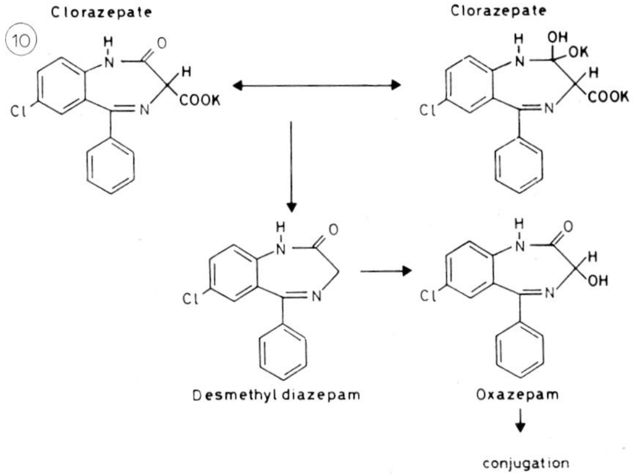

Fig. 10. Metabolic pathways of clorazepate.

Clorazepate

Metabolism in man: clorazepate (CZP), when given orally, is rapidly converted in the stomach into *N*-desmethyldiazepam, which is then absorbed. When given parenterally, CZP is biotransformed into desmethyldiazepam, the process having a half-life of about 2 hours (Rey et al., 1979). Figure 10 shows CZP and its active metabolites.

54

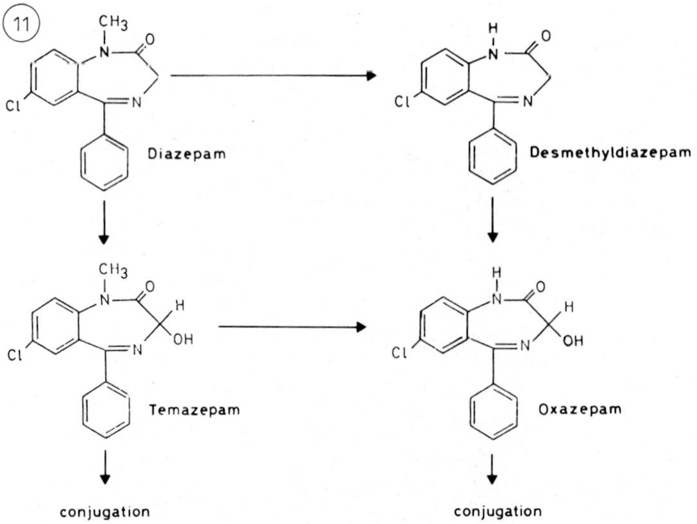

Fig. 11. Metabolic pathways of diazepam.

Clinically relevant remarks: CZP is substantially a pro-drug for *N*-desmethyldia-
zepam.

Diazepam

Metabolism in man: diazepam (DZ) follows two main metabolic pathways (Fig.
11): *N*-desmethylation to desmethyldiazepam and further hydroxylation to oxazepam, and 2) hydroxylation to temazepam and then desmethylation to oxazepam
or direct conjugation (Garattini et al., 1973).

Clinically relevant remarks: DZ is one of the most widely used BDZ thoughout
the Western World (market data), and probably the most thoroughly studied.
During chronic treatment its desmethylated active derivative, nordiazepam, accumulates in the body. The elimination half-life of both DZ and nordiazepam is
prolonged in the elderly, the newborn and in severe liver disease like cirrhosis and
acute and chronic viral hepatitis (Morselli et al., 1973; Mandelli et al., 1978).
Administration of DZ to pregnant women leads to rapid distribution to the foetal
compartment, and accumulation of both DZ and nordiazepam could cause prolonged sedation in the newborn; no major complications are to be expected following a single dose of DZ during labour (Mandelli et al., 1978).

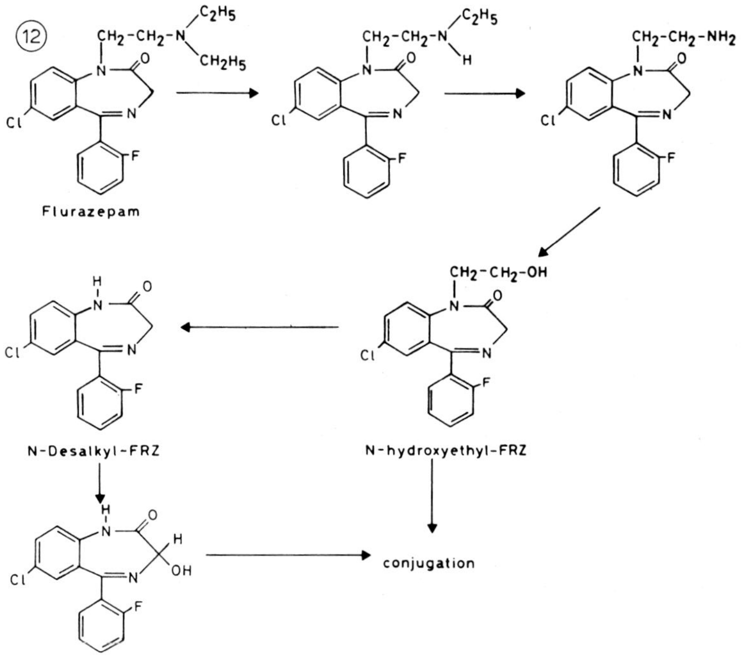

Fig. 12. Metabolic pathways of flurazepam (FRZ) (after Greenblatt et al., 1975).

Flurazepam

Metabolism in man: flurazepam (FRZ) metabolic transformation is shown in Fig. 12. After oral administration, FRZ undergoes major 'first pass' metabolism in the small intestine wall and the liver (Mahon et al., 1977) resulting in removal of one or both -C_2H_5 groups from the side-chain nitrogen. Unmodified FRZ is detectable only in trace amounts in the systemic circulation.

Clinically relevant remarks: oxidation to the hydroxyethyl derivative is an important step in the elimination pathway of FRZ since the glucuronide and sulfate are the main metabolites (up to 92%) found in human urine in the 48 hours after an oral dose. Within that time up to 56% of an oral dose is excreted, but during chronic treatment the *N*-unsubstituted metabolite, *N*-desalkyl FRZ, accumulates in the body and is eliminated with a half-life of 41–100 hours. These facts explain the inclusion of FRZ in the pronordiazepam-like group.

Fosazepam

Metabolism in man: fosazepam (FSZ) is a BDZ for which published data is very

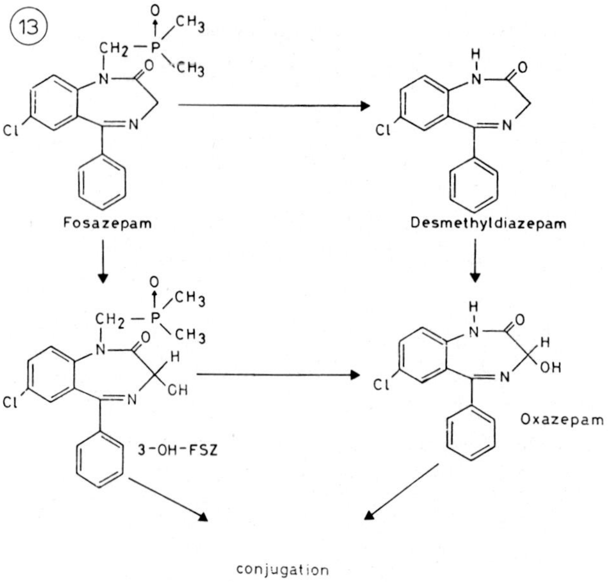

Fig. 13. Metabolic pathways of fosazepam (FSZ) (after Allen and Oswald, 1976).

scarce; its metabolism is shown in Fig. 13. FSZ is rapidly converted ($t\frac{1}{2} = 2$ hours) to 1) the hydroxylated derivative or 2) the *N*-unsubstituted derivative. The former may be directly conjugated or further biotransformed to oxazepam, and the latter follows the pathways of desmethyldiazepam metabolism.

Clinically relevant remarks: *N*-desmethyldiazepam formation is reported to be the fate of at least 25% of the dose of the parent compound and accounts for inclusion of FSZ in the pro-nordiazepam group.

Medazepam

Metabolism in man: medazepam (MDZ) differs from the other 1,4-BDZ in that it lacks the keto group at position 2. Its metabolism is shown in Fig. 14; MDZ is 1) first demethylated and then oxidized to desmethyldiazepam or 2) oxidized to diazepam. It then follows the metabolic pathways previously described for *N*-desmethyldiazepam and diazepam respectively.

Clinically relevant remarks: as with the other pro-nordiazepam compounds, after chronic treatment with MDZ, desmethyldiazepam is the active compound accumulating and persisting in the body.

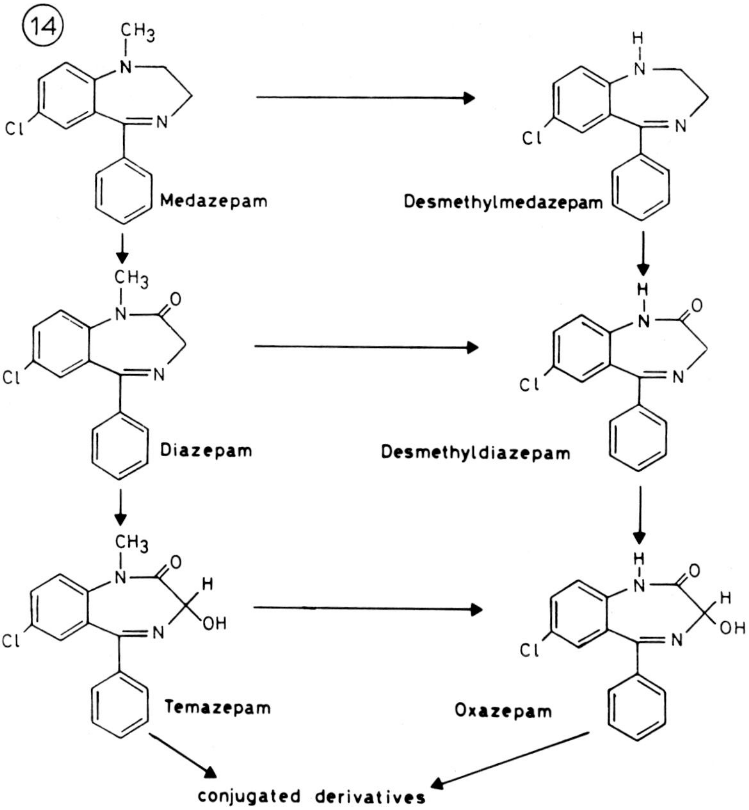

Fig. 14. Metabolic pathways of medazepam (after Schwartz, 1973).

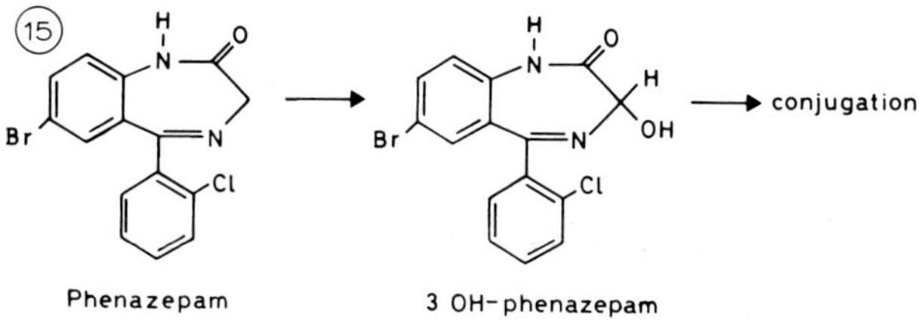

Fig. 15. Metabolic pathways of phenazepam (after Zherdev et al., 1981).

Phenazepam

Metabolism in man: phenazepam (PHZ) is a 1,4-BDZ for which published data is very scarce. Its metabolism and kinetics have been studied by Zherdev et al. (1981) and its biotransformation pathway is shown in Fig. 15.

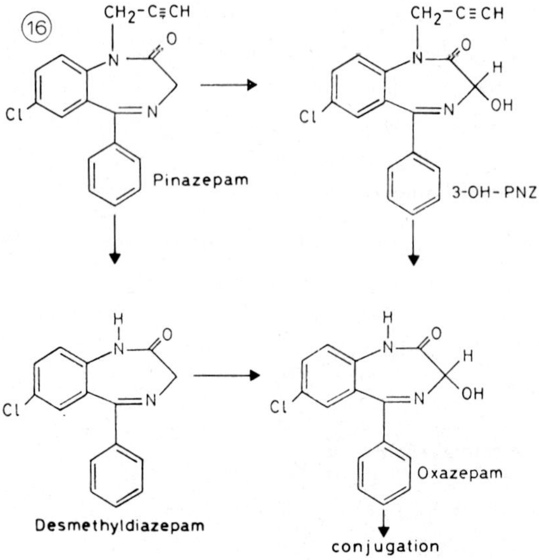

Fig. 16. Metabolic pathways of pinazepam (PNZ).

Clinically relevant remarks: PHZ metabolism recalls that of *o*-chloro-*N*-desme-thyldiazepam. Hydroxylation at position 3 takes place with a halflife of about 60 hours, justifying the inclusion of PHZ in the pro-nordiazepam-like group.

Pinazepam

Metabolism in man: pinazepam (PNZ) metabolism is shown in Fig. 16. PNZ is mainly metabolized through the formation of *N*-desmethyldiazepam and its hydroxylation to oxazepam. The conjugated form of the latter compound consti-tutes 88% of human urine metabolites (Garattini et al., 1977).

Clinically relevant remarks: PNZ is substantially a pro-drug for *N*-desmethyl diazepam.

Prazepam

Metabolism in man: prazepam (PRZ) undergoes almost complete removal of the cyclo-propylmethyl *N*-substituent before reaching the systemic circulation. The 'first pass' metabolism yields *N*-desmethyldiazepam (see Fig. 17).

Clinically relevant remarks: PRZ can be considered a drug precursor of *N*-desmethyldiazepam.

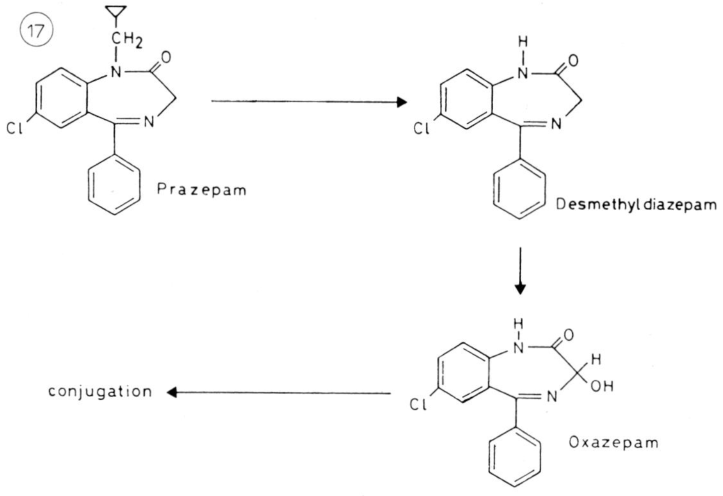

Fig. 17. Metabolic pathways of prazepam (after Greenblatt and Shader, 1978).

OXAZEPAM-LIKE BENZODIAZEPINES

Considered here are those compounds that share with oxazepam the characteristic of a -OH group at position 3. As a consequence BDZ in this group are readily conjugated and eliminated with a half-life usually shorter than 24 hours. Furthermore, BDZ in this group are not transformed into active metabolites with a longer half-life than the parent compound and a once-a-day regimen gives rise to no significant accumulation of metabolites or parent compound (Greenblatt, 1981).

Finally, the elimination rate of oxazepam-like BDZ does not seem to be influenced by older age or liver disease. For oxazepam-like compounds it has been shown in animals in entero-hepatic circulation (Bertagni et al., 1972, 1978). The importance of this process in man is largely unknown.

Oxazepam and lorazepam

Metabolism in man: oxazepam (OXZ) and lorazepam (LRZ) are discussed together because of the similarity of their metabolic fate. These two compounds are the most widely studied in the oxazepam-like BDZ group. OXZ and LRZ are directly conjugated with glucuronic acid yielding inactive metabolites which are excreted in the urine (Fig. 18) (Greenblatt, 1981). Minor metabolites have been identified, but their relevance seems to be practically nil.

Clinically relevant remarks: OXZ and LRZ are probably the most used BDZ in

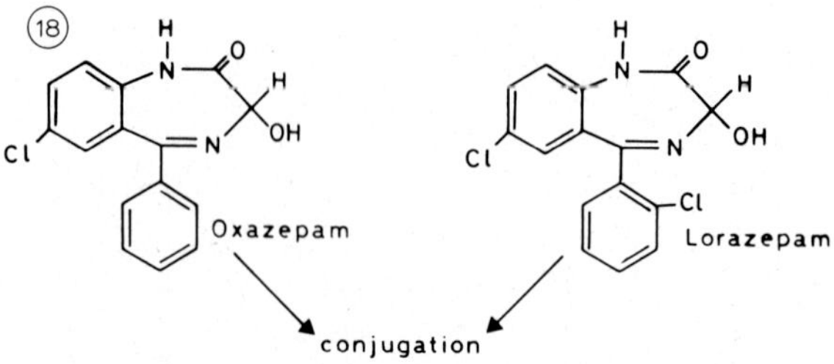

Fig. 18. Metabolic pathways of oxazepam and lorazepam (after Greenblatt, 1981).

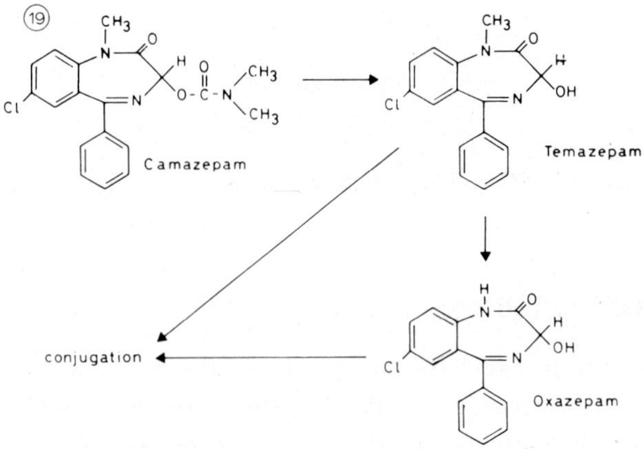

Fig. 19. Metabolic pathways of camazepam.

the OXZ-like group. They have been suggested as the BDZ of choice in elderly patients and those with severe liver disease since no relevant modification of their elimination rate has been observed in such patients (Bellantuono et al., 1980; Greenblatt, 1981). The elimination half-life of OXZ usually ranges from 5 to 15 hours and that of LRZ from 8 to 25 hours (Greenblatt, 1981).

Camazepam

Metabolism in man: Temazepam and oxazepam glucuronides are present in human urine after an oral dose of camazepam (CMZ), but no detectable blood levels of the unconjugated drugs were observed, indicating that after hydrolysis of the ester bond TMZ and OXZ formed are promptly conjugated and eliminated (Fig. 19) (Garattini et al., 1977).

Clinically relevant remarks: the elimination half-life of CMZ is about 20 hours.

Lormetazepam

Metabolism in man: lormetazepam (LMT) metabolism is shown in Fig. 20. The main metabolic attack is direct conjugation of LMT since less than 6% of the total dose is found in the form of the desmethylated derivative lorazepam.

Clinically relevant remarks: clinical studies on LMT are at present limited. LMT elimination half-life has been reported to be about 13 hours (Hümpel et al., 1980).

Temazepam

Metabolism in man: temazepam (TMZ), also called methyloxazepam or 3-OH-diazepam, is metabolized following the pathways shown in Fig. 21. TMZ is partly directly conjugated and partly *N*-desmethylated to yield oxazepam.

Clinically relevant remarks: elimination half-life of TMZ is about 8 hours (Fuccella et al., 1977). No accumulation of TMZ or active metabolites should occur on a once-a-day regimen as utilized for the treatment of insomnia.

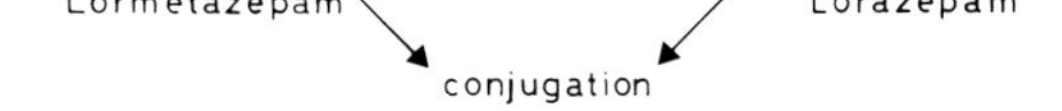

Fig. 20. Metabolic pathways of lormetazepam (after Hümpel et al., 1979, 1980).

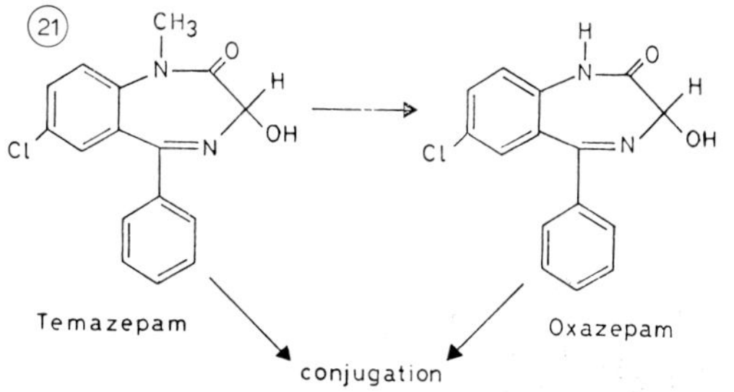

Fig. 21. Metabolic pathways of temazepam.

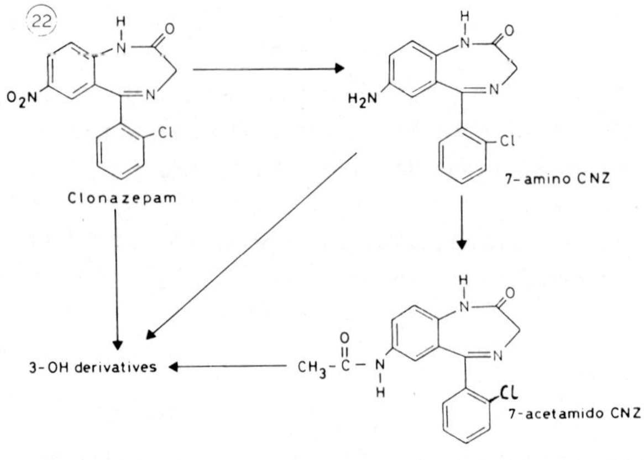

62

Fig. 22. Metabolic pathways of clonazepam (CNZ) (after Pinder et al., 1976).

NITROBENZODIAZEPINES

A characteristic common to all the compounds in this group is a -NO$_2$ substituent at position 7. The nitro-group is the point of major metabolic attack.

Clonazepam

Metabolism in man: clonazepam (CNZ) metabolism is shown in Fig. 22. The most important step in man is reduction to 7-amino-CNZ and its further acetylation. Only trace amounts of 3-OH derivatives can be detected in the urine.

Clinically relevant remarks: CNZ is a BDZ not frequently used for the treatment of anxiety states and insomnia but only as an antiepileptic drug. The clinical relevance of the formation of the 7-amino derivative is not yet understood (Lai et al., 1979), but the 7-amino derivative of flunitrazepam is known to be active (see below).

Flunitrazepam

Metabolism in man: flunitrazepam (FNT) metabolism is shown in Fig. 23. FNT may undergo 1) desmethylation yielding desmethyl FNT or 2) reduction of the nitro group yielding 7-amino FNT. These are the two main metabolites detectable in human plasma after single or multiple oral doses of FNT (Breimer, 1979).

Clinically relevant remarks: both 7-amino-FNT and desmethyl-FNT are active and their elimination half-life is similar to that of the parent compound (15–30

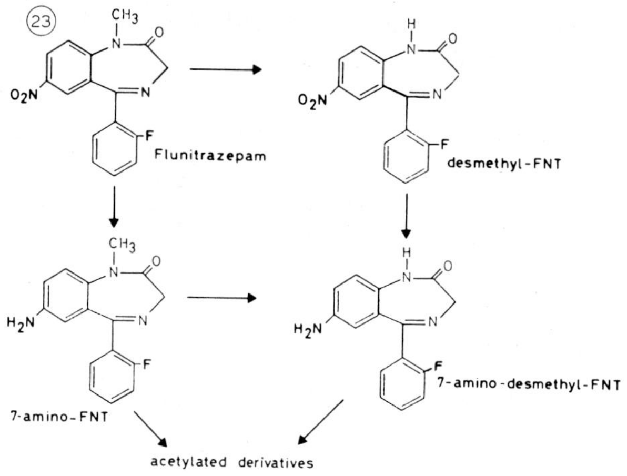

Fig. 23. Metabolic pathways of flunitrazepam (FNT) (after Breimer, 1979).

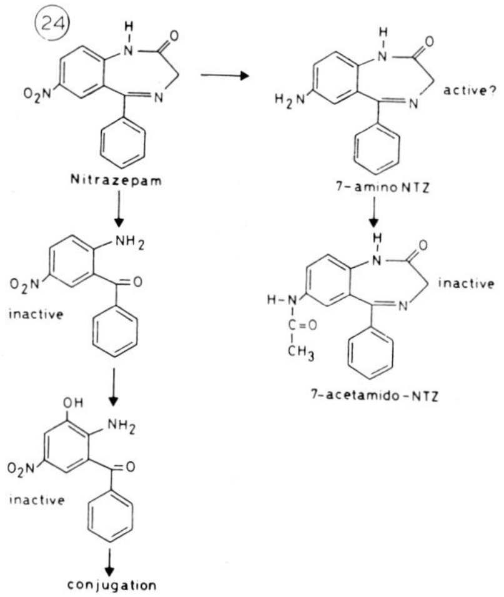

Fig. 24. Metabolic pathways of nitrazepam (NTZ) (after Rieder and Wendt, 1973).

hours) (Breimer, 1979). For this reason accumulation may occur during chronic treatment, even with a once-a-day regimen.

Nitrazepam

Metabolism in man: nitrazepam (NTZ) metabolism is shown in Fig. 24. Two main pathways have been postulated for NTZ biotransformation: 1) reduction of the 7-NO_2 group to 7-amino-NTZ and its further acetylation yielding 7-acetamido-NTZ which is the prevailing metabolite in man (Rieder and Wendt, 1973); 2) cleavage of the 7-atom ring to form benzophenone derivatives.

Clinically relevant remarks: NTZ elimination half-life is influenced by age, the average value being around 28 hours for young volunteers and 40 hours for older patients (Kangas et al., 1979). NTZ has been proposed for anticonvulsant therapy but has now been almost completely abandoned (Browne and Penry, 1973).

TRIAZOLO-BENZODIAZEPINES

Triazolo-benzodiazepines are relatively new among the BDZ. Clinical information on these compounds is less abundant than for the other BDZ. The best known of this series, triazolam, has been the topic of an interesting debate about the efficiency and reliability of existing adverse reaction notification systems; for details see WHO (1980) and Dukes (1980).

Triazolam

Metabolism in man: triazolam (TRZ) postulated metabolism is shown in Fig. 25. Hydroxylation of the methyl substituent at position 1 is the major pathway, 69% of human urinary metabolites being 1-hydroxymethyl-TRZ. The 4-hydroxylated derivative accounts for 11% of urinary metabolites. Other metabolites are various hydroxylated or poly-hydroxylated derivatives (Eberts et al., 1981).

Clinically relevant remarks: TRZ is considered the shortest-acting BDZ avail-

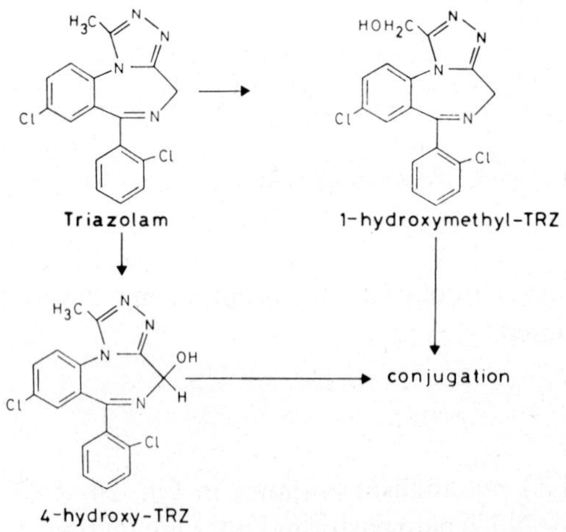

Fig. 25. Metabolic pathways of triazolam (TRZ) (after Eberts et al., 1979, 1981).

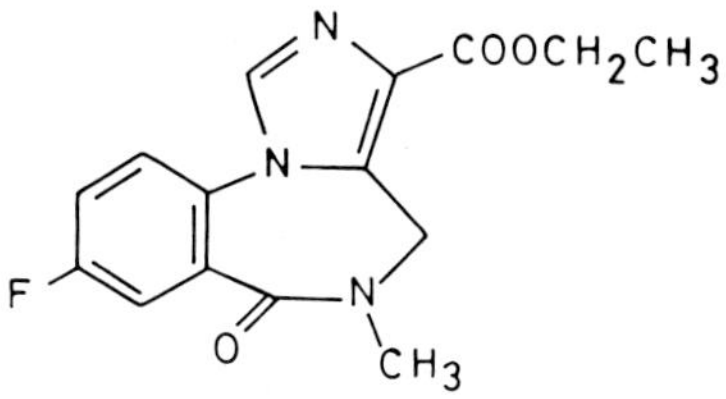

Ro 15-1788

Fig. 26. Structure of Ro 15-1788, ethyl-8-fluoro-5,6-dihydro-5-methyl-6-oxo-4H-imidazo(1,5-a)
(1,4) benzodiazepine-3-carboxylate.

able, its elimination half-life being reportedly 2.2–4.5 hours. Its two major metabolites have an elimination half-life of about 4 hours, but it is not clear whether
they are of clinical importance (see Pakes et al., 1981). No accumulation of TRZ
or its metabolites is believed to occur during prolonged treatment (Editorial,
1979).

ANTAGONISTS OF THE BENZODIAZEPINES

The benzodiazepines are thought to act through facilitation of inhibitory GABA-
ergic synaptic transmission (Haefely et al., 1975), following interaction between
the active drug and a specific neuronal membrane receptor (Möhler and Okada,
1978). Several imidazodiazepines inhibit the specific high-affinity binding of ^{3}H-
diazepam to brain synaptosomal fractions without producing in vivo any of the
typical benzodiazepine effects (Hunkeler et al., 1981). Between these compounds
Ro 15-1788 (Fig. 26) has been found, in tolerance studies in man, to be well
tolerated when given at single oral doses up to 200 mg and to be devoid of any
demonstrable intrinsic pharmacological activity (Darragh et al., 1981).

Furthermore, Ro 15-1788 has been shown by psychometric evaluation to antagonize the central effects of a benzodiazepine in healthy volunteers (Darragh et
al., 1981).

Much more investigation is requested to clarify the pharmacology of compounds like Ro 15-1788 which could be useful both clinically (as in the reversal of
benzodiazepine overdosage effects) and in basic research.

CONCLUSIONS

In the light of the relevant information available to date about BDZ metabolism,
the picture may now be sufficiently clear to permit the following conclusions:

– some currently marketed BDZ are probably only drug precursors for others,
  already known active compounds;

TABLE 2

Proposed classification of the benzodiazepines.

Class	Common characteristics	Compounds	
1) Pro-nordiazepam-like compounds	Limiting step is hydroxylation at position 3	a) pro-drugs	Clorazepate Prazepam
	Active metabolites with elimination half-life longer than 40 hrs Accumulation of active compounds may occur even on a once-a-day regimen	b) compounds with peculiar chemical differences	Chlordesmethyldiazepam Clobazam* Flurazepam Phenazepam Triflubazam
		c) other drugs	Chlordiazepoxide Desmethyldiazepam Diazepam Fosazepam Medazepam Pinazepam
2) Oxazepam-like compounds	Active metabolites either have an elimination half-life not longer than that of the parent compound or are not formed at all Elimination half-life shorter than 24 hrs		Camazepam Lorazepam Lormetazepam Oxazepam Temazepam
3) Nitro-BDZ	Inactivation via reduction of nitro group Elimination half-life between 24 and 48 hrs		Clonazepam Flunitrazepam Nitrazepam
4) Triazolo-BDZ	Very short elimination half-life (up to 5 hrs)		Triazolam

* See section on Clobazam.

- many BDZ undergo very similar metabolic transformation pathways, yielding the same active metabolites and with virtually identical elimination half-lives. This helps explain similarities rather than differences between the 'different' compounds;
- the study of metabolism might play a key role for investigating and possibly clarifying slight differences which may be encountered in clinical practice regarding the incidence of side effects related or not with particular physiological conditions or disease states;
- classification of BDZ on kinetic metabolic considerations might follow the lines proposed in Table 2. A challenge for this classification is bromazepam which undergoes hydroxylation at position 3 like all the pro-nordiazepam compounds but, unlike them, is eliminated with the relatively short half-life of about 20 hours.

REFERENCES

Allen, S. and Oswald, I.   (1976)   Anxiety and sleep after fosazepam. Br. J. Clin. Pharmacol. 3, 165–168.

Arnold. E.   (1975)   A simple method for determing diazepam and its major metabolites in biological fluids: application in bioavailability studies. Acta Pharmacol. Toxicol. 36, 335–352.

Bellantuono, C., Reggi, V., Tognoni, G. and Garattini, S.   (1980)   Benzodiazepines: clinical pharmacology and therapeutic use. Drugs 19, 195–219.

Belvedere, G., Tognoni, G., Frigerio, A. and Morselli, P. L.   (1972)   A specific, rapid and sensitive method for gas-chromatographic determination of methyl-oxazepam in small samples of blood. Anal. Lett. 5, 531–541.

Bertagni, P., Marcucci, F., Mussini, E. and Garattini, S.   (1972)   Biliary excretion of conjugated hydroxyl benzodiazepines after administration of several benzodiazepines to rats, guinea pigs, and mice. J. Pharm. Sci. 61, 965–966.

Bertagni, P., Bianchi, R., Marcucci F., Mussini, E. and Garattini, S.   (1978)   The enterohepatic circulation of oxazepam-O-glucuronide in guinea pigs. J. Pharm. Pharmacol. 30, 185–186.

Breimer, D. D.   (1979)   Pharmacokinetics and metabolism of various benzodiazepines used as hypnotics. Br. J. Clin. Pharmacol. 8, 7S-13S.

Browne, T. R. and Penry, J. K.   (1973)   Benzodiazepines in the treatment of epilepsy. A review. Epilepsia 14, 277–310.

Caccia, S., Ballabio, M., Guiso, G. and Zanini, M. G.   (1979)   Gas-liquid chromatographic determination of clobazam and N-desmethylclobazam in plasma. J. Chromatogr. 164, 100–105.

Caccia, S. Guiso, G. and Garattini, S.   (1980)   Brain concentrations of clobazam and N-desmethylclobazam and antileptazol activity. J. Pharm. Pharmacol. 32, 295–296.

Dal Bo, L., Marcucci, F., Mussini, E., Perbellini, D., Castellani, A. and Fresia, P.   (1980)   Plasma levels of chlorodesmethyldiazepam in humans. Biopharm. Drug Dispos. 1, 123–126.

Darragh, A., Lambe, R., Scully, M. and Brick, I.   (1981)   Investigation in man of the efficacy of a benzodiazepine antagonist, Ro 15-1788. Lancet 2, 8–10.

De Silva, J. A. F. and Puglisi, C. V.   (1970)   Determination of medazepam (nobrium) diazepam (valium) and their major biotransformation products in blood and urine by electron capture gas-liquid chromatography. Anal. Chem. 42, 1725–1736.

De Silva, J. A. F. and Strojny, N.   (1971)   Determination of flurazepam and its major biotransfor-

68

mation products in blood and urine by spectrophotofluorometry and spectrophotometry. J. Pharm. Sci. 60, 1303–1314.

De Silva, J. A. F., Bekersky, I. and Brooks, M. A. (1974a) Electron-capture GLC determination of blood levels of 7-chloro-1,3-dihydro-5-(2´-chlorophenyl)-2H-1, 4-benzodiazepin-2-one in humans and its urinary excretion as lorazepam determined by differential pulse polarography. J. Pharm. Sci. 63, 1943–1945.

De Silva, J. A. F., Puglisi, C. V. and Munno, N. (1974b) Determination of clonazepam and fluni-trazepam in blood and urine by electron-capture GLC. J. Pharm. Sci. 63, 520–527.

Dukes, M. N. G. (1980) The van der Kroef syndrome. In: M. N. G. Dukes (Ed.), Side Effects of Drugs, Annual 4, Excerpta Medica, Amsterdam, pp. V–IX.

Eberts, Jr., F. S., Philopoulos, Y. and Vliek, R. W. (1979) Disposition of ^{14}C-triazolam, a short-acting hypnotic, in man. Pharmacologist 21, 168.

Eberts, Jr., F. R., Philopoulos, Y., Reineke, L. M. and Vliek, R. W. (1981) Triazolam disposition. Clin. Pharmacol. Ther. 29, 81–93.

Editorial (1979) Two more benzodiazepines. Drug Ther. Bull. 17, 65–66.

Fuccella, L. M., Bolcioni, G., Tamassia, V., Ferrario, L. and Tognoni, G. (1977) Human pharmacokinetics and bioavailability of temazepam administered in soft gelatin capsules. Eur. J. Clin. Pharmacol. 12, 383–386.

Garattini, S., Marcucci, F. and Mussini, E. (1969) Gas chromatographic analysis of benzodiazepines. In: R. Porter (Ed.), Ciba Foundation Symposium on Gas Chromatography in Biology and Medicine. Churchill, London, pp. 161–172.

Garattini, S., Mussini, E., Marcucci, F. and Guaitani, A. (1973) Metabolic studies on benzodiazepines in various animal species. In: S. Garattini, E. Mussini and L. O. Randall (Eds.), The Benzodiazepines. Raven Press, New York, pp. 75–97.

Garattini, S., Marcucci, F. and Mussini, E. (1977) The metabolism and pharmacokinetics of selected benzodiazepines. In: E. Usdin and I. S. Forrest (Eds.), Psychotherapeutic Drugs, Part. II, Applications. M. Dekker, New York, pp. 1039–1087.

Greenblatt, D. J. (1981) Clinical pharmacokinetics of oxazepam and lorazepam. Clin. Pharmacokinet. 6, 89–105.

Greenblatt, D. J. and Shader, R. I. (1974) Benzodiazepines in Clinical Practice. Raven Press, New York.

Greenblatt, D. J. and Shader, R. I. (1978) Prazepam and lorazepam, two new benzodiazepines. N. Engl. J. Med. 299, 1342–1344.

Greenblatt, D. J., Shader, R. I. and Koch-Weser, J. (1975) Flurazepam hydrochloride. Clin. Pharmacol. Ther. 17, 1–14.

Greenblatt, D. J., Shader, R. I., MacLeod, S. M. and Sellers, E. M. (1978a) Clinical pharmacokinetics of chlordiazepoxide. Clin. Pharmacokinet. 3, 381–394.

Greenblatt, D. J., Franke, K. and Shader, R. I. (1978b) Analysis of lorazepam and its glucuronide metabolite by electron-capture gas-liquid chromatography: use in pharmacokinetic studies of lorazepam. J. Chromatogr. 146, 311–320.

Haefely, W., Kulcsàr, A., Möhler, H., Pieri, L., Polc, P. and Schaffner, R. (1975) Possible involvement of GABA in the central actions of benzodiazepines. In: E. Costa and P. Greengard (Eds.), Mechanism of Action of Benzodiazepines. Raven Press, New York, pp. 131–151.

Hümpel, M., Illi, V., Milius, W., Wendt, H. and Kurowski M. (1979) The pharmacokinetics and biotransformation of the new benzodiazepine lormetazepam in humans. I. Absorption, distribution, elimination and metabolism of lormetazepam-5-[14]C. Eur. J. Drug Metab. Pharmacokinet. 4, 237–243.

Hümpel, M., Nieuweboer, B., Milius, W., Hanke, H. and Wendt, H. (1980) Kinetics and biotransformation of lormetazepam. Clin. Pharmacol. Ther. 28, 673–679.

Hunkeler, W., Möhler, H., Pieri, L., Polc, P., Bonetti, E. P., Cumin, R., Schaffner, R. and Haefely, W. (1981) Selective antagonists of benzodiazepines. Nature 290, 514–516.

Kangas, L. (1977) Comparison of two gas-liquid chromatographic methods for plasma nitrazepam determination. J. Chromatogr. 136, 259–270.

Kangas, L., Iisalo, E., Kanto, J., Lehtinen, V., Pynnönen, S., Ruikka, I., Salminen, J., Sillanpää, M. and Syvälahti, E. (1979) Human pharmacokinetics of nitrazepam: effect of age and diseases. Eur. J. Clin. Pharmacol. 15, 163–170.

Kaplan, S. A., Jack, M. L., Weinfeld, R. E., Glover, W., Weissman, L. and Cotler, S. (1976) Biopharmaceutical and clinical pharmacokinetic profile of bromazepam. J. Pharmacokinet. Biopharm. 7, 87–95.

Klotz, U. (1981) Determination of bromazepam by gas-liquid chromatography and its application for pharmacokinetic studies in man. J. Chromatogr. 222, 501–506.

Lader, M. (1976) Antianxiety drugs: Clinical pharmacology and therapeutic use. Drugs 12, 362–373.

Lai, A. A., Min, B. H., Garland, W. A. and Levy, R. H. (1979) Kinetics of biotransformation of clonazepam to its 7-amino metabolite in the monkey. J. Pharmacokinet. Biopharm. 7, 87–95.

Lanzoni, J., Airoldi, L., Marcucci, F. and Mussini, E. (1979) Gas chromatographic determination of chlorodesmethyldiazepam and lorazepam in rats and mice. J. Chromatogr. 168, 260–265.

Mahon, W. A., Inaba, T. and Stone, R. M. (1977) Metabolism of flurazepam by the small intestine. Clin. Pharmacol. Ther. 22, 228–233.

Mandelli, M., Tognoni, G. and Garattini, S. (1978) Clinical pharmacokinetics of diazepam. Clin. Pharmacokinet. 3, 72–91.

Marcucci, F., Guaitani, A., Kvetina, J., Mussini, E. and Garattini, S. (1968) Species difference in diazepam metabolism and anticonvulsant effect. Eur. J. Pharmacol. 4, 467–470.

Marcucci, F., Mussini, E., Cotellessa, L., Ghirardi, P., Parenti, M., Riva, R. and Salvá, P. (1978) Distribution of camazepam in rats and mice. J. Pharm. Sci. 67, 1470–1471.

Möhler, H. and Okada, T. (1978) Benzodiazepine receptor: demonstration in the central nervous system. Science 198, 849–851.

Morselli, P. L., Principi, N., Tognoni, G., Reali, E., Belvedere, G., Standen, S. M. and Sereni, F. (1973) Diazepam elimination in premature and full term infants, and children. J. Perinat. Med. 1, 133–141.

Nau, H., Brendel, K. and Liddiard, C. (1979) Benzodiazepine metabolism in cultures of isolated hepatocytes and liver fragments of human fetus. Drug Metab. Rev. 9, 131–146.

Pakes, G. E., Brogden, R. N., Heel, R. C., Speight, T. M. and Avery, G. S. (1981) Triazolam: a review of its pharmacological properties and therapeutic efficacy in patients with insomnia. Drugs 22, 81–110.

Pinder, R. M., Brogden, R. N., Speight, T. M. and Avery, G. S. (1976) Clonazepam: a review of its pharmacological properties and therapeutic efficacy in epilepsy. Drugs 12, 321–361.

Rey, E., d'Athis, Ph., Giraux, P., de Lauture, D., Turquais, J. M., Chavinie, J. and Olive, G. (1979) Pharmacokinetics of clorazepate in pregnant and non-pregnant women. Eur. J. Clin. Pharmacol. 15, 175–180.

Rieder, J. and Wendt, G. (1973) Pharmacokinetics and metabolism of the hypnotic nitrazepam. In: S. Garattini, E. Mussini and L. O. Randall (Eds.), The Benzodiazepines. Raven Press, New York, pp. 99–127.

Sellers, E. M. (1978) Clinical pharmacology and therapeutics of benzodiazepines. Can. Med. Assoc. J. 118, 1533–1538.

Schwartz, M. A. (1973) Pathways of metabolism of the benzodiazepines. In: S. Garattini, E. Mussini and L. O. Randall (Eds.), The Benzodiazepines. Raven Press, New York, pp. 53–74.

Sternbach, L. H. (1973) Chemistry of 1,4-benzodiazepines and some aspects of the structure-activity relationship. In: S. Garattini, E. Mussini and L. O. Randall (Eds.), The Benzodiazepines. Raven Press, New York, pp. 1–26.

Trebbi, A., Gervasi, G. B. and Comi, V. (1975) Determination of pinazepam and its metabolites in serum, urine and brain by gas-liquid chromatography and mass spectrometry. J. Chromatogr. 110, 309–319.

Volz, M., Christ, O., Kellner, H. M., Kuch, H., Fehlhaber, H. W., Gantz, D., Hajdu, P. and Cavagna, F. (1979) Kinetics and metabolism of clobazam in animals and man. Br. J. Clin. Pharmacol. 7, 41S–50S.

W.H.O. (1980) Drug Information. January–March, pp. 12–13.

Zherdev, V. P., Caccia, S., Garattini, S. and Ekonomov, A. L. (1981) Species differences in phenazepam kinetics and metabolism. Eur. J. Drug Metab. Pharmacokinet. (in press).

Burrows/Norman/Davies (eds) Antianxiety agents
© *Elsevier Science Publishers B.V., 1984*

Chapter 5

Measurement of antianxiety drugs in biological samples

KAY P. MAGUIRE

and

ANN FULTON

Department of Psychiatry, University of Melbourne, Australia

INTRODUCTION

Amongst the large number of drugs that have been used for treating anxiety, e.g. the barbiturates, meprobamate, some phenothiazines and a number of tricyclic antidepressants, the benzodiazepine class of drugs is now the most frequently prescribed. This popularity is due to a number of factors: their long half-lives leading to prolonged duration of action without frequent dosages; their lack of liver enzyme inducing activity; the low incidence of dependence and tolerance associated with their use; and most importantly, their safety in overdosage.

As the use of the benzodiazepines became general, the development and refinement of methods for their identification and measurement kept pace. At the present time, any one of a large battery of techniques may be selected and applied, depending on the drug concentration to be measured and the specificity and sensitivity desired. Whatever the method chosen (excepting perhaps for radioimmunoassay) the first step is common and compulsory – the extraction of the drugs from plasma, urine or other biological medium.

EXTRACTION OF SAMPLES

The interference due to various proteins and lipids present in the biological medium can generally be eliminated by extraction of the drugs from an alkalinized sample into an organic phase (such as ethyl acetate, diethyl ether, chloroform, etc.). When large samples of plasma must be extracted from to improve sensitivity, back extraction of the organic phase into acid, followed by re-extraction of the neutralized acid with fresh organic solvent, may often be necessary. For more efficient sample clean-up, protein precipitation prior to extraction may be practised. This is effected by gentle warming of the sample with acid or by salt saturation. A comprehensive review of extraction conditions for the benzodiazepines and their metabolites has been provided by De Silva et al. (1976).

MEASUREMENT OF BENZODIAZEPINE CONCENTRATIONS OF $\geqslant \mu g/ml$

When samples containing high concentrations of the benzodiazepine drugs are to be measured, as following overdosage, in toxicological studies or after chronic daily administrations of 30 mg or more, the range of methods applicable is wide indeed.

Spectrophotometry

By application of Beer's Law to the absorption maximum (around 250 nm) of these molecules, the benzodiazepine content of a sample can be determined. Alternatively, the drugs may be hydrolysed to an aromatic amine, diazotized and coupled to N-(1-naphthyl)ethylenediamine (the Bratton-Marshall reaction, 1939) to form an intensely coloured dye, thus allowing the drug to be assayed colorimetrically. These two methods will yield the total benzodiazepine content, but will not distinguish between parent drug and metabolite levels.

Specificity is less of a problem using fluorometric techniques. Chlordiazepoxide and its desmethyl metabolite (Koechlin and D'Arconte, 1963), flurazepam and its metabolites (De Silva and Strojny, 1971), nitrazepam and its two metabolites (Rieder, 1973), have all been measured as the fluorophore formed after acid hydrolysis, or after hydrolysis and reaction with dimethyl formamide, or after irradiation of the drug molecule with ultra violet light. Conversion to the 9-acridanone has been used as a screening method for the detection of diazepam, chlordiazepoxide, oxazepam, clorazepate and their major metabolites in blood and urine (Valentour et al., 1975).

Thin-layer chromatography

By application of this method, the various benzodiazepines may be separated from each other, from their metabolites and then identified, as well as quantitated. Wouters et al. (1979) advocated the simultaneous running of plates in three mobile systems for the routine identification of 19 commonly used benzodiazepine drugs.

After development of the chromatogram the spots can be located under ultra violet light or with spray reagents, eluted and quantitated by any suitable method. The article by Clifford and Franklin-Smyth (1974) should be consulted for an extensive review of thin-layer separation of the benzodiazepines.

Differential pulse polarography

Although there have been many reports of the determination of the benzodiazepine drugs from their cathodic reduction (e.g. medazepam, Oelschlager and Oehr, 1970; oxazepam, Oelschlager et al., 1969; chlordiazepoxide, Hackman et al., 1974; clorazepate, Hanna et al., 1978), this method of analysis has not been widely applied, probably since it has little to recommend it above the other available methods.

MEASUREMENT OF BENZODIAZEPINE CONCENTRATIONS OF ≤ng/ml

After acute administration, or chronic administration of doses <20 mg daily, the plasma levels of the benzodiazepines are often no higher than ng/ml concentrations. In order to measure such quantities, methods of great sensitivity and accuracy must be applied. This is especially true for measuring the new potent benzodiazepines of extremely short half-lives, such as triazolam (Halcion: Upjohn) and midazolam (Roche).

The methods which fulfil these conditions are: gas-liquid chromatography (including gas chromatography-mass spectrometry), high pressure liquid chromatography, radioimmunoassay, and radioreceptor assay.

Gas-liquid chromatography (GLC)

The most commonly used method of benzodiazepine analysis, GLC, may be used to separate and detect the drugs as the unchanged molecule (Berlin et al., 1972; Greaves, 1974; Haidukewych et al., 1980) after acid hydrolysis of the benzodiazepines to the benzophenones (Beharrell et al., 1972; Knowles and Ruelius, 1972) or after derivatization with acetic anhydride (Gelbke and Schlicht, 1978), with silylating agents (De Silva et al., 1976), and alkylating agents (Vessman et al., 1977;

Sun and Hoffman, 1978).
The electron-capture detector has found a wide application for benzodiazepine analysis, due to its sensitivity. The flame-ionization detector is also frequently used. Its poorer sensitivity compared with the former kind of detector, is compensated for by its less rigorous need for meticulous sample clean-up. The nitrogen-phosphorus detector can yield sensitivity levels comparable to the electron-capture detector, however, it has not yet been as popularly exploited.

GLC coupled to a mass spectrometer as the detection device is an extremely specific technique with better sensitivity than GLC alone, but the price of the equipment is prohibitive. A number of studies has applied this method to identify benzodiazepine metabolites (Forgione et al., 1971; Trebbi et al., 1975; Clatworthy et al., 1977; Miwa et al., 1981) and to pharmacokinetic investigations in humans (Higuchi et al., 1979).

High pressure liquid chromatography (HPLC)

HPLC has one major advantage over GLC techniques in that the analysis is carried out at room temperature. This is particularly useful for the thermally labile compounds such as chlordiazepoxide and its metabolites (Skellern et al., 1978). A simple one-step extraction allows for a short analysis time and adequate specificity and reproducibility have been demonstrated (Mackichan et al., 1979; Wallace et al., 1979). Sensitivity at present may not be as good as GLC with electron-capture detection but comparison with the latter method for diazepam and desmethyldiazepam has shown good agreement (Raisys et al., 1980). Further advances in HPLC technology will probably lead to this technique becoming more widespread.

Radioimmunoassay (RIA)

RIA procedures have been developed for a limited number of benzodiazepine drugs: diazepam (Peskar and Spector, 1973; Bourne et al., 1978; Dixon and Crews, 1978), chlordiazepoxide (Dixon et al., 1975, 1979) and flunitrazepam (Dixon et al., 1981). This mode of estimation is sensitive, inexpensive and rapid, especially when prior extraction is not necessary. Specificity may be a problem as metabolites may cross react with antisera produced against the parent molecule. Paradoxically, for those benzodiazepines which do not have active metabolites, e.g. oxazepam and lorazepam, no antisera have yet been successfully developed.

A commercial enzyme immunoassay kit (Syva Corporation) is now available, based on an antiserum which cross reacts to the same extent with both diazepam and desmethyldiazepam. Total diazepam and desmethyldiazepam concentrations correlated well with both GLC-electron capture and HPLC (Wallace et al., 1980).

Radioreceptor assay

This method is akin to the RIA method, differing in that the antiserum is replaced by the high affinity ^{3}H-diazepam binding sites (Braestrup et al., 1977; Mohler and Okada, 1977) found in mammalian brains. Sample extraction or protein precipitation is necessary before the assay proper, and total concentrations, including those of the active metabolites, are quantitated in terms of equivalents of the drug with which the standard curve was set up.

A quick and inexpensive procedure, the radioreceptor assay is ideal where only sensitivity, and not specificity, is demanded (Hunt et al., 1979; Owen et al., 1979; Skolnick et al., 1979).

SUMMARY

A wide range of analytical techniques is available for the quantitation of benzodiazepine concentrations in biological samples. For toxicological or overdosage studies where concentrations are high, spectrophotometry, thin-layer chromatography, polarography or fluorimetry may suffice. For measurement of concentrations in the ng/ml range, gas-liquid chromatography, high pressure liquid chromatography, radioimmunoassay and radioreceptor assay have the required sensitivity. For precise separate quantitation of parent drug and metabolites, either gas-liquid chromatography or high pressure liquid chromatography are most suitable. If rapid screening is required and specificity is not important, e.g. for compliance testing, radioimmunoassay (or enzyme immunoassay) and radioreceptor techniques are ideal. Gas chromatography-mass spectrometry has its place in characterization of metabolites and pharmacokinetic studies where even better sensitivity is required.

REFERENCES

Beharrell, G. P., Hailey, D. M. and McLaurin, M. K. (1972) Determination of nitrazepam (Mogadon) in plasma by electron capture gas-liquid chromatography. J. Chromatogr. 70, 45–52.

Berlin, A., Siwers, B., Agurell, S., Hjort, A., Sjoqvist, F. and Strom, S. (1972) Determination of bioavailability of diazepam in various formulations from steady-state plasma concentrations data. Clin. Pharmacol. Ther. 13, 733–744.

Berry, D. J. (1971) The cathode-ray polarographic determination of diazepam 7-chloro-1, 3-dihydro-1-methyl-5-phenyl-2H-1, 4-benzodiazepine-2-one, in human plasma. Clin. Chim. Acta 32, 235–241.

Bourne, R. C., Robinson, J. D. and Teale, J. D. (1978). A simple radioimmunoassay for plasma diazepam and its application to single dose studies in man. Br. J. Clin. Pharmacol. 63, 371P.

Braestrup, C., Albrechtsen, A. and Squires, R. F. (1977) High densities of benzodiazepine receptors in human cortical areas. Nature 269, 702–704.

Bratton, A. C. and Marshall, E. K. (1939) A new coupling component for sulfanilamide determination. J. Biol. Chem. 128, 537–550.

76

Clatworthy, A. J., Jones, L.V. and Whitehouse, M. J.   (1977). The gas chromatography mass spectrometry of the major metabolites of flurazepam. Biomed. Mass Spectrom. 4, 248–254.

Clifford, J. M. and Franklin-Smyth, W.   (1974). The determination of some 1, 4-benzodiazepines and their metabolites in body fluids: a review. Analyst 99, 241–272.

De Silva, J. A. F. and Strojny, N.   (1971)   Determination of flurazepam and its major biotransformation products in blood and urine by spectrophoto-fluorometry and spectrophotometry. J. Pharm. Sci. 60, 1303–1314.

De Silva, J. A., Bekersky, I., Puglisi, C. V., Brooks, M. A. and Weinfeld, R. E.   (1976)   Determination of 1,4-benzodiazepines and their 2-ones in blood by electron-capture gas-liquid chromatography. Anal. Chem. 48, 10–19.

Dixon, W. R. and Crews, T.   (1978)   Diazepam: determination in micro samples of blood, plasma and saliva by radioimmunoassay. J. Anal. Toxicol. 2, 210–213.

Dixon, W. R., Earley, J. and Postma, E.   (1975)   Radioimmunoassay of chlordiazepoxide in plasma. J. Pharm, Sci. 64, 937–939.

Dixon, W. R., Lucek, R., Earley, J. and Perry, C.   (1979)   Chlordiazepoxide: a new, more sensitive and specific radioimmunoassay. J. Pharm. Sci. 68, 261.

Dixon, W. R., Glover, W. and Earley, J.   (1981)   Specific radioimmunoassay for flunitrazepam. J. Pharm. Sci. 70, 230–231.

Forgione, A., Martelli, P., Marcucci, F., Fanelli, R., Mussini, E. and Jommi, G. C.   (1971)   Gas-liquid chromatography and mass-spectrometry of various benzodiazepines. J. Chromatogr. 59, 163–168.

Gelbke, H. P. and Schlicht, H. J.   (1978)   Formation of thermally stable derivatives of chlordiazepoxide and its desmethyl metabolite for GLC. J. Pharm. Sci. 67, 1176–1177.

Greaves, M. S.   (1974)   Quantitative determination of medazepam, diazepam and nitrazepam in whole blood by flame-ionization gas-liquid chromatography. Clin. Chem. 20, 141–147.

Hackman, M. R., Brooks, M. A. and De Silva, J. A.   (1974)   Determination of chlordiazepoxide hydrochloride (Librium) and its major metabolites in plasma by differential pulse polarography. Anal. Chem. 46, 1075–1082.

Haidukewych, D., Rodin, E. A. and Davenport, R.   (1980)   Monitoring clorazepate dipotassium as desmethyldiazepam in plasma by electron-capture gas-liquid chromatography. Clin. Chem. 26, 142–144.

Hanna, S., Diana, F., Slevinski, J., Veronich, K. and Lachman, L.   (1978)   Differential pulse polarographic determination of clorazepate monopotassium and dipotassium. J. Pharm. Sci. 67, 1723–1725.

Higuchi, S., Urabe, H. and Shiobara, Y.   (1979)   Simplified determination of lorazepam and oxazepam in biological fluids by gas chromatography-mass spectrometry. J. Chromatogr. 164, 55–61.

Hunt, P., Husson, J. M. and Raynaud, J. P.   (1979)   A radioreceptor assay for benzodiazepines. J. Pharm. Pharmacol. 31, 448–451.

Knowles, J. A. and Ruelius, H. W.   (1972)   Absorption and excretion of 7-chloro-1, 3-dihydro-3-hydroxy-5-phenyl-2H-1, 4-benzodiazepin-2-one (oxazepam) in humans: determination of the drug by gas-liquid chromatography with electron capture detection. Arnzeim. Forsch. 22, 687–692.

Koechlin, B. A. and D'Arconte, L.   (1963)   Determination of chlordiazepoxide (Librium) and of a metabolite of lactam character in plasma of humans, dogs and rats by a specific spectrofluorometric micro method. Anal. Biochem. 5, 195–207.

Mackichan, J. J., Jusko, W. J., Duffner, P. K. and Cohen, M. E.   (1979)   Liquid-chromatographic assay of diazepam and its major metabolites in plasma. Clin. Chem. 25, 856–859.

Miwa, B. J., Garland, W. A., and Blumenthal, P.   (1981)   Determination of flurazepam in human plasma by gas chromatography-electron capture negative chemical ionization mass spectrometry. Anal. Chem. 53, 793–797.

Mohler, H. and Okada, T.   (1977)   Benzodiazepine receptor: demonstration in the central nervous system. Science 198, 849–851.

Oelschlager, H. and Oehr, H. P.   (1970)   Polarographic determination of medazepam (Nobrium), XII: drug analysis by polarography and oscillopolarography. Pharm. Acta Helv. 45: 708–716.

Oelschlager, H., Volke, J., Lim, C. T. and Spang, R.   (1969)   Reduction of oxazepam on Hg-drip-electrode, X: drug analysis by polarography and oscillopolarography. Arch. Pharm. 302, 946–951.

Owen, F., Lofthouse, R. and Bourne, R. C.   (1979)   A radioceptor assay for diazepam and its metabolites in serum. Clin. Chim. Acta 93, 305–310.

Peskar, B. and Spector, S.   (1973)   Quantitative determination of diazepam in blood by radioimmunoassay. J Pharmacol. Exp. Ther. 186, 167–172.

Raisys, V. A., Friel, P. N., Graaff, P. R., Opheim, K. E. and Wilensky, A. J.   (1980). High performance liquid chromatographic and gas-liquid chromatographic determination of diazepam and nordiazepam in plasma, J. Chromatogr. 183, 441–448.

Rieder, J.   (1973)   A fluorimetric method for determining nitrazepam and the sum of its main metabolites in plasma and urine. Arzneim. Forsch. 23, 207–211.

Skellern, G. G., Meier, J., Knight, B. I. and Whiting, B.   (1978)   The application of HPLC to the determination of some 1,4 benzodiazepines and their metabolites in plasma. Br. J. Clin. Pharmacol. 5, 483–487.

Skolnick, P., Goodwin, F. K. and Paul, S. M.   (1979)   A rapid and sensitive radioreceptor assay for benzodiazepines in plasma. Arch. Gen. Psychiatry 36, 78–80.

Sun, S. R. and Hoffman, D. J.   (1978)   Rapid GLC determination of chlordiazepoxide and metabolites in serum using on-column methylation. J. Pharm. Sci. 67, 1647–1648.

Trebbi, A., Gervasi, G. B. and Comi, V.   (1975)   Determination of pinazepam and its metabolites in serum, urine, and brain by gas-liquid chromatography and mass spectrometry. J. Chromatogr. 110, 309–319.

Valentour, J. C., Montforte, J. R., Lorenzo, B. and Sunshine, I.   (1975)   Fluorometric screening method for detecting benzodiazepines in blood and urine. Clin. Chem. 21, 1976–1979.

Vessman, J., Johansson, M., Magnusson, P. and Stromberg, S.   (1977)   Determination of intact oxazepam by electron capture gas chromatography after an extractive alkylation reaction. Anal. Chem. 49, 1545–1549.

Wallace, J. E., Schwertner, H. A. and Shimak, E. L.   (1979)   Analysis for diazepam and nordiazepam by electron capture-gas chromatography and liquid chromatography. Clin. Chem. 25, 1296–1300.

Wallace, J. E., Harris, S. C. and Shimek, E. L.   (1980)   Evaluation of an enzyme immunoassay for determining diazepam and nordiazepam in serum and urine. Clin. Chem. 26, 1905–1907.

Wouters, I., Roets, E. and Hoogmartens, J.,   (1979)   Thin layer chromatographic identification of nineteen benzodiazepine derivatives. J. Chromatogr. 179, 381–389.

Burrows/Norman/Davies (eds) Antianxiety agents
© *Elsevier Science Publishers B.V., 1984*

Chapter 6

Benzodiazepine pharmacokinetics: An overview

DAVID J. GREENBLATT, MARCIA DIVOLL,
DARRELL R. ABERNETHY, HERMANN R. OCHS

and

RICHARD I. SHADER

*Division of Clinical Pharmacology, Departments of Psychiatry and Medicine, Tufts University
School of Medicine and New England Medical Center Hospital, Boston, and the Medizinische
Universitätsklinik, University of Bonn, Bonn-Venusberg, F.R.G.*

INTRODUCTION

Benzodiazepines are the most widely used group of medications for treatment of anxiety and sleep disorders in clinical practice. Controlled studies of benzodiazepines have taught us a great deal about the nature and characteristics of these syndromes and their possible response to drug treatment. Benzodiazepines have also proved highly valuable for studies of drug metabolism in humans. All benzodiazepines are structurally similar, but their pathways of metabolism differ considerably, thereby allowing this group of drugs to serve as models to evaluate metabolic capacity and factors altering biotransformation activity. Finally, benzodiazepines have become highly valuable tools for neuropharmacologists involved in neuroreceptor research, since specific brain binding sites for benzodiazepines have been identified (Tallman et al., 1980).

80

METHODS FOR CATEGORIZING BENZODIAZEPINES

No single approach to classification will adequately explain or categorize all similarities and differences among benzodiazepines. For example, the intensity and duration of clinical activity of a single oral dose of a benzodiazepine are determined by different factors than those related to activity during and after multiple doses. Likewise, drug elimination rate depends in part, but not entirely, on the particular drug's pathway of hepatic biotransformation (i.e. oxidation versus conjugation). The following classification schemes incorporate the major pharmacokinetic and metabolic properties of benzodiazepines.

Onset and duration of action after single doses

Drug absorption rate is a major determinant of the rate of onset of activity after a single oral dose (Bliding, 1974; Greenblatt et al., 1977; Shader et al., 1978) (Fig. 1; Table 1). Rapidly absorbed benzodiazepines, such as diazepam and clorazepate (Fig. 2), reach the systemic circulation rapidly and cause clinical effects of rapid onset after a single oral dose. Conversely, slowly absorbed benzodiazepines such as prazepam, oxazepam, and temazepam, have a slower onset of action after single oral doses. Chlordiazepoxide and lorazepam fall in between these two extremes. Absorption rates of benzodiazepines are determined by the physicochemical properties of the drug itself, together with the pharmaceutical characteristics of the tablet or capsule preparation. Circumstances of drug administration may also influence rate of absorption. A drug is absorbed most rapidly when given on an empty stomach. Coadministration of food or aluminium-containing antacids will reduce the rate of gastric emptying and thereby reduce drug absorption rate and the onset and intensity of clinical effects (Greenblatt et al., 1976, 1977, 1978a; Shader et al., 1978).

   The duration of action of a single dose, on the other hand, is determined mainly by drug distribution. After peak plasma diazepam concentrations are attained following a single dose, the drug is rapidly and extensively distributed to body

KINETIC DETERMINANTS OF CLINICAL ACTION

ABSORPTION DISTRIBUTION ELIMINATION

Single-dose effects
Onset of action   +
Duration of action   +   +

Multiple-dose effects
Cumulative sedation   +
Post-drug phenomena   +

Fig. 1.

TABLE 1

Time of peak plasma concentration following single oral doses of various benzodiazepines administered to healthy volunteers in the fasting state.

Drug	Dosage form*	Time of peak concentration (hr)	
		Mean	Range
Diazepam	Tablet (Valium, Roche)	0.88	(0.08–2.5)
Clorazepate (yielding desmethyldiazepam)	Capsule (Tranxene, Abbott)	1.18	(0.5–2.5)
Lorazepam	Tablet (Ativan, Wyeth)	1.88	(0.5–6.0)
Oxazepam	Tablet (Serax, Wyeth)	2.31	(0.5–6.0)
Temazepam	Capsule (Restoril, Sandoz)	2.46	(0.75–4.0)
Prazepam (yielding desmethyldiazepam)	Tablet (Verstran, Warner-Lambert)	7.8	(2.5–4.0)

* American trade name and manufacturer shown in parentheses.

tissues due to its very high lipid solubility (Fig. 3). The distributional fall in plasma levels may lead to a rapid termination of clinical effects, even though diazepam's elimination half-life is long. Conversely, less extensively distributed benzodiazepines such as lorazepam may have a longer duration of action after a single dose because effective plasma concentrations persist longer (Ameer and Greenblatt, 1981). Thus, elimination half-life does not necessarily predict clinical duration of action after a single dose, since distribution rather than rate of elimination generally determines duration of action. Short half-life benzodiazepines such as triazolam, midazolam and brotizolam are special cases, since their very rapid rate of elimination may terminate clinical action.

Structural configuration (Fig. 4)

2-Keto derivatives. Diazepam is the most familiar of the '2-keto' benzodiazepines (Mandelli et al., 1978), which also include desmethyldiazepam, desalkylflurazepam, halazepam, and several other experimental drugs. The major characteristics

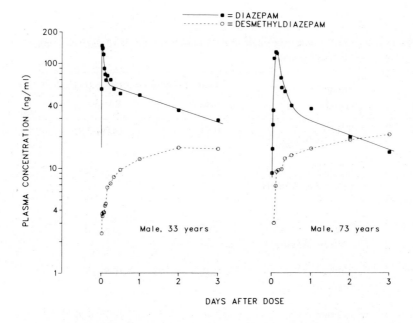

Fig. 2. Plasma concentrations of diazepam and its major metabolite, desmethyldiazepam, following single 5 mg oral doses of diazepam administered to fasting male volunteers. Solid line represents pharmacokinetic function for diazepam.

of this category of benzodiazepines are their long values of elimination half-life, and their oxidative hepatic biotransformation pathway, often leading to pharmacologically active metabolites.

3-Hydroxy. Oxazepam, lorazepam and temazepam are the most important 3-hydroxy benzodiazepines. These drugs have short to intermediate half-life values (Divoll et al., 1981; Greenblatt, 1981) and are biotransformed by conjugation rather than oxidation. The 3-hydroxy substitution of these benzodiazepines allows direct conjugation to glucuronic acid, yielding pharmacologically inactive water-soluble glucuronide metabolites.

7-Nitro. The anticonvulsant clonazepam is the only 7-nitro benzodiazepine available in the United States. In Europe, nitrazepam is extensively used as a hypnotic (Kangas and Breimer, 1981), and flunitrazepam as an anesthetic induction agent and a hypnotic (Kanto et al., 1981). These drugs have intermediate half-life values and are biotransformed in part or entirely by nitroreduction.

Triazolo and imidazo. Triazolam is an ultra-short acting hypnotic (Eberts et al., 1981), while alprazolam is an anxiolytic-antidepressant agent (Cohn, 1981).

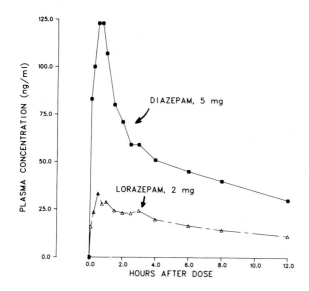

Fig. 3. Plasma concentrations of diazepam and lorazepam in a healthy male volunteer who received a single deltoid intramuscular injection of both drugs on two occasions. Note the rapid distributional decline in plasma diazepam concentrations after the peak is reached. This pattern is not observed for lorazepam.

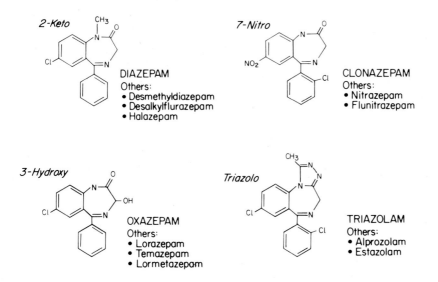

Fig. 4. Structural categories of benzodiazepines.

Estazolam (Allen et al., 1979) is used as a hypnotic drug in Japan and parts of Europe. Closely related to the triazolo compounds is the imidazo derivative midazolam, another ultra-short half-life benzodiazepine, which is an ultra-short acting induction agent and hypnotic (Greenblatt et al., 1981d; Smith et al., 1981). All of the drugs in this category are transformed by oxidative reactions.

Chlordiazepoxide. Chlordiazepoxide was the first benzodiazepine derivative to become available in 1960 (Greenblatt et al., 1978b). It is structurally unique, having 2-methylamino and 4-nitrone substituents that are not shared by any other benzodiazepine. Chlordiazepoxide is an oxidized benzodiazepine, transformed to a series of active metabolites. The most important of these are desmethylchlordiazepoxide and demoxepam. Desmethyldiazepam and oxazepam may also appear in blood during long-term chlordiazepoxide therapy.

Metabolic pathway and rate of elimination

Oxidation. Many benzodiazepines are biotransformed by oxidative reactions in the liver, primarily *N*-demethylation or hydroxylation (Fig. 5), and the process of oxidation often yields pharmacologically active compounds. Two benzodiazepines – clorazepate and prazepam – are prodrugs or drug precursors, being almost completely transformed to desmethyldiazepam before reaching the systemic circulation. Flurazepam also serves mainly as a precursor for desalkylflurazepam. Oxidized benzodiazepines vary widely in their elimination half-lives, and oxidative pathways may be influenced by such factors as old age, liver disease, or coadministration of other drugs that may induce or impair hepatic oxidizing capacity (Shader et al., 1977, 1981; Roberts et al., 1978; Allen et al., 1980; Greenblatt et al., 1980a, 1981a, b) (Fig. 6).

BENZODIAZEPINES METABOLIZED BY OXIDATION

Parent Compound	Active Substances Present in Blood	Overall Rate of Elimination
Chlordiazepoxide	Chlordiazepoxide Desmethylchlordiazepoxide Demoxepam	Intermediate to Slow
Diazepam	Diazepam Desmethyldiazepam	Slow
[Clorazepate]	Desmethyldiazepam	Slow
[Prazepam]	Desmethyldiazepam	Slow
[Flurazepam]	Desalkylflurazepam	Slow
Clobazam	Clobazam Desmethylclobazam	Slow
Alprazolam	Alprazolam	Intermediate
Triazolam	Triazolam	Very Rapid

[ ] indicate prodrugs

Fig. 5.

PLASMA DIAZEPAM CONCENTRATION (ng/ml)
500
200
100
50
20
10
5
2
1
Male, 79 years
Male, 30 years
0
1
2
3
4
5
6
7
DAYS AFTER DOSE

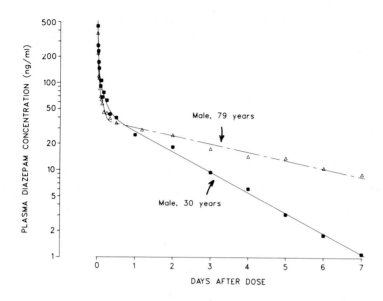

Fig. 6. Plasma diazepam concentrations following single intravenous doses administered to young and elderly male volunteers. Lines represent pharmacokinetic functions (desmethyldiazepam concentrations not shown).

Conjugation. Unlike oxidized benzodiazepines, conjugated benzodiazepines do not have active metabolites (Fig. 7). Only the parent compounds account for clinical activity, and the overall rate of elimination is in the short to intermediate range. Unlike oxidative processes, conjugation tends to be less influenced by aging, liver disease, and drug interactions (Shull et al., 1976; Kraus et al., 1978; Greenblatt et al., 1979, 1980b; Divoll et al., 1981).

Nitroreduction. Benzodiazepines with nitro substituents in the 7-position are biotransformed by reduction, forming 7-amino derivatives, then acetylated to 7-acetamino analogues (Kangas and Breimer, 1981). Both metabolites are inactive.

BENZODIAZEPINES METABOLIZED BY CONJUGATION

Parent Compound	Active Substances Present in Blood	Overall Rate of Elimination
Oxazepam	Oxazepam	Rapid
Lorazepam	Lorazepam	Intermediate
Temazepam	Temazepam	Intermediate

Fig. 7.

The metabolic pathway of flunitrazepam is more complex, involving both oxidative N-demethylation to yield desmethylflunitrazepam, as well as reduction of the nitro group. Nitrazepam, clonazepam, and flunitrazepam have half-live values in the intermediate range.

PHARMACOKINETIC PROPERTIES OF SPECIFIC BENZODIAZEPINES

Diazepam

Diazepam is initially biotransformed by the oxidative step of N-demethylation yielding desmethyldiazepam. This metabolite is oxidized by hydroxylation at the 3-position, yielding oxazepam which is then conjugated to form the final metabolite, oxazepam glucuronide. Diazepam and desmethyldiazepam are the principal active substances appearing in blood (Greenblatt et al., 1981c). Oxazepam and temazepam (formed by a minor parallel pathway) are found only in very low concentrations, since both are conjugated and excreted almost as rapidly as they are formed.

The slow rate of diazepam elimination implies that drug accumulation will be slow and extensive during multiple dose therapy (Fig. 8). Desmethyldiazepam also accumulates, but at an even slower rate. Typically 5 days to 2 weeks are required for both compounds to reach their steady-state values, at which time desmethyldiazepam levels are usually equal to or exceed concentrations of the parent drug (Greenblatt et al., 1981c). After abrupt termination of dosage, diazepam washes out from the body at a rate that is correspondingly slow. Desmethyldiazepam disappears more slowly than the parent compound, and both can be detected in plasma for many days after the last dose.

Since diazepam clearance is impaired in old age (Greenblatt et al., 1980a; Macklon et al., 1980), particularly in elderly males, accumulation will be greater during multiple dose therapy in elderly individuals. A need for reduced dosage of diazepam should therefore be anticipated in the elderly population.

Desmethyldiazepam

Desmethyldiazepam is an extremely important benzodiazepine, since many other benzodiazepines are transformed into it. Desmethyldiazepam is a minor metabolite of chlordiazepoxide and a major metabolite of medazepam, a drug used in Europe. Desmethyldiazepam is the major metabolite of diazepam, and also is the principal active substance appearing in blood allowing administration of its two precursor compounds, prazepam and clorazepate. Finally, several other investigational benzodiazepines (halazepam, fosazepam, clazepam, ketazolam) also yield desmethyldiazepam as a metabolic intermediate. Once formed, desmethyldiaze-

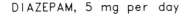

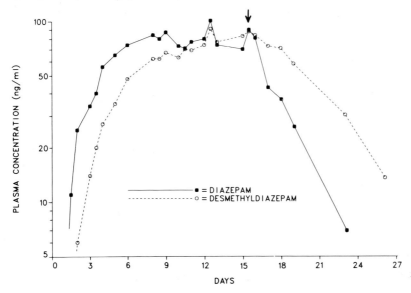

Fig. 8. Plasma concentrations of diazepam and its major metabolite, desmethyldiazepam, in a volunteer who ingested 5 mg of diazepam daily for 15 consecutive days, then abruptly terminated treatment (arrow). Plasma levels were measured during and after the period of dosage.

pam is hydroxylated to form oxazepam, and thereafter appears in the urine as oxazepam glucuronide. Since desmethyldiazepam has an extremely long elimination half-life, then any drug that is transformed into it must also effectively act as a substance with a long half-life that will accumulate during multiple dosage. Furthermore, desmethyldiazepam, since it is transformed by oxidation, will have a prolonged elimination half-life and reduced total clearance in elderly males (Allen et al., 1980; Shader et al., 1981).

Although both prazepam and clorazepate yield desmethyldiazepam as the final product in the systemic circulation, the rate at which these two processes occur is different. In the case of clorazepate, desmethyldiazepam appears in blood very rapidly, whereas for prazepam, desmethyldiazepam appears slowly. The perception of clinical effects after single oral doses therefore may differ greatly between these two compounds.

Flurazepam

Flurazepam is the most widely used hypnotic agent in the United States. Metabolism of flurazepam appears to proceed by stepwise degradation of the *N*-alkyl

88

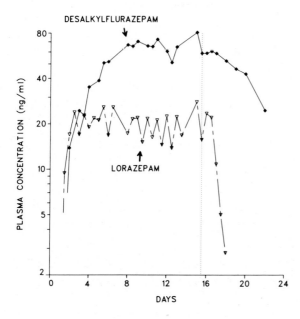

Fig. 9. A healthy volunteer female subject participated in two different pharmacokinetic studies on two occasions several months apart. One study involved ingestion of lorazepam, 3 mg daily, for 15 consecutive days. In the other study, 15 mg of flurazepam was ingested for 15 consecutive nights. Plasma concentrations of lorazepam and of desalkylflurazepam (the principal active metabolite formed from flurazepam, as in Fig. 5) were measured during the 15-day period of dosage, and following drug discontinuation (vertical dotted line).

side chain. Two of these transformation products (hydroxyethyl and aldehyde derivatives) appear rapidly in plasma after a single oral dose, then disappear within 12 hours. In fact, flurazepam itself is essentially undetectable (Miwa et al., 1981). The principal metabolite, N-desalkylflurazepam, appears more slowly and has a long elimination half-life ranging from 40 to more than 200 hours in healthy persons (Greenblatt et al., 1981a). As in the case of other oxidized benzodiazepines, the half-life of desalkylflurazepam becomes significantly prolonged with age in men.

Consistent with its long elimination half-life, desalkylflurazepam accumulates slowly during multiple dosage with flurazepam, reaches steady-state, then washes out slowly after termination of dosage (Fig. 9). The pattern of drug accumulation and washout is similar to that observed with diazepam, desmethyldiazepam, clobazam, or other slowly eliminated benzodiazepines.

Triazolam, midazolam, and alprazolam

All of these benzodiazepine derivatives are biotransformed by oxidative reactions mainly involving hydroxylation. Half-life values for triazolam and midazolam are in the 'very short' range of 6 hours or less, and therefore will be essentially nonaccumulating during multiple dosage (Eberts et al., 1981; Greenblatt et al., 1981d, e). Alprazolam has a half-life range of 6 to 15 hours, and appears to have anxiolytic and antidepressant properties (Cohn, 1981).

Clobazam

Clobazam structurally differs from other 1,4-benzodiazepines, having instead a 1,5-benzodiazepine configuration. However, its metabolic pathway is similar to that of diazepam, proceeded by N-demethylation to yield the pharmacologically active metabolite, desmethylclobazam. Clobazam is effectively a long half-life, accumulating benzodiazepine. Furthermore, its clearance is reduced and half-life prolonged in elderly as opposed to young males (Greenblatt et al., 1981b).

Conjugated benzodiazepines: Oxazepam, lorazepam, and temazepam

The 3-hydroxy benzodiazepine derivatives oxazepam, lorazepam, and temazepam are directly conjugated to glucuronic acid, yielding pharmacologically inactive, water-soluble glucuronide conjugates that are excreted in urine (Greenblatt, 1981). Up to 90% of a single dose of these three drugs can be recovered in the urine as glucuronide conjugates.

Values of elimination half-life for conjugated benzodiazepines are in the short to intermediate range. Oxazepam half-life ranges from 5 to 12 hours (mean: 8 hours) (Greenblatt et al., 1980b; Ochs et al., 1981). For temazepam and lorazepam, the usual range is 8 to 24 hours, with a mean of 15 hours (Greenblatt et al., 1979; Divoll et al., 1981). The relatively slow rate of gastrointestinal absorption of oxazepam and temazepam is of considerable importance (Table 1), since the onset of action of a single dose will be relatively slow. These two drugs probably are not ideal for sleep disturbances characterized primarily by difficulty in falling asleep. If administered for sleep latency insomnia, oxazepam and temazepam are best given on an empty stomach, 1–2 hours before bedtime.

Compared to oxidation, drug conjugation is a relatively 'nonsusceptible' metabolic pathway, being minimally influenced by age and liver disease (Shull et al., 1976; Kraus et al., 1978; Greenblatt et al., 1979, 1980b; Divoll et al., 1981; Greenblatt, 1981; Ochs et al., 1981). Because conjugated benzodiazepines have shorter elimination half-life values than most oxidized benzodiazepines, there is less accumulation during multiple dosage (Fig. 9).

POTENTIAL CLINICAL IMPLICATIONS OF DRUG ACCUMULATION

The rate of drug accumulation during multiple dosage is governed mainly by elimination half-life, and the extent of accumulation by total metabolic clearance. Accumulation may be important in terms of cumulative sedative or antianxiety effects during the period of drug administration, as well as the rate of termination of drug effects after the drug is discontinued (Fig. 10).

For short-acting drugs, accumulation is minimal since each dose is largely eliminated before the next one is given. This has potential benefits and disadvantages. The likelihood of residual daytime effects or cumulative sedation tends to be reduced and drug disappearance is essentially complete within 1 to 2 days of the last dose (Fig. 9). However, the rapid elimination of active substances following termination of dosage may lead to rapid recrudescence of clinical symptoms (Kales et al., 1979; Nicholson, 1980). For long-acting benzodiazepines, the situation is reversed. There is slow and extensive accumulation during the period of dosage, because the elimination half-life exceeds the dosage interval. At the termination of dosage, washout of active substances is correspondingly slow (Figs. 8 and 9). This profile also has benefits and disadvantages. Long-acting drugs may lead to cumulative sedative and performance impairing effects (Church and Johnson, 1979), although this may be partially or completely offset by adaptation or tolerance. On the other hand, such drugs can be given on a once daily basis due to their persistence throughout the day. The slow washout of active compounds after the final dose tends to reduce or minimize symptom recrudescence or 'rebound' problems associated with drug discontinuation. Based on knowledge of half-life values for individual benzodiazepines, clinicians should be in a position to anticipate profiles of drug accumulation.

	Elimination Half-Life	
Multiple-Dose Kinetics	Short	Long
Rate of Accumulation	Rapid	Slow
Extent of Accumulation	Minimal	Extensive
Post-Dosage Washout	Rapid	Slow

Fig. 10. Influence of elimination half-life on kinetic behavior during and after multiple-dose drug administration.

ACKNOWLEDGEMENTS

This work was supported in part by Grants MH-34223, GM-07611, and AM-32050 from the United States Public Health Service; and by Grant Oc 10/6-3 from Deutsche Forschungsgemeinschaft, Bonn-Bad Godesberg, West Germany.

REFERENCES

Allen, M. D., Greenblatt, D. J. and Arnold, J. D. (1979) Single and multiple dose kinetics of estazolam, a triazolo benzodiazepine. Psychopharmacology 66, 267–274.

Allen, M. D., Greenblatt, D. J., Harmatz, J. S. and Shader, R. I. (1980) Desmethyldiazepam kinetics in the elderly after oral prazepam. Clin. Pharmacol. Ther. 28, 196–202.

Ameer, B. and Greenblatt, D. J. (1981) Lorazepam: a review of its clinical pharmacological properties and therapeutic uses. Drugs 21, 161–200.

Bliding, A. (1974) Effect of different rates of absorption of two benzodiazepines on subjective and objective parameters. Eur. J. Clin. Pharmacol. 7, 201–211.

Church, M. W. and Johnson, L. C. (1979) Mood and performance of poor sleepers during repeated use of flurazepam. Psychopharmacology 61, 309–316.

Cohn, J. B. (1981) Multicenter double-blind efficacy and safety study comparing alprazolam, diazepam and placebo in clinically anxious patients. J. Clin. Psychiatry 42, 347–351.

Divoll, M., Greenblatt, D. J., Harmatz, J. S. and Shader, R. I. (1981) Effect of age and gender on disposition of temazepam. J. Pharmaceut. Sci. 70, 1104–1107.

Eberts, F. S., Philopoulos, Y., Reineke, L. M. and Vliek, R. W. (1981) Triazolam disposition. Clin. Pharmacol. Ther. 29: 81–83.

Greenblatt, D. J. (1981) Clinical pharmacokinetics of oxazepam and lorazepam. Clin. Pharmacokinet. 6, 89–105.

Greenblatt, D. J., Shader, R. I., Harmatz, J. S., Franke, K. and Koch-Weser, J. (1976) Influence of magnesium and aluminum hydroxide mixture on chlordiazepoxide absorption. Clin. Pharmacol. Ther. 19, 234–239.

Greenblatt, D. J., Shader, R. I., Harmatz, J. S., Franke, K. and Koch-Weser, J. (1977) Absorption rate, blood concentrations, and early response to oral chlordiazepoxide. Am. J. Psychiatry 134, 559–562.

Greenblatt, D. J., Allen, M. D., MacLaughlin, D. S., Harmatz, J. S. and Shader, R. I. (1978a) Diazepam absorption: effect of antacids and food. Clin. Pharmacol. Ther. 24: 600–609.

Greenblatt, D. J., Shader, R. I., MacLeod, S. M. and Sellers, E. M. (1978b) Clinical pharmacokinetics of chlordiazepoxide. Clin. Pharmacokinet. 3, 381–394.

Greenblatt, D. J., Allen, M. D., Locniskar, A., Harmatz, J. S. and Shader, R.I. (1979) Lorazepam kinetics in the elderly. Clin. Pharmacol. Ther. 26, 103–113.

Greenblatt, D. J., Allen, M. D., Harmatz, J. S. and Shader, R. I. (1980a) Diazepam disposition determinants. Clin. Pharmacol. Ther. 27, 301–312.

Greenblatt, D. J., Divoll, M., Harmatz, J. S. and Shader, R. I. (1980b) Oxazepam kinetics: effects of age and sex. J. Pharmacol. Exper. Ther. 215, 86–91.

Greenblatt, D. J., Divoll, M., Harmatz, J. S., MacLaughlin, D. S. and Shader, R. I. (1981a) Kinetics and clinical effects of flurazepam in young and elderly noninsomniacs. Clin. Pharmacol. Ther. 30, 475–486.

Greenblatt, D. J., Divoll, M., Puri, S. K., Ho, I., Zinny, M. A. and Shader, R. I. (1981b) Clobazam kinetics in the elderly. Br. J. Clin. Pharmacol. 12, 631–636.

Greenblatt, D. J., Laughren, T. P., Allen, M. D., Harmatz, J. S. and Shader, R. I. (1981c) Plasma diazepam and desmethyldiazepam concentrations during long-term diazepam therapy. Br. J. Clin. Pharmacol. 11, 35–40.

Greenblatt, D. J., Locniskar, A., Ochs, H. R. and Lauven, P. M. (1981d) Automated gas chromatography for studies of midazolam pharmacokinetics. Anesthesiology 55, 176–179.

Greenblatt, D. J., Divoll, M., Moschitto, L. J. and Shader, R. I. (1981e) Electron-capture gas chromatographic analysis of the triazolobenzodiazepines alprazolam and triazolam. J. Chromatogr. 225, 202-207.

92

Greenblatt, D. J., Shader, R. I. and Abernethy, D. R. (1983a) Current status of benzodiazepines. N. Engl. J. Med. 309, 354–358, 410–416.

Greenblatt, D. J., Divoll, M., Abernethy, D. R., Ochs, H. R. and Shader, R. I. (1983b) Clinical pharmacokinetics of the newer benzodiazepines. Clin. Pharmacokinet. 8, 233–253.

Kales, A., Scharf, M. B., Kales, J. D. and Soldatos, C. R. (1979) Rebound insomnia: a potential hazard following withdrawal of certain benzodiazepines. J. Am. Med. Assoc. 241, 1692–1695.

Kangas, L. and Breimer, D. D. (1981) Clinical pharmacokinetics of nitrazepam. Clin. Pharmacokinet. 6, 346–366.

Kanto, J., Kangas, L., Aaltonen, L. and Hilke, H. (1981) Effect of age on the pharmacokinetics and sedative effect of flunitrazepam. Int. J. Clin. Pharmacol. 19, 400–404.

Kraus, J. W., Desmond, P. V., Marshall, J. P., Johnson, R. F., Schenker, S. and Wilkinson, G. R. (1978) Effects of aging and liver disease on disposition of lorazepam. Clin. Pharmacol. Ther. 24, 411–419.

Macklon, A. F., Barton, M., James, O. and Rawlins, M. D. (1980) The effect of age on the pharmacokinetics of diazepam. Clin. Sci. 59, 479–483.

Mandelli, M., Tognoni, G. and Garattini, S. (1978) Clinical pharmacokinetics of diazepam. Clin. Pharmacokinet. 3, 72–91.

Miwa, B. J., Garland, W. A. and Blumenthal, P. (1981) Determination of flurazepam in human plasma by gas chromatography-electron capture negative chemical ionization mass spectrometry. Analyt. Chem. 53, 793–797.

Nicholson, A. N. (1980) Hypnotics: Rebound insomnia and residual sequelae. Br. J. Clin. Pharmacol. 9, 223–225.

Ochs, H. R., Greenblatt, D. J. and Otten, H. (1981) Disposition of oxazepam in relation to age, sex, and cigarette smoking. Klin. Wochenschr. 59, 899–903.

Roberts, R. K., Wilkinson, G. R., Branch, R. A. and Schenker, S. (1978) Effect of age and parenchymal liver disease on the disposition and elimination of chlordiazepoxide (Librium). Gastroenterology 75, 479–485.

Shader, R. I., Greenblatt, D. J., Harmatz, J. S., Franke, K. and Koch-Weser, J. (1977) Absorption and disposition of chlordiazepoxide in young and elderly male volunteers. J. Clin. Pharmacol. 17, 709–718.

Shader, R. I., Georgotas, A., Greenblatt, D. J., Harmatz, J. S. and Allen, M. D. (1978) Impaired absorption of desmethyldiazepam from clorazepate by magnesium aluminium hydroxide. Clin. Pharmacol. Ther. 24, 308–315.

Shader, R. I., Greenblatt, D. J. Ciraulo, D. A., Divoll, M., Harmatz, J. S. and Georgotas, A. (1981) Effect of age and sex on disposition of desmethyldiazepam formed from its precursor clorazepate. Psychopharmacology 75, 193–197.

Shull, H. J., Wilkinson, G. R., Johnson, R. and Schenker, S. (1976) Normal disposition of oxazepam in acute viral hepatitis and cirrhosis. Ann. Int. Med. 84, 420–425.

Smith, M. T., Eadie, M. J. and Brophy, T. O. (1981) The pharmacokinetics of midazolam in man. Eur. J. Clin. Pharmacol. 19, 271–278.

Tallman, J. F., Paul, S. M., Skolnick, P. and Gallagher, D. W. (1980) Receptors for the age of anxiety: pharmacology of the benzodiazepines. Science 207, 274–281.

Usdin, E., Skolnick, P., Tallman, J. F., Greenblatt, D. J. and Paul, S. M. (1983) (Eds) Pharmacology of Benzadiozepines. MacMillan, London.

Burrows/Norman/Davies (eds) Antianxiety agents
© *Elsevier Science Publishers B.V., 1984*

Chapter 7

Benzodiazepine plasma concentrations and anxiolytic response

TREVOR R. NORMAN

and

GRAHAM D. BURROWS

Department of Psychiatry, University of Melbourne, Australia

INTRODUCTION

Since their introduction, the benzodiazepines (see Table 1) have been the first choice for the treatment of morbid anxiety states. In addition to their anxiolytic effect they possess muscle relaxant, anticonvulsant and sedative-hypnotic properties, as well as being safe on overdosage. Controlled clinical comparisons of benzodiazepine anxiolytics have consistently demonstrated their efficacy compared with a placebo in anxious non-psychotic patients (Greenblatt and Shader, 1974). No differences between drugs with regard to clinical efficacy has been demonstrated in most comparative studies (e.g. Burrows et al., 1977; Kanto et al., 1979). The British Committee on the Review of Medicines (CRM) found no evidence for the preferential use of any particular benzodiazepine in anxiety or insomnia (CRM, 1980). Pharmacokinetic studies have demonstrated clinically meaningful differences between the benzodiazepines with respect to their rate and route of elimination and the presence or absence of active metabolites (Shader and Greenblatt, 1977). The role of plasma monitoring in benzodiazepine therapy is discussed here, with particular emphasis on the relationship between steady-state drug concentrations in plasma and clinical effect. Pharmacokinetics are not discussed here since they have been described in this volume (see Chapter 6) and elsewhere at length (Greenblatt et al., 1978; Mandelli et al., 1978; Fulton et al., 1981; Greenblatt et al., 1981b).

BENZODIAZEPINE PLASMA CONCENTRATIONS

Repeated administration of a standard dose of a benzodiazepine has been shown to result in a wide inter-individual variation of plasma drug concentrations. For example, Zingales (1973) observed marked variation in diazepam concentrations in patients receiving the same dose of drug. Similarly, Rutherford et al. (1978) and Greenblatt et al. (1981a) found large inter-individual variations of diazepam concentrations during chronic dosing. Kanto and colleagues (1974) showed a decrease in steady-state concentrations of diazepam over a 6-week period, suggesting self-induction of metabolism. Long-term therapy with diazepam leads to accumulation in the blood of both diazepam and its major metabolite, N-desmethyldiazepam (Klotz et al., 1976; Bond et al., 1977; Rutherford et al., 1978; Greenblatt et al., 1981a). With other benzodiazepines, a similar pattern of parent drug and metabolite accumulation may be expected on chronic dosing. Steady-state concentrations of chlordiazepoxide, desmethylchlordiazepoxide and demoxepam are achieved with long-term administration (Bond et al., 1977; Boxenbaum et al., 1977; Greenblatt et al., 1978; Lin and Friedel, 1979). Lorazepam and oxazepam, which are without active metabolites, also achieve steady-state concentrations on chronic oral administration (Alvan et al., 1977; Greenblatt et al., 1977a). The large inter-individual variability in plasma benzodiazepine concentrations has been attributed to differences in genetic and environmental factors, age, sex, diet (Breimer et al., 1980; Greenblatt and Shader, 1980). In addition, disease states, particularly renal and hepatic diseases, can alter the pharmacokinetics of the benzodiazepines (Sellers et al., 1977; Mandelli et al., 1978; Greenblatt, 1981). Few clinically significant interactions occur between the benzodiazepines and other drugs, the most important being with alcohol (Seppala et al., 1979). This possibly represents a pharmacodynamic rather than pharmacokinetic interaction, although plasma drug concentrations are elevated (Linnoila et al., 1974; MacLeod et al., 1977).

The benzodiazepines are highly protein bound, greater than 90 % in blood plasma (Van der Kleijn et al., 1971; Boxenbaum et al., 1977; Abel et al., 1979). Since the free-drug concentration is pharmacologically active, changes in protein binding of 1–2 % may have profound effects on the free-drug fraction. Present analytical techniques determine total (free + protein bound) plasma drug concentrations, so that differences in protein binding are rarely considered in drug concentration-effect relationships.

PLASMA CONCENTRATION – CLINICAL RESPONSE RELATIONSHIPS

The relationship between plasma concentration and clinical effect of the benzodiazepines has not been widely investigated, despite the availability of reliable assay methods and objective anxiety rating scales. A summary of studies is presented in Table 1, and some individual studies described below.

Diazepam

Plasma concentration – anxiolytic effect.   A double-blind comparison of diazepam and placebo was carried out in a group of 30 inpatients in 'acute clinical anxiety states' (Dasberg et al., 1974). Patients were matched for age, sex, diagnosis, duration of the present illness and previous treatment. After a 2 day drug-free period, each patient in the diazepam group received 20 mg/day orally for 5 days. Plasma samples were taken 2 hours after the morning dose and diazepam and nordiazepam levels determined by gas chromatography. Patient improvement was judged from changes in the Hamilton anxiety rating score and a patient-rated scale; the three main symptoms.

A significant correlation between plasma diazepam concentration and improvement on patient-rated symptoms was obtained. A significant positive correlation between nordiazepam concentration and improvement in gastrointestinal symptoms was found. Nordiazepam levels were negatively correlated with autonomic nervous system symptoms, with patients whose nordiazepam levels exceeded 300 μg/l, having more complaints of dry mouth, flushing, pallor, perspiration, giddiness and tremor. On the basis of the results presented by these authors, their conclusion that the minimum effective plasma diazepam level is 400 μg/l on day 5 of treatment appears to be unjustified. No correlation of plasma level with overall clinical improvement was presented. For some symptoms of anxiety, a minimum effective plasma level for improvement has been demonstrated. Robin et al., (1974) compared the effects of diazepam, clorazepate and placebo in a double-blind crossover trial. Eleven patients completed 2 weeks treatment of each drug. No other drugs were allowed during the trial period. Clinical progress was assessed at fortnightly intervals using a visual analogue scale, symptom rating test, global rating and three target symptoms selected by each patient. Plasma concentrations of diazepam and nordiazepam were measured after each interview. Each patient received 15 mg/day of diazepam or 22.5 mg/day of clorazepate (i.e. equivalent doses). A significant improvement in anxiety scores over pretreatment scores was noted. The active compounds were superior to placebo and equivalent to each other in anxiolytic effects. A negative correlation between plasma nordiazepam concentration and the symptom rating test score was obtained for individual patients, but not for the whole group. No relationship was found for plasma diazepam or total benzodiazepine concentration and clinical response.

TABLE 1

Plasma levels and clinical response of benzodiazepine antianxiety agents.

Author	Diagnosis	Dosage, other drugs	Clinical Assessment	Relationship
CHLORDIAZEPOXIDE				
Gottschalk and Kaplan (1972)	Anxiety	25 mg single oral dose; no other drugs	Speech content analysis	Plasma levels 0.70 μg/ml; greatest reduction in anxiety and hostility scores
Bond et al. (1977)	Anxiety	10–50 mg/d for 2–4 wks; mean dose 28 mg/d; no other drugs	H.A.R.S.*; self-rating scales	No relationship
Greenblatt et al. (1977)	Volunteer study	25 mg single oral dose; no other drugs	Visual analogue scale	Significant correlation between total drug concentration and some items of analogue scale
Lin and Friedel (1979)	Anxiety	30–60 mg/d for 1 wk; mean dose 55 mg/d; no other drugs	Hopkins symptoms checklist; H.A.R.S.	Significant correlation between clinical response and metabolite concentrations
DIAZEPAM				
Dasberg et al. (1974)	Acute anxiety	20 mg/d for 5 days. Chloral hydrate as needed	H.A.R.S.: self-rating scale	Some correlations of various symptoms and plasma DZ or NDZ. Minimum 400 ng/ml DZ for improvement
Robin et al. (1974)	Persistent anxiety states	15 mg/d for 2 wks; no other drugs	H.A.R.S.: visual analogue scale; symptom-rating test; global rating	Significant correlation between plasma NDZ and clinical response for individuals
Bianchi et al. (1974)	Anxious neurotics	Up to 20 mg/d for 3 wks; no other drugs	H.A.R.S.: Zung self-rating depression scale; Physical symptoms inventory	A low 2 hr plasma DZ level after a single oral 10 mg dose correlated highly with good clinical response

Reference	Condition	Dose	Measure	Result
Kanto et al. (1974)	Anxiety neurosis	15 mg/d for 5–24 wks; no other drugs	Taylor manifest anxiety scale	No simple relationship
Smith et al. (1976)	Anxiety	0.3 mg/kg single oral dose; no other drugs	Taylor manifest anxiety scale; symptom distress checklist	No simple relationship
Bond et al. (1977)	Anxiety	2–20 mg/d for 2–4 wks; mean dose 11 mg/d; no other drugs	H.A.R.S.; self-rating scale	No relationship
Tansella et al. (1978)	Anxiety states	16–42 mg/d for 1 wk; mean dose 26 mg/d; no other drugs	H.A.R.S.; Morbid anxiety inventory scale	No relationship
Gottschalk and Cohn (1978)	Alcohol withdrawal	10 mg/d	Speech content analysis	A non-significant tendency for higher plasma levels to be associated with a decrease in anxiety scores
NORDIAZEPAM				
Robin et al. (1974)	Persistent anxiety states	22.5 mg clorazepate/d for 2 wks; no other drugs	H.A.R.S.; visual analogue scale; symptom-rating test; global rating	Significant correlation between plasma NDZ and clinical response for individuals
Tansella et al. (1975)	Anxiety neurosis and insomnia	10 mg/d or 20 mg/d for 1 wk; no other drugs	H.A.R.S.; self-rating scales	No relationship
Tognoni et al. (1975)	Anxiety and depression	20–30 mg/d for 10 days; Nortriptyline 75–100 mg/d	Visual analogue scale; nurses' observations	No relationship
MEDAZEPAM				
Bond et al. (1977)	Anxiety	10–50 mg/d for 2–4 wks; mean dose 27 mg/d; no other drugs	H.A.R.S.; self-rating scales	No relationship
KETAZOLAM				
Gottschalk and Cohn (1978)	Alcohol withdrawal	50–3000 mg/d for 21 days	5 min speech content analysis	No significant correlation between blood and anxiety or hostility levels

* Hamilton anxiety rating score.

Bianchi et al. (1974) studied a group of 25 anxious neurotic patients who received varying doses (mean 21 mg/day) of diazepam for 3 weeks. No other drugs were allowed during the trial period. Patients' improvement was monitored using weekly Hamilton anxiety rating scores, Zung self-rating scores and changes in the physical symptoms inventory. Patients received an initial single oral dose of 5 mg of diazepam and plasma levels were measured by gas chromatography 1 and 2 hours after the dose. The authors report a significant correlation between the 2-hour plasma diazepam level and the steady-state level achieved (although steady-state levels were not reported) and the best clinical response was achieved in patients with a low 2-hour plasma level. No steady-state levels of diazepam or its metabolites were reported and the correlation between clinical response after 1, 2 or 3 weeks was not examined.

Kanto et al. (1974) studied the anxiolytic effects of 15 mg/day of diazepam in 12 outpatients over a period of 5–24 weeks. Clinical state was assessed at the beginning of therapy and after one month's treatment using the Taylor manifest anxiety scale. Plasma levels of diazepam, nordiazepam and oxazepam were measured at weekly intervals using gas chromatography. Steady-state levels of diazepam and nordiazepam were not reached, but tended to decrease with time. Free oxazepam was found in some, but not all patients, in negligible quantities. No simple correlation between plasma levels and clinical response was found.

Bond et al. (1977) examined the relationship between diazepam plasma levels and clinical effects in 19 anxious patients. Diazepam dosage ranged from 2 to 20 mg/day (mean 11 mg/day) and each patient was treated from 2 to 4 weeks. Plasma diazepam levels ranged from 70 to 392 μg/l and plasma nordiazepam from 83 to 1070 μg/l. No relationship was found between the plasma concentration of either drug and clinical effect or between total benzodiazepine concentration and clinical effect.

A study in 24 inpatients with severe morbid anxiety was carried out by Tansella et al. (1978). After a 4 to 7 day washout period each patient received, under double-blind conditions, diazepam, amylobarbitone sodium or placebo for one week. Clinical assessment was based on the Hamilton rating scale for anxiety and the morbid anxiety inventory, which were rated at the end of the washout period and after each week of treatment. The mean dosage of diazepam was 26 mg/day (range 16–42 mg/day). Plasma samples were collected on days 2, 4 and 7 of each treatment, 11 hours after the last dose. Diazepam and its major metabolite nordiazepam were measured by gas chromatography. After one week of treatment the mean diazepam level was 741 μg/l (range 280–2083 μg/l) and the mean nordiazepam level was 761 μg/l (range 338–1039 μg/l). No correlation was found between plasma diazepam or nordiazepam and clinical response. This study was in agreement with that of Bond et al.. (1977). It should be borne in mind that steady-state levels of diazepam and nordiazepam were not achieved in this study. Additionally, the random allocation of some patients to amylobarbitone first was shown by the authors to affect the levels of diazepam and nordiazepam achieved.

Gottschalk and Cohn (1978) studied 10 chronic alcoholic patients undergoing alcohol withdrawal who each received 10 mg of diazepam at night. Anxiety scores were assessed from speech content analysis and blood samples were drawn 12 hours after the last dose of diazepam, for diazepam and nordiazepam plasma level determinations, on these days. There was a significant negative correlation between hostility scores and diazepam or nordiazepam plasma levels. Although there was a tendency for higher plasma levels to be associated with a decrease in anxiety scores, this relationship did not reach statistical significance. The details of this trial were not presented so it is not clear for how long diazepam was administered, if plasma levels reached steady state, if other drugs were administered concomitantly or if a placebo period was included. Direct comparisons of this trial with the others described may not be valid since the study populations (anxious inpatients or outpatients and chronic alcoholics) were different.

Plasma concentration – acute effects. A group of 20 anxious patients were studied after single oral doses of diazepam or placebo in a randomized double-blind trial (Smith et al., 1976). The Taylor manifest anxiety scale and the symptom distress checklist were used to assess anxiety levels at baseline 1, 2, 3 and 6 hours after drug administration. Plasma and red blood cell levels of diazepam were measured by gas chromatography at 1, 3 and 6 hours after drug ingestion. No simple relationship between effects on mood and plasma or red blood cell levels of diazepam was observed. The effects of diazepam on anxiety, sedation, or the greatest mood change score, in individuals, was not related to peak blood level, fall in blood level or diazepam half-life. Nordiazepam levels were not reported in this study. Some other studies, as discussed above, have shown this is an important determinant of the action of diazepam.

Studies of the effects of diazepam administered to healthy volunteers have described the physiological and psychological results after different dosage formulations. In two papers, Hillestad et al. (1974a,b) examined the effect of single and repeated doses of diazepam in volunteers. In both studies there was a close correlation between serum levels and effects on sleepiness, ability to perform mental arithmetic tasks, blurred vision, co-ordination, systolic blood pressure, heart and respiration rate. The significance of these findings for the treatment of anxious patients is to show that certain clinical effects are more pronounced with high diazepam levels, but that patients can expect to develop a tolerance to these effects during chronic dosage. Bliding (1974) compared the effects of different doses of diazepam and oxazepam on subjective side effects, pulse rates and performance in psychometric tests in six volunteers. In this single dose study, subjective and objective effects were greater during periods of rising serum concentration. It is suggested that drugs which are rapidly absorbed may offer a greater risk of habituation. Independent evidence to support this thesis is at present lacking. A positive correlation between plasma levels of diazepam and subjective sedatory effect was found in 10 volunteers after 5 mg of diazepam administered orally, intramuscularly or rectally (Kanto, 1975). This result has been confirmed by Ghoneim et al. (1975) after intravenous administration of 10- or 20-mg doses of diazepam to 10 volunteers. Positive correlations were also found with fuzziness, mental slowness, weakness, clumsiness and lethargy as assessed by a subjective rating questionnaire. Baird and Hailey (1972) noted pronounced drowsiness 10–15 mins after the administration of diazepam to volunteers, which was followed by recovery at 2 hours. Subsequently, subjects reported a recurrence of symptoms at 6 hours, which was associated with an increase in diazepam and desmethyldiazepam plasma levels. This double-peak phenomenon is commonly observed in benzodiazepine kinetic studies and has been explained by Wilensky et al. (1978) as an effect of food or due to enterohepatic recycling. Two other studies have shown no relationship between plasma diazepam concentration and central nervous system depression (Reidenberg et al., 1978) or objectively and subjectively measured parameters, e.g. sedation, excitement, dizziness, blood pressure, pulse rate (Kanto et al., 1979).

Fink and co-workers (1976) examined the relationship between blood concentration and EEG effects following a single oral dose of diazepam in male volunteers. Significant changes in EEG beta activity were associated with blood levels of 100 ng/ml of diazepam. EEG changes paralleled changes in the concentration of diazepam in the blood. A significant correlation between blood levels and increased EEG beta activity was observed.

Chlordiazepoxide

Gottschalk and co-workers (Gottschalk and Kaplan, 1972; Gottschalk et al., 1973) reported the relationship between plasma levels of chlordiazepoxide and clinical response. A single oral dose of 25 mg of chlordiazepoxide or placebo was administered in a randomized double–blind trial to 18 anxious subjects who had fasted for 10–12 hours and plasma levels were determined 1–2 hours after the dose. Anxiety and hostility scores were measured from speech content analysis. No statistically significant differences between placebo and chlordiazepoxide were demonstrated for the group as a whole using the anxiety scale. For 11 patients, whose chlordiazepoxide plasma level exceeded 0.70 μg/ml, there was a tendency for plasma level to be associated with decrease in anxiety score. Hostility scores decreased more with chlordiazepoxide than with placebo. Significant correlations for plasma level and hostility scores were found for the 11 subjects with the highest concentrations.

Greenblatt et al. (1977b) administered single oral doses of chlordiazepoxide to 10 volunteers, once with water and once with an antacid. Both studies were placebo controlled. Subjective feelings were recorded using visual analogue scales. Changes in subjective ratings of 'feeling spaced out' and 'thinking slowed down' showed significant correlation with the blood concentration of chlordiazepoxide plus desmethylchlordiazepoxide at 30 mins. No correlation was found at later times. The subjective effects were greatest when the drug was given with water and absorption was rapid. The findings suggest an effect of absorption rate on the psychological effect of single oral doses, but probably have little relevance to the chronic dosing situation.

Bond et al. (1977) compared the anxiolytic effects of chlordiazepoxide and placebo in a group of 20 patients, who received an average dose of 28 mg/day (range 10–50 mg/day) for 2–4 weeks. Clinical changes in anxiety levels were assessed using the Hamilton anxiety and self-rating scales and steady-state concentrations of chlordiazepoxide and its major metabolites desmethylchlordiazepoxide and demoxepam were determined by spectrofluorimetry. There was no relationship between clinical anxiolytic effect and the plasma level of the parent drug or any of its metabolites.

In a double-blind crossover study of chlordiazepoxide and placebo, 15 patients received both substances for one week each (Lin and Friedel, 1979). The Hopkins symptom checklist and the Hamilton anxiety rating scale were administered to each patient before and at the end of each week of treatment. Plasma levels of chlordiazepoxide, desmethylchlordiazepoxide and demoxepam were determined by spectrofluorimetry. There was no correlation between anxiolytic effect and the plasma concentration of chlordiazepoxide. A significant correlation between the change in Hamilton score and the plasma level of desmethylchloridazepoxide was observed. Changes in the items of somatic anxiety on the Hamilton scale were negatively correlated with plasma levels of desmethylchlordiazepoxide and demoxepam.

Other benzodiazepines

A few studies have reported the anxiolytic effects of other benzodiazepines in relation to their plasma concentrations. In the study described above, Robin et al. (1974) found no relationship between plasma nordiazepam concentrations, after clorazepate administration, and anxiolytic effects for the group of patients studied, but was able to demonstrate a within-patient relationship. Tansella et al. (1975) similarly found no relationship between plasma levels of nordiazepam and clinical response in 30 patients with anxiety neurosis and insomnia.

In a study of 15 anxious depressed patients, no relationship was found between plasma levels of nordiazepam and anxiolytic response (Tognoni et al., 1975). After a placebo period of one week, all patients received 20–30 mg/day of N-desmethyldiazepam and 75–100 mg/day of nortriptyline. Plasma concentrations were determined by gas chromatography on days 5 and 10. Anxiety ratings were recorded with self-rating scales or by nurses' observation scales during the 10 days of treatment. Since two drugs were co-administered, it is difficult to decide which drug gave the therapeutic response. Also the problem of interactions between these two compounds has not been investigated and may additionally have affected the clinical outcome.

In a study of medazepam in 19 patients, Bond et al. (1977) were unable to demonstrate any relationship between plasma concentrations and anxiolytic effect as assessed by the Hamilton anxiety rating scale. Mean medazepam dosage was 27 mg/day (range 10–50 mg) administered on a flexible schedule over 2–4 weeks. Ketazolam (50–300 mg/day) was administered to 10 chronic alcoholic patients undergoing treatment for alcohol withdrawal (Gottschalk and Cohn, 1978). Anxiety levels were assessed by 5 mins speech content analysis. Plasma levels of ketazolam and its desmethyl metabolite were measured by gas chromatography after 21 days of chronic drug administration. No significant correlation between plasma levels and clinical response was observed.

ROUTINE MONITORING OF BENZODIAZEPINE PLASMA CONCENTRATIONS?

In the management of patients with anxiety states and receiving benzodiazepines, the question of routine plasma drug monitoring arises. The review of the literature, as presented, indicates that no consensus exists concerning the relationship between anxiolytic effect and drug concentration. Only a limited data base, drawn from studies with differing protocols, is available. Further studies exploring this relationship are required. In such studies careful consideration should be given to the type of patients studied, to drug assay methodology and to the use of standardized rating scales. The presence of active drug metabolites should also be taken into account; the inclusion of a placebo period should be mandatory; the use of other psychotropics excluded; the length of drug treatment should be sufficient for clinical response to be anticipated. Such studies, given an adequate number of patients, will clarify the situation regarding the range of benzodiazepine concentrations necessary for clinical response. Currently there is no indication for routine monitoring of benzodiazepine plasma concentrations in anxiety states.

In certain situations monitoring can be justified. As a check on the patient compliance, plasma concentrations determined at the same time post-dose and 3–4 days apart should be within 10–15 % of each other. In patients experiencing severe side effects, a high plasma level would suggest the need to lower the dose. Clearly in these situations the peak of the plasma concentration, which occurs 2–3 hours after the dose, should be avoided for a meaningful result. Trough concentrations, occurring 10–15 hours after the dose, are more representative of the pseudo steady-state value. Monitoring is often advisable in patients with renal or hepatic disease, where high plasma concentrations are liable to develop due to a diminished ability to excrete or metabolize the drugs. A similar situation pertains to elderly patients, who generally have an increased susceptibility to the side effects of drugs. Where these patients are experiencing severe side effects a plasma drug concentration may be a valuable aid. Plasma concentrations after overdoses are not related to the ultimate clinical outcome (Divoll et al., 1981) nor are they related to electrocardiographic parameters (Norman and Burrows, 1984). In these cases monitoring is clearly irrelevant.

Routine monitoring of the benzodiazepines is unnecessary in most circumstances. Effective patient management can be gauged from careful clinical observations. In some specific instances monitoring may be of benefit to the patient.

REFERENCES

Abel, J. G., Sellers, E. M., Naranjo, C. A., Shaw, J., Kadar, D. and Romach, M. K. (1979) Inter and intra subject variation in diazepam free fraction. Clin. Pharmacol. Ther. 26, 247–255.

Alvan, G., Siwers, B. and Vessman, J. (1977) Pharmacokinetics of oxazepam in healthy volunteers. Acta. Pharmacol. Toxicol. (Suppl. 1) 40, 52–62.

Baird, E. S. and Hailey, D. M. (1972) Delayed recovery from a sedative correlation of the plasma levels of diazepam with clinical effects after oral and intravenous administration. Br. J. Anaesth. 44, 803–808.

Bianchi, G. N., Fennessy, M. R., Phillips, J. and Everitt, B. S. (1974) Plasma levels of diazepam as a therapeutic predictor in anxiety states. Psychopharmacologia (Berl.) 35, 113–122.

Bliding, A. (1974) Effects of different rates of absorption of two benzodiazepines on subjective and objective parameters. Significance for clinical use and risk of abuse. Eur. J. Clin. Pharmacol. 7, 201–211.

Bond, A. J., Hailey, D. M. and Lader, M. H. (1977) Plasma concentrations of benzodiazepines. Br. J. Clin. Pharmacol. 4, 51–56.

Boxenbaum, H. G., Geitner, K. A., Jack, M. L., Dixon, W. R., Spiegel, H. E., Symington, J., Christian, R., Moore, J. D., Weissman, L. and Kaplan, S. A. (1977) Pharmacokinetic and biopharmaceutic profile of chlordiazepoxide HCl in healthy subjects: single dose studies by intravenous, intramuscular and oral routes. J. Pharmacokinet. Biopharm. 5, 3–23.

Breimer, D. D., Jochemsen, R. and van Albert, H. H. (1980) Pharmacokinetics of benzodiazepines: short acting versus long acting. Arzneim. Forsch. 30, 875–881.

Burrows, G. D., Dumovic, P., Smith, J. A., Norman, T. and Maguire, K. (1977) A controlled comparative trial of clorazepate (Tranxene) and diazepam (Valium) for anxiety. Med. J. Aust. 2, 525–528.

Committee on the Review of Medicines (1980) Systematic review of the benzodiazepines. Br. Med. J. 280, 910–912.

Dasberg, H. H., van der Kleijn, E., Guelen, P. J. R. and van Praag, H. M. (1974) Plasma concentrations of diazepam and of its metabolite N-desmethyldiazepam in relation to anxiolytic effect. Clin. Pharmacol. Ther. 15, 473–483.

Divoll, M., Greenblatt, D. J., Lacasse, Y. and Shader, R. I. (1981) Benzodiazepine overdosage: plasma concentration and clinical outcome. Psychopharmacologia 73, 381–383.

Fink, M., Irwin, P., Weinfeld, R. E., Schwartz, M. A. and Conney, A. H. (1976) Blood levels and electroencephalographic effects of diazepam and bromazepam. Clin. Pharmacol. Ther. 20, 184–191.

Fulton, A., Maguire, K. P., Norman, T. R. and Wurm, J. M. E. (1981) Benzodiazepine pharmacokinetics, plasma levels and clinical response. In: G.D. Burrows and T.R. Norman (Eds), Psychotropic Drugs: Plasma Concentration and Clinical Response. Marcel Dekker, New York, pp. 361–400.

Ghoneim, M. M., Mewaldt, S. P. and Ambre, J. (1975) Plasma levels of diazepam and mood ratings. Anesth. Analg. 54, 173–177.

Gottschalk, L. A. and Cohn, J. B. (1978) The relationship of diazepam and ketazolam blood levels to anxiety and hostility in chronic alcoholics. Psychopharmacologia Bull. 14, 39–43.

Gottschalk, L. A. and Kaplan, S. A. (1972) Chlordiazepoxide plasma levels and clinical responses. Compr. Psychiatry 13, 519–527.

Gottschalk, L. A., Noble, E. P., Stolzoff, G. E., Bates, D. E., Coble, C. G., Uliana, R. L., Birch, H. and Fleming, E. W. (1973) Relationships of chlordiazepoxide blood levels to psychological and biochemical responses. In: S. Garattini, E. Mussini and L. O. Randall (Eds), The Benzodiazepines. Raven Press, New York, pp. 257–278.

Greenblatt, D. J. (1981) Clinical pharmacokinetics of oxazepam and lorazepam. Clin. Pharmacokinet. 6, 89–105.

Greenblatt, D. J. and Shader, R. I. (1974) Benzodiazepines in Clinical Practice. Raven Press, New York.

Greenblatt, D. J. and Shader, R. I. (1980) Effects of age and other drugs on benzodiazepine kinetics. Arzneim. Forsch. 30, 886–890.

Greenblatt, D. J., Comer, W. H., Elliott, H. Wl., Shader, R. I., Knowles, J. A. and Ruelius, H. W. (1977a) Clinical pharmacokinetics of lorazepam. III. Intravenous injection. J. Clin. Pharmacokinet 17, 490–494.

Greenblatt, D. J., Shader, R. I., Harmatz, J. S., Franke, K. and Koch-Weser, J. (1977b) Absorption rate, blood concentrations, and early response to oral chlordiazepoxide. Am. J. Psychiatry 134, 559–562.

Greenblatt, D. J., Shader, R. I., MacLeod, S. M. and Sellers, E. M. (1978) Clinical pharmacokinetics of chlordiazepoxide. Clin. Pharmacokinet. 3, 381–394.

Greenblatt, D. J., Laughren, T. P., Allen, M. D., Harmatz, J. S. and Shader, R. I. (1981a) Plasma diazepam and desmethyldiazepam concentrations during long-term diazepam therapy. Br. J. Clin. Pharmacol. 11, 35–40.

Greenblatt, D. J., Shader, R. I., Divoll, M. and Harmatz, J. S. (1981b) Benzodiazepines: a summary of pharmacokinetic properties. Br. J. Clin. Pharmacol. 11, 11S–16S.

Hillestad, L., Hansen, T., Melsom, H. and Drivenes, A. (1974a) Diazepam metabolism in normal man. I. Serum concentrations and clinical effects after intravenous, intramuscular, and oral administration. Clin. Pharmacol. Ther. 16, 479–484.

Hillestad, L., Hansen, T. and Melsom, H. (1974b) Diazepam metabolism in normal man. II. Serum concentrations and clinical effect after oral administration and cumulation. Clin. Pharmacol. Ther. 16, 485–489.

Kanto, J. (1975) Plasma concentrations of diazepam and its metabolites after peroral, intramuscular and rectal administration. Correlation between plasma concentration and sedatory effect of diazepam. Int. J. Clin. Pharmacol. 12, 427–432.

Kanto, J., Iisalo, E., Lehtinen, V. and Salminen, J. (1974) The concentrations of diazepam and its metabolites in the plasma after an acute and chronic administration. Psychopharmacologia (Berl.) 36, 123–131.

Kanto, J., Iisalo, E. u. M., Hovi-Viander, M. and Kangas, L. (1979) A comparative study on the clinical effects of oxazepam and diazepam. Relationship between plasma level and effect. Int. J. Clin. Pharmacol. Biopharm. 17, 26–31.

Klotz, U., Antonin, K. L. and Biek, P. R. (1976) Pharmacokinetics and plasma binding of diazepam in man, dog, rabbit, guinea pig and rat. J. Pharmacol. Exp. Ther. 199, 67–73.

Lin, K. M., and Friedel, R. O. (1979) Relationship of plasma levels of chlordiazepoxide and metabolites to clinical response. Am. J. Psychiatry 136, 18–23.

Linnoila, M., Otterstrom, S. and Anttila, M. (1974) Serum chlordiazepoxide, diazepam and thioridazine concentrations after the simultaneous ingestion of alcohol or placebo drink. Ann. Clin. Res. 6, 4–6.

MacLeod, S. M., Giles, H. G., Patzalek, G., Thiessen, J. J. and Sellers, E. M. (1977) Diazepam actions and plasma concentrations following ethanol ingestion. Eur. J. Clin. Pharmacol. 11, 345–349.

Mandelli, M., Tognoni, G. and Garattini, S. (1978) Clinical pharmacokinetics of diazepam. Clin. Pharmacokinet. 3, 72–91.

Norman, T. R. and Burrows, G. D. (1984) Plasma concentrations of benzodiazepines – a review of clinical findings and implications. Prog. Neurol. Psychopharmacol. (in press).

Reidenberg, M., Levy, M., Warner, H., Coutinho, C. B., Schwartz, M. A., Yu, G. and Cheripko, J. (1978) Relationship between diazepam dose, plasma level, age, and central nervous system depression. Clin. Pharmacol. Ther. 23, 371–374.

Robin, A., Curry, S. H. and Whelpton, R. (1974) Clinical and biochemical comparison of clorazepate and diazepam. Psychol. Med. 4, 388–392.

Rutherford, D. M., Okoko, A. and Tyrer, P. J. (1978) Plasma concentrations of diazepam and N-desmethyldiazepam during chronic diazepam therapy. Br. J. Clin. Pharmacol. 6, 69–73.

Sellers, E. M., MacLeod, S. M., Greenblatt, D. J. and Giles, H. G. (1977) Influence of disulfiram and disease on benzodiazepine disposition. Clin. Pharmacol. Ther. 21, 117.

Seppala, T., Linnoila, M. and Mattila, M. J. (1979) Drugs, alcohol and driving. Drugs 17, 389–408.

Shader, R. I. and Greenblatt, D. J. (1977) Clinical implications of benzodiazepine pharmacokinetics. Am. J. Psychiatry 134, 652–655.

Smith, R. C., Dekirmenjian, H., Davis, J., Casper, R., Gosenfeld, L. and Tsai, C. (1976) Blood level, mood and MHPG responses to diazepam in man. In: L. Gottschalk and S. Merlis (Eds), Pharmacokinetics of Psychoactive Drugs. Spectrum, New York, pp. 141–156.

Tansella, M., Siciliani, O., Burti, L., Schiavoni, M., Zimmermann-Tansella, Ch., Gerna, M., Tognoni, G. and Morselli, P. L. (1975) N-desmethyldiazepam and amylobarbitone sodium as hypnotics in anxious patients. Plasma levels, clinical efficacy and residual effects. Psychopharmacologia (Berl.) 41, 81–85.

Tansella, M., Zimmerman-Tansella, Ch., Ferrario, L., Preziati, L., Tognoni, G. and Lader, M. (1978) Plasma concentrations of diazepam, nordiazepam and amylobarbitone after short term treatment of anxious patients. Pharmakopsychiatry 11, 68–75.

Tognoni, G., Gomeni, R., DeMaio, D., Alberti, G. D., Franciosi, P., and Scieghi, G. (1975) Pharmacokinetics of N-desmethyldiazepam in patients suffering from insomnia and treated with nortriptyline. Br. J. Clin. Pharmacol. 2, 227–232.

Van der Kleijn, E., Van Rossum, J. M., Muskens, E. T. J. M. and Rijntjes, N. V. M. (1971) Pharmacokinetics of diazepam in dogs, mice and humans. Acta Pharmacol Toxicol. 29 (Suppl. 3), 109–127.

Wilensky, A. J., Levy, R. H., Troupin, A. S., Moretti-Ojemann, L. and Friel, P. (1978) Clorazepate kinetics in treated epileptics. Clin. Pharmacol. Ther. 24, 22–30.

Zingales, I. A. (1973) Diazepam metabolism during chronic medication; unbound fraction in plasma, erythrocytes and urine. J. Chromatogr. 75, 55–78.

Burrows/Norman/Davies (eds) Antianxiety agents
© *Elsevier Science Publishers B.V., 1984*

Chapter 8

Clinical aspects of antianxiety agents

LEO E. HOLLISTER

*Veterans Administration Medical Center and Department of Psychiatry and
Pharmacology, Stanford University School of Medicine, Stanford, California, U.S.A.*

Current classification of anxiety disorders

The diagnostic rubrics for anxiety disorders have changed remarkably in the United States as a result of the current version of the Diagnostic and Statistical Manual of Mental Disorders (DSM III). What is now called generalized anxiety disorder is what was formerly called anxiety state or anxiety neurosis. Some patients with this disorder were subject to acute, overwhelming attacks of anxiety, now referred to as panic disorder. Panic disorder may also be associated with phobic disorders, but whether the phobia causes the panic or is the result of behaviour designed to avoid its precipitation is still unclear. Obsessive-compulsive disorder, always known to overlap with phobic disorders, is now also included within the framework of anxiety disorders. Post-traumatic stress disorders round out the classification.

Antianxiety drugs in the present context of anxiety disorders

The place of drug treatment in this motley group of disorders is in a state of flux. Most authorities would agree that antianxiety drugs are clearly indicated for patients with generalized anxiety disorder. If one views panic attacks as possibly an exaggeration of the same disorder, it is possible that such drugs might be useful in this situation, possibly requiring much larger doses than conventionally used.

For the phobic and obsessive-compulsive disorders, much more success has been reported from treatment with antidepressants, either tricyclics or monoamine oxidase (MAO) inhibitors, which has raised the question of whether these disorders are more closely associated with depression.

When we speak of antianxiety drugs, we do not refer to their use in each of the anxiety disorders as they are now defined, but rather in the more limited sense of treating for generalized anxiety disorder. The latter may be considered to be primary, that is, without any obvious precipitating cause, or secondary, usually to some concurrent physical illness or adverse life event.

TYPES OF ANTIANXIETY DRUGS

Various classes

Many types of agents can be used for, or have been promoted for, the treatment of anxiety. At present seven different chemical classes of such drugs can be described (Table 1). One group, exemplified by barbiturates, meprobamate and its congeners, and benzodiazepines, has a profile of pharmacologic actions resembling that of conventional 'sedative-hypnotics': sedation proceeding to hypnosis, muscle relaxation, anticonvulsant action, tolerance development, and potential for either psychological or physical dependence.

A second group of antianxiety agents was named 'sedative-autonomic' for lack of a better term. This term indicates that they differ from the sedative-hypnotics in having variable effects on the peripheral autonomic nervous system, such as anticholinergic or alpha-adrenergic blocking actions. In addition, the sedation they produce is qualitatively different from that of the sedative-hypnotics. Sedative-autonomic drugs include various sedative antihistamines, some of which are sold without prescription as sedatives or hypnotics, antipsychotic drugs in small doses, and some of the more sedative tricyclic antidepressants. These drugs also differ from the sedative-hypnotic group in increasing muscle tone, lowering convulsive thresholds, and having a minimal predisposition for producing tolerance of dependence. A third group, still small, is exemplifed by buspirone, which may be a weak neuroleptic.

Dominance of benzodiazepines

The displacement of the barbiturates and meprobamate-like drugs by benzodiazepines is probably justified. Why is it that more recent competitors of the sedative-autonomic type constitute so little threat to their dominance? The main reason is that patients find the qualitatively different sedation and autonomic side effects of sedative-autonomic drugs rather unpleasant. The same reasons that make these drugs less acceptable to patients also make them less likely to be

TABLE 1

Seven classes of antianxiety drugs.

Sedative-hypnotic	Sedative-autonomic
BARBITURATES	**DIPHENYLMETHANE ANTIHISTAMINES**
butabarbital sodium phenobarbital	diphenhydramine hydroxyzine
GLYCEROL DERIVATIVES	**ANTIPSYCHOTICS**
meprobamate tybamate	acetophenazine haloperidol trifluoperazine
BENZODIAZEPINES	**TRICYCLIC ANTIDEPRESSANTS**
alprazolam chlordiazepoxide chlorazepate dipotassium diazepam halazepam lorazepam oxazepam	amitriptyline doxepin **WEAK NEUROLEPTIC?** buspirone

abused. The lack of abuse potential of the sedative-autonomics has been used in their promotion, but most physicians as well as patients seem to be willing to accept a small risk of dependence rather than to accept the disadvantages of the sedative-autonomic class.

Proliferation of benzodiazepines

A great number of active benzodiazepines are possible on the basis of chemical variations. The basic benzodiazepine nucleus has been substituted at several positions to produce compounds with varying degrees of pharmacological potency, as shown in Fig. 1. Whether or not the spectrum of pharmacologic activity varies as much is still an unsettled question. Nonetheless, drugs have been promoted for different indications on the basis of chemical differences. For instance, flurazepam and temazepam are promoted only as hypnotics, clonazepam only as an anticonvulsant, but diazepam as an antianxiety drug, a muscle relaxant, an anticonvulsant and an anaesthetic.

110

Possible explanation for benzodiazepine dominance

Although differences among sedative-hypnotic and sedative-autonomic drugs are more often of degree than type, they may help to determine one's choice of a drug. Both in terms of favourable and unfavourable attributes, benzodiazepines seem to have the edge over the other classes of sedatives.

The ratio between antianxiety and sedative effects is believed to be higher with meprobamate and the benzodiazepines than with the others, although such an assertion is exceedingly difficult to prove. Muscle relaxation is also greater with the benzodiazepines, especially as compared with the sedative-autonomic drugs, which may actually increase muscle tone. On a theoretical basis, at least, one could argue that skeletal muscle relaxation may contribute to the relief of anxiety.

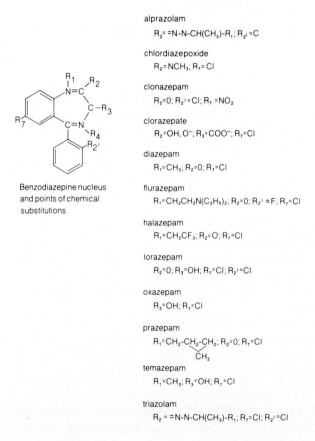

Benzodiazepine nucleus and points of chemical substitutions

alprazolam
$R_2 = =N-N-CH(CH_3)-R_1; R_{2'} =C$

chlordiazepoxide
$R_2 = NCH_3; R_7 = Cl$

clonazepam
$R_2 = 0; R_{2'} = Cl; R_7 = NO_2$

clorazepate
$R_2 = OH, O^-; R_3 = COO^-; R_7 = Cl$

diazepam
$R_1 = CH_3; R_2 = 0; R_7 = Cl$

flurazepam
$R_1 = CH_2CH_2N(C_2H_5)_2; R_2 = 0; R_{2'} = F; R_7 = Cl$

halazepam
$R_1 = CH_2CF_3; R_2 = O; R_7 = Cl$

lorazepam
$R_2 = 0; R_3 = OH; R_7 = Cl; R_{2'} = Cl$

oxazepam
$R_3 = OH; R_7 = Cl$

prazepam
$R_1 = CH_2-CH_2-CH_2; R_2 = 0; R_7 = Cl$
        CH_2

temazepam
$R_1 = CH_3; R_3 = OH; R_7 = Cl$

triazolam
$R_2 = =N-N-CH(CH_3)-R_1; R_7 = Cl; R_{2'} = Cl$

Fig. 1. Structural relationship of various benzodiazepines. Differences in pharmacokinetic aspects are more evident than pharmacodynamic actions. The uses for which drugs are promoted often have little bearing on either.

A long duration of action is desirable in most cases. It decreases the frequency of drug administration and inhibits reinforcement of drug-taking, it produces more sustained therapeutic effects, and it tends to maintain therapeutic benefits briefly even after discontinuation of drug use. Thus, most benzodiazepines have an advantage on most favourable attributes of these drugs.

An unfavourable attribute of a drug is the ability to induce drug-metabolizing enzymes. Clinically significant interactions with other drugs may ensue, as well as loss of the drug's effect. The benzodiazepines are conspicuously better than other sedative-hypnotics in this regard. Except for meprobamate, tolerance and physical dependence with all drugs of this type are mild and infrequent when they are used as medically prescribed. Although most psychoactive drugs affect the normal sleep pattern, the degree of departure is least with the benzodiazepines. This group is also the safest in suicide potential; it is virtually impossible to cause death by taking these drugs alone. The tricyclics are exceedingly hazardous as suicidal agents, although antipsychotics are safer. Thus, benzodiazepines seem to possess fewer unfavourable attributes than do other sedatives.

PHARMACOLOGIC ACTION

The benzodiazepine receptor

The discovery in 1977 of specific receptors for benzodiazepines in the brain of various mammals has triggered a tremendous amount of investigation into the modes of action of these drugs (Mohler and Okada, 1977; Squires and Braestrup, 1977). Intensive subsequent investigation has led to the idea that benzodiazepine receptors are functionally linked to receptors for γ-aminobutyric acid (GABA) and to a chloride ion channel. GABA is a widely distributed inhibitory neurotransmitter which probably works by opening the chloride ion channel, allowing more chloride ions to enter the cell and causing hyperpolarization and decreasing firing. Benzodiazepines augment further this action of GABA (Tallman et al., 1980). The in vitro affinity of various benzodiazepines to bind to these receptors parallels their clinical potency, lending additional credence to the idea that their actions are mediated by these receptors.

Following the analogy of the opiate receptor (1971–1973) and the rapid subsequent discovery of endogenous ligands for this receptor (1975–1980), it seems logical that an endogenous ligand may be found for the benzodiazepine receptor. A number of purines, such as inosine, hypoxanthine, and adenosine, as well as the non-purine, nicotinamide, has been proposed as possible endogenous ligands. Most bind rather weakly, but the case is growing that adenosine may be involved (Wu et al., 1981).

A practical outcome of this type of research is that a specific antagonist for benzodiazepines has been developed. Such a drug should be useful not only in the laboratory but also in clinical situations of drug overdose (Möhler and Richards, 1981).

Neurotransmitters

Evidence regarding the effect of benzodiazepines on various neurotransmitters, such as dopamine, serotonin and norepinephrine, is contradictory. The most persuasive evidence is that benzodiazepines augment the natural inhibitory function of gamma-aminobutyric acid (GABA) (Costa and Guidotti, 1979). Besides reducing the firing rate of neurons, this action may be reflected secondarily in other neurotransmitter systems. For instance, release of serotonin might be inhibited in the brain's punishment system and thereby disinhibit suppressed reward-seeking behaviour. Increased GABA activity might also be pertinent to the anticonvulsant and muscle-relaxant effect of these drugs.

Neurophysiological studies

These drugs could be active in various major integrating systems of the brain. An effect on the reticular activating system might permit more selective monitoring of incoming signals, perhaps decreasing the signal/noise ratio. An effect on the limbic system might diminish the affective tone of incoming messages. An effect on the hypothalamic-pituitary-endocrine and sympathetic nervous system might diminish the bodily responses to stress. Most of these mechanisms have been hypothesized for other psychotherapeutic drugs, so that it is difficult to be sure whether or not any of them is germane to this particular group of drugs.

Behavioural studies

Behavioural pharmacologists have been clever in devising several paradigms of conflict behaviour, which seem to have some relevance to what is encountered in real life (Geller et al., 1962). One such conflict situation puts a hungry rat in a cage rigged so that if the animal presses a lever that delivers a food pellet it will also receive a foot-shock. Fear of punishment predominates, so the animal will prefer to remain hungry rather than to press the lever for more food. Benzodiazepines mitigate the fear-conditioned behaviour so that the animal will seek the reward in the face of certain punishment. This behaviour is retained during chronic treatment with these drugs, while behavioural signs of sedation and ataxia rapidly disappear due to the development of tolerance to these unwanted effects. Thus, the 'antianxiety' effects of these drugs can be separated from their purely sedative actions.

Implications for a biological basis for anxiety

If endogenous ligands for benzodiazepines exist, they may be either of two types. One might mimic the action of benzodiazepines and possibly function as a coping mechanism against stress. Another might bind to the receptor but produce anxiety rather than inhibit it. Such a material, beta-carboline-3-carboxylic acid ester, has been found to be anxiogenic (File et al., 1982). Such beta-carbolines could easily be produced in the brain and could function in this fashion. Thus, aberrations in either of these mechanisms, either due to deficient production of some 'endogenous benzodiazepine' or overproduction of some endogenous 'anxiogenic' might provide a biological basis for anxiety. Such abnormalities would not be expected to occur frequently. However, patients showing high clinical levels of 'trait' anxiety, that is, an excessive proneness to become anxious when placed under stress are also uncommon. Finally, use patterns of these drugs suggest that relatively few patients, probably no more than 6% of the adult population, use these drugs chronically, and possibly fewer still use them solely for relief of anxiety (Balter et al., 1974). These notions are still hypothetical, but they are potentially testable.

METABOLISM AND KINETICS

Metabolism

Four routes of metabolism, dealkylation, oxidation, reduction and glucuronidation, account for the principal metabolic pathways of various benzodiazepines. Several routes may be employed with some compounds, producing a succession of active metabolites. Some of the metabolic interrelationships between various commonly used benzodiazepines are shown in Fig. 2. Chlordiazepoxide, for instance, undergoes first dealkylation, then oxidation and reduction to form a common metabolite of many of these agents, *N*-desmethyldiazepam (nordiazepam).

Some drugs on the market are essentially pro-drugs for nordiazepam, very quickly being converted from the parent compound to that active metabolite. This may occur either by dealkylation (prazepam) or by hydrolysis (clorazepate dipotassium). Drugs that have a hydroxy-group at the 3-position form no active metabolites but are directly conjugated.

Kinetics

The pharmacokinetic parameters of various benzodiazepines are summarized in Table 2. Much more information is available about some of the older agents than the newer ones. An extensive literature has developed regarding the kinetics of benzodiazepines and has been reviewed elsewhere (Greenblatt et al., 1981).

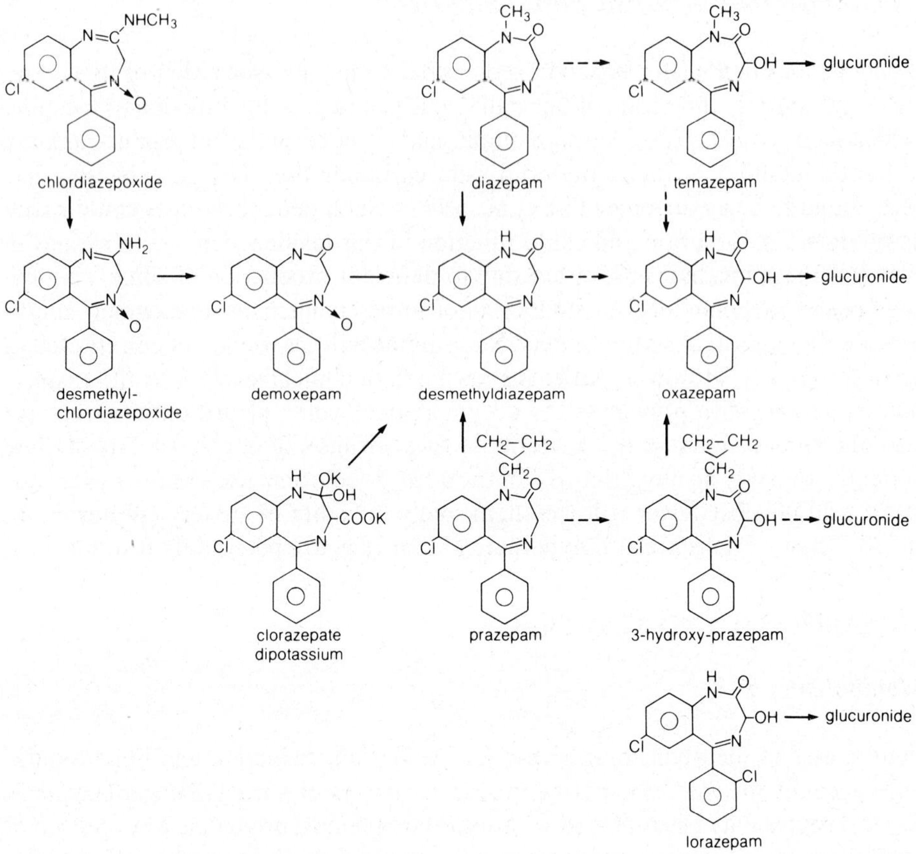

Fig. 2. Metabolic pathways for various types of benzodiazepines. The central position of *N*-desmethyl-diazepam (nordiazepam) is evident.

Kinetic differences and choice of drug. As the pharmacological spectrum of action of various benzodiazepines is not much different, one drug from another, do differences in pharmacokinetics suggest specific indications for certain compounds? Diazepam's rapid onset of action when given orally, as well as its long duration of action through its major metabolite, seem to make it the most ideal.

CLINICAL USE

General considerations

Despite their wide popularity, antianxiety drugs continue to be controversial. Many believe that such great dependence on drug therapy for symptoms that

TABLE 2

Pharmacokinetic parameters of benzodiazepines.

Drug	$t_{1/2}b$ (hrs)	Vd (L/Kg)	Protein binding	Active metabolites	$t_{1/2}b$ (hrs)	Ther. Conc. (ng/ml)
Very-Short						
triazolam	2–8	1.1	89	7-α-hydroxy	3–10	
Short						
alprazolam	6–20					
lorazepam	9–22	0.7–1.0	85	none		
oxazepam	6–24	0.6–1.6	86	none		
temazepam	5–20	0.8	76	oxazepam		
Intermediate						
chlordiazepoxide	7–15	0.3–0.6	93	desmethyl-demoxepam	14–46	750
diazepam	14–90	0.7–2.6	94–98	nordiazepam	30–200	400–600
halazepam		1.0–1.3	98.6	nordiazepam	30–200	
Long						
clorazepate	–	1.0–1.3	98.6	nordiazepam	30–200	430
prazepam	–	1.0–1.3	98.6	nordiazepam	30–200	430
Very-Long						
flurazepam	very short	3.4		desmethyl	40–100	
				hydroxyethyl	6–7	

seem to be rooted in life experience may deny patients the benefits of other treatments, particularly psychotherapy, which is a more specific and permanent treatment. Although the efficacy of these drugs for relieving symptoms of anxiety is generally accepted, many doubt that the benefits of drug therapy are very great. Finally, the rapid increase in nonmedical use of mind-altering drugs has led to concerns that overenthusiastic prescribing of these drugs may contribute to this problem.

The best epidemiological study of the use of antianxiety drugs is now several years old. As the number of prescriptions for these drugs has probably declined during the intervening period, the findings of this study probably still reflect current patterns. In 1971, households chosen by usual sampling techniques in the United States as well as in nine European countries, were asked about their use of antianxiety drugs (Balter et al., 1974). The two major questions were whether any adult member (over age 18 years) had used such a drug in the preceding 12 months and if so, whether the use had been for as long as one month. The highest overall use of antianxiety drugs was in Belgium, where 16.8 % of adults queried had used such a drug on at least one occasion in the preceding year; only 9.7 % answered positively to this question in Spain. Other data from the United States indicated a figure of 15 %. One month or more of chronic use of these agents followed a similar pattern with a maximum of 8.6 % and a minimum of 3.4 % of adults using these drugs in this manner. In the United States such use was reported by 6 % of those surveyed. Those persons who had used them were quite positive in their opinions about the benefits derived; 77 % claiming 'substantial benefit'.

What emerged from these data was the remarkable fact that medical use of sedative-hypnotics is not out of hand, but seems to have stabilized at a reasonable level. Further, despite vast cultural, political, and economic differences between developed countries, use of these agents is remarkably comparable within a rather narrow rank. This use pattern suggests that a relatively small proportion of the population perceives a need for these drugs and benefit from their use. Further analysis of the data from this survey indicate that physicians prescribe these drugs in a medical model, the rate of prescription increasing proportional to the degree of 'life stress' or psychic distress' reported by the patients (Mellinger et al., 1978). Actually the number of persons with high levels of stress was considerably greater than the number who take drugs, indicating that many persons are able to cope with stress without the use of drugs at all.

INDICATIONS

Anxiety

We have already mentioned that the feeling of nervousness or constant worry of uncertain cause, which is termed 'anxiety', is a prime indication for the antianxiety drugs. They are especially valuable when symptoms are severe, rather than when they are relatively mild. These drugs are most valuable when agitation or severe apprehension is also present. Concomitant depression is not a contraindication, but should alert one to the possibility that the patient may be primarily depressed rather than anxious. Failure to respond to an antianxiety drug, or the apparent precipitation of depression during treatment with one, makes a depression probable. As anxiety is a nonspecific symptom, it may be the early sign of other serious emotional disorders, such as schizophrenia. Again, failure to respond should alert one to diagnostic reconsideration. Usually, given the proper dose of drugs one would expect to see some positive response within the first week of treatment, even though optimal effects may not be obtained for 3 weeks.

Insomnia

The hypnotic effect of these drugs is simply an extension of their sedative action. Some drugs are promoted primarily as hypnotics while others do not even mention such use. Those drugs currently used as hypnotics include flurazepam, temazepam and triazolam, but virtually all of the benzodiazepines could be used for this purpose. Flurazepam is generally considered to be a long-acting drug based on the half-life of its desalkyl metabolite. However, much of its hypnotic action may be ascribed to its hydroxyethyl metabolite, which has a much shorter span of action. Temazepam has an intermediate duration of action, while triazolam is very short-acting. The question of rebound anxiety and insomnia after discontinuation of short-acting hypnotics has been raised, but this might only be a problem when these drugs have been used chronically without interruption, as they rarely should be (Kales et al., 1983).

Muscle spasticity

Diazepam has been widely used for treating muscle spasm associated with disseminated sclerosis, tetanus, cerebral palsy or stroke. Although some debate still exists about the concept of a centrally-acting muscle relaxant, many persons still believing that muscle relaxation is secondary to sedation, diazepam could have a specific action. Its GABA-enhancing effect might enhance the presynaptic inhibition of motor neurons in the spinal cord and decrease their firing rate.

The use of antianxiety drugs, including meprobamate-like drugs such as methocarbamol, for treating simple muscle strains should be discouraged. Judicious use of local physical measures and adequate doses of aspirin are more to the point.

Status epilepticus

Diazepam given intravenously has been the drug of choice for the treatment of status epilepticus. Due to rapid entry of the drug into brain, control is readily attained. Sustained control requires a subsequent loading dose of phenytoin. Some benzodiazepines, such as clonazepam or clorazepate dipotassium have been promoted for limited use in convulsive disorders. A comparison between clorazepate dipotassium and phenobarbital for maintenance treatment of epilepticus showed a preference on the part of patients for the former drug (Wilensky et al., 1981).

Alcohol withdrawal

Alcohol withdrawal is best treated with benzodiazepines because: they have pharmacological properties that are similar to alcohol, and, thus, are reasonable substitutes; they are effective anticonvulsants, affording protection against this frequent complication of alcohol withdrawal; they are not harmful, as phenothia-zines, sedative antihistaminics, or barbiturates can be and they are not noxious, as is paraldehyde. Paraldehyde was compared with diazepam in treating patients with severe delirium tremens (Thompson et al., 1975). Giving diazepam in initial doses of 10 mg intravenously followed by 5 mg every 5 min until the patients were calm yet awake was rapidly effective. Oral doses achieve the same ends. Following initial loading with diazepam, subsequent doses may not be required due to the long plasma half-life of the major metabolite, nordiazepam.

Anaesthetic or induction agent

Diazepam and lorazepam have been used as intravenous anaesthetics or induction agents. Sufficient anaesthesia may be obtained from these drugs alone for brief operative procedures such as electric cardioversion, endoscopic procedures, dental surgery, reductions of minor fractures, and so forth. Both also have been used orally as preoperative medications and were superior to a barbiturate for this purpose (Wilson and Ellis, 1973). Lorazepam may produce more anterograde amnesia than diazepam.

DOSES, DOSAGE, DURATION

Both peak plasma concentrations of benzodiazepines following single doses as well as steady-state concentrations following long-term doses show a variability among different persons ranging from 2- to 6-fold. Aside from that, people vary greatly in their pharmacodynamic responses to these drugs. Thus, it is clear that picking the same dose for everyone, or even the median dose suggested on the package label, is a poor way to judge doses.

How can one arrive at a proper dose for a patient clinically, assuming that plasma concentrations as a control are not easily or readily available and may have questionable significance in any case? A reasonable approach would be establish the minimally effective hypnotic dose of the drug. Initial doses of the drug would be given 2 to 3 hours before bedtime, while patients are still active, and they would be instructed to look for enforced sleepiness, deeper than usual sleep, and a mini-mally discernible degree of 'hangover'. When this dose had been found, it could be assumed to provide the desired effects of the drug. Thus, one would start with the lowest available dose unit of a particular drug (probably with even less if the tablet can be cracked) and double the dose on successive nights until the above criteria have been met. Doses used during the day would be taken as needed, usually one-third to one-fourth the nighttime dose.

The range of clinical doses for various types of antianxiety drugs is shown in Table 3.

TABLE 3

Dose guide for antianxiety drugs.

	Typical initial dose (mg)	Range of daily doses	Dose units for oral administration (mg)
BENZODIAZEPINES			
alprazolam	0.5	1–4	0.25,0.50,1.0
chlordiazepoxide hydrochloride	10.0	15–100	5,10,25
clorazepate dipotassium	7.5	15–60	3.75,7.5,15.0
diazepam	5.0	6–80	2.5,10.0
halazepam	20.0	40–160	20,40
lorazepam	0.5	2–4	0.5,1.0,2.0
oxazepam	15.0	10–60	10,15,30
prazepam	10.0	20–40	5,10

Dosage schedules

Drugs with a slow disappearance rate are well suited to single daily dosage. Such a dosage schedule is desirable for antianxiety drugs, as one does not wish unduly to emphasize drug-taking. The most appropriate time to give the single dose would be in the evening, when one can take advantage of the hypnotic effects of these drugs. A patient with anxiety so severe that drug treatment is required would commonly also have some difficulty sleeping. Further, it does not make much pharmacologic sense to instruct patients to take a sedative right after their morning stimulant – coffee. The 'daytime hangover', which is inevitable with these long-acting drugs, provides precisely the degree of mild sedation compatible with unimpaired daily activities and relief of troublesome symptoms. Fractional doses of drug may be used as needed for particular daytime stress.

Short-acting drugs probably require dosing several times a day. For some patients, the placebo effect of taking medication frequently may be important, so that not all patients should be placed on once-daily dosage, regardless of the type of drug they have been prescribed.

Flexible dosage schedules are acceptable to patients. In one study, patients were instructed to ask for counseling and/or diazepam as their symptoms required. The use of drug was reduced over what it would have been had a standard, equally divided dose order for drug been carried out (Winstead et al., 1974). In a survey of chronic users of diazepam (median duration more than 5 years) in which steady-state plasma concentrations of diazepam/nordiazepam were measured, about one-third of patients had concentrations so low as to cast doubt on their adhering to the prescribed dosage pattern. Many of them were in a range that would be considered subtherapeutic, suggesting that the drug was being taken on an 'as needed' basis. None of the patients appeared to be abusing the drug (Hollister et al., 1981).

Duration of treatment

Anxiety is often episodic, waxing and waning with changes in one's life. In such cases, treatment might follow the course, with drugs being used only when symptoms are discomforting or disabling, and not indefinitely. Such episodes of treatment might be limited to a week or two. If anxiety is relieved, it might remain so without drugs. The knowledge that relief is available may sustain the patient over subsequent periods.

The proposal for brief, interrupted courses of treatment should be made at the onset of treatment. It is virtually impossible to make this proposal after the patient has been under treatment for several weeks or months and feels fine. Arguments that might be used to persuade patients to follow this course are that tolerance may develop to the effects of the drug, larger doses might be needed and the patient may be at risk for becoming dependent. Although these arguments are not very sound from a scientific basis, patients have become so fearful of becoming dependent on drugs that they can be persuasive.

Despite these injunctions, some patients may find that their symptoms return promptly when the drug is stopped and will wish to take it without interruption. If the dose can be kept at minimal levels, no great harm comes from this procedure. Nonetheless, periodic breaks in the treatment programme should be scheduled to ascertain that the drug is still needed and that withdrawal symptoms associated with 'therapeutic-dose dependence' are not evident.

NEW APPROACHES

Many clinicians now combine beta-adrenoreceptor blocking drugs, such as propranolol, with benzodiazepines. The former drugs allay the somatic aspects of anxiety and the latter are more specific for the psychic components. In this sense, the beta-blockers may be considered as 'benzodiazepine-sparing' agents. Although the practice is widespread, experimental validation of its benefit is lacking.

Preliminary experience with a variant of the butyrophenone structure, buspirone, showed it to be as effective as diazepam in treating anxious patients. An excellent antidepressant effect was claimed as well. It remains to be seen whether subsequent experience will be as favourable (Goldberg and Finnerty, 1979). Buspirone is of particular interest in that it does not act through the benzodiazepine receptor or through any GABA-ergic mechanism. It seems to possess both agonist and antagonist actions for dopamine. This novel action raises the possibility that dopamine may play a role in the treatment of anxiety (Taylor et al., 1982).

The recent renewal of interest in clonidine as a psychotherapeutic drug has led to its reappraisal as an antianxiety agent. A double-blind crossover design in 23 patients treated with clonidine or placebo showed that the drug was effective in those patients who could tolerate it, 17 % of patients becoming worse. The main effect of this drug, unlike propranolol, was relief of the psychic but not the somatic symptoms of anxiety (Hoehn-Saric et al., 1981).

NON-PHARMACOLOGICAL TREATMENTS

Anxiety is often related to life experiences. Psychotherapy and altering the environment may be more to the point than are drugs in treating anxiety. Some purists have maintained that it is impossible to have effective psychotherapy in the presence of drug treatment, as the presence of anxiety is a motivating force for psychotherapy. However, little proof exists for this assertion.

No one has tried yet to exploit fully the interaction of metapharmacological influences and antianxiety drugs. From what we know already, it would seem reasonable to try to maximize the patient's belief in the treatment. On the other hand, some patients, who react to anxiety by extroverted behaviour and physical activity, tolerate sedative drugs poorly. Such patients often complain of being made more anxious by sedatives, and should be treated with smaller than usual dose, if at all.

Non-pharmacologic approaches to treatment that are currently being used include biofeedback of various kinds, autogenic training (a form of self-hypnosis), various relaxation techniques, and massage. With the exception of a modern technology in the case of biofeedback, virtually all of these techniques are quite old. Enthusiastic advocates come largely from a self-selected group, so that it is difficult to compare these approaches with the use of drugs.

Two non-pharmacological treatments that have much to commend them (they are as effective as any others and have the virtue of being cheap) are exercise and meditation. Exercise can be of any type, from running or walking to swimming or bicycling. Preferably, it should be taken several hours before bedtime. All it costs is calories, something most of us can easily spare. Meditation requires nothing more than a quiet place and some time. No one need pay for a custom-made nonsense syllable as a mantra, as any simple word, such as 'one' will do when repeated endlessly.

SUMMARY PRINCIPLES OF USE

Some general principles of use of these drugs, based on the foregoing discussion are listed in Table 4.

122

TABLE 4

Summary principles in use of antianxiety drugs.

1) Use only for good reasons – severe symptoms, disability, discomfort.

2) Be aware that anxiety is a symptom; try to make a diagnosis before treating.

3) Consider non-drug therapies – 'psychotherapy', environmental manipulations, exercise, meditation.

4) Propose brief interrupted courses of treatment at the onset.

5) Titrate doses to the needs of individual patients; avoid oversedation.

6) Constantly assess efficacy – poor efficacy, possibly another diagnosis.

7) Avoid in those with history of alcohol or drug abuse – may wish to use a sedative antihistamine.

8) Warn patients about interactions with alcohol and other depressants; to use drugs only for themselves.

9) Limit number of refills; amounts should be consonant with dosage schedule.

10) Discontinue gradually if the patient has been on therapeutic doses for more than one month.

SIDE EFFECTS AND COMPLICATIONS

Sedation

Oversedation is the most common side effect of antianxiety drugs. Directing patients to take the largest dose in the evening hours converts this effect from something harmful to something beneficial. Patients should be warned about the possibility of sedation from any dose take during the day. Usually it will be the greatest 1–2 hours after the drug is taken. Activities that would be dangerous, such as driving an automobile, or making critical judgements should be deferred.

Tolerance/dependence

Tolerance to a drug, during which doses must be increased to obtain the same effects as previously experienced, is the usual prelude to dependence. Although tolerance develops to the sedative effects of benzodiazepines quite readily, it may develop only slowly and to a small degree to the antianxiety action.

The key to the development of tolerance is chronic, uninterrupted use of the drug; thus, the fashion in which these drugs are commonly used makes tolerance scarcely avoidable. The recommendation given before using of these drugs in brief, interrupted courses has the potential for minimizing or avoiding the development of tolerance.

Physical dependence undoubtedly occurs with the benzodiazepines. The author's study showed that it could occur with high multiples of the usual daily dose both from chlordiazepoxide and from diazepam (Hollister et al., 1961, 1963). Since these early experimental studies in man, a number of clinical reports of spontaneous dependence on benzodiazepines has appeared. The total number of such reports of physical dependence has been remarkably small considering the enormous amount of use of these drugs during the past two decades.

Normally one associates withdrawal reactions to sedatives or other drugs with excessive doses over substantial time periods. It may very well be that the interaction is between dose and time so that as the latter becomes longer the dose becomes less. Discontinuation of chlordiazepoxide 45 mg/day in patients who had been treated with this dose for several months produced minor withdrawal symptoms that seemed clearly to be distinguishable from mere return of anxiety (Covi et al., 1973). Subsequently, a number of other cases of withdrawal from therapeutic doses of diazepam has been reported, most of which are included in the review of such reports mentioned above (Marks, 1978). A patient who had been treated with 30–45 mg/day of diazepam for 20 months and which was suddenly stopped, showed a clearcut withdrawal reaction. Precipitous weight loss and orthostatic tachycardia accompanied the typical dysphoria of withdrawal, which occurred between the fifth and ninth days after discontinuation of the drug (Pevnick et al., 1978). In other cases, the withdrawal reaction under these circumstances has been markedly protracted, though mild.

The concept of dependence from sedative drugs given at therapeutic doses is still relatively new. The mechanism of action is not clear (Schopf, 1983). One might speculate that in the case of drugs that act on receptors, such as the benzodiazepines, prolonged use may cause subsensitivity of receptors. When the drug is withdrawn, the response to any endogenous ligand might be reduced. Further, the possibility exists that patients who require these drugs on a continuing basis could be deficient in such endogenous ligands. Thus, such patients might not be protected against sudden withdrawal of the drug as well as others. Of course, all of this speculation has no substantial evidence as yet to support it.

Hostility and depression

Outbursts of aggressive or hostile behaviour during treatment with various benzodiazepines have been rare, but were described quite early in their history. One can only conclude that these episodes represent a release of personality characteristics in much the same way that alcohol is notorious in this respect.

Depression in patients on these drugs is more than likely coincidental, as nothing in their known pharmacological actions should be intrinsically depressogenic. As anxiety and depression are inextricable, it is possible that many patients are treated with antianxiety drugs who are basically depressed. Depression becomes unmasked as the anxiety is relieved.

Dysmorphogenesis

This issue is continually raised with all drugs and has been with the benzodiazepines. It is not yet resolved, as the possible risks are so small as to be unlikely to be detected clinically. Whenever there is doubt, it is wise to be prudent; drugs of any sort should be used only when imperative if the patient is known to be pregnant. If they have been used in a pregnant patient, they should be discontinued whenever possible as soon as the pregnancy is discovered.

OVERDOSES

The safety of benzodiazepines in overdose cannot be surpassed. Between 1962 and 1975, 773 patients with acute overdoses of drug were admitted to the Massachusetts General Hospital. Benzodiazepine derivatives were involved overall in 99 patients, or 13 %, with a gradually increasing proportion over the years. Only 12 intoxications were with benzodiazepines alone and none of these patients were seriously ill or needed assisted respiration. When benzodiazepines were combined with other drugs, the attendant problems were virtually what might have been expected from the types and amounts of other drugs present (Greenblatt et al., 1977).

An extensive survey of 27 medical examiner or coroner offices in the United States and Canada was conducted during the latter part of 1976. The combined jurisdictional population of these sites was 79.2 million people. Diazepam was found to be present on toxicological analysis in 1,239 cases of death. Drugs alone caused death in 914 cases; the remaining 375 fatalities were due to other causes. Only two patients died after having taken only diazepam (Finkle et al., 1980). Considering that one is always at some risk of death whenever one is comatose and treatment is delayed, this minute number of deaths is probably the irreducible minimum for drug overdoses.

REFERENCES

Balter, M. B., Levine, J. and Manheimer, D. I. (1974) Cross-national study of the extent of antian-xiety/sedative drug use. N. Engl. J. Med. 290, 769–774.

Costa, E. and Guidotti, A. (1979) Molecular mechanisms in the receptor action of benzodiaze-pines. Ann. Rev. Pharmacol. Toxicol. 19, 531–545.

Covi, L., Lipman, R. S., Pattison, J. H., Derogatis, L. and Uhlenhuth, E. D. (1973) Length of treatment with anxiolytic sedatives and response to their sudden withdrawal. Acta Psychiatr. Scand. 49, 51–64.

File, S. E., Lister, R. G. and Nutt, D. J. (1982) The anxiogenic action of benzodiazepine antagon-ists. Neuropharmacology 21, 1033–1037.

Finkle, B. S., McCloskey, K. L. and Goodman, L. S. (1980) Diazepam and drug associated deaths in a United States and Canada survey. J. Am.Med. Assoc. 242, 429–434.

Geller, I., Kulak, Jr., J. T. and Seifter, J. (1962) The effects of chlordiazepoxide and clorpromazine on a punishment discrimination. Psychopharmacologia 3, 374–385.

Goldberg, H. L. and Finnerty, R. J. (1979) The comparative efficacy of buspirone and diazepam in the treatment of anxiety. Am. J. Psychiatry 136, 1184–1187.

Greenblatt, D. J., Allen, M. D., Noel, B. S. N. and Shader, R. I. (1977) Special article: acute overdosage with benzodiazepine derivatives. Clin. Pharmacol. Ther. 21, 497–514.

Greenblatt, D. J., Shader, R. I., Divoll, M. and Harmatz, J. S. (1981) Benzodiazepines: a summa-ry of pharmacokinetic properties. Br.J. Clin. Pharmacol. 11, 118–168.

Hoehn-Saric, R., Merchant, A. F., Keyser, M. L. and Smith, V. K. (1981) Effects of clonidine on anxiety disorders. Arch. Gen. Psychiatry 38, 1278–1282.

Hollister, L. E., Motzenbecker, F. P. and Degan, R. O. (1961) Withdrawal reactions from chlo-rdiazepoxide (Librium). Psychopharmacologia 2, 63–68.

Hollister, L. E., Bennett, J. L., Kimbell, Jr., I., Savage, C. and Overall, J. E. (1963) Diazepam in newly admitted schizophrenics. Dis. Nerv. Syst. 24, 1–4.

Hollister, L. E., Conley, F. K., Britt, R. H. and Shuer, L. (1981) Long-term use of diazepam. J. Am. Med. Assoc. 246, 1568–1570.

Kales, A., Soldatos, C. R., Bixler, E. O. and Kales J. D. (1983) Early morning insomnia with rapidly eliminated benzodiazepines. Science 230, 95–97.

Marks, J. (1978) The Benzodiazepines: Use, Misuse, Abuse. MTP Press, Ltd., Lancaster, England. p.111.

Mellinger, G. D., Balter, M. B., Manheimer, D. I., Cisin, I. H. and Parry, H. I. (1978) Psychic distress, life crisis, and use of psychotherapeutic medications. National household survey. Arch. Gen. Psychiatry 35, 1045–1052.

Mohler, H. and Okada, T. (1977) Benzodiazepine receptor: demonstration in the central nervous system. Science 198, 849–851.

Mohler, H. and Richards, J. G. (1981) Agonist and antagonist benzodiazepine receptor inter-action in vitro. Nature 294, 763–765.

Pevnick, J. S., Jasinski, D. R. and Haertzen, C. A. (1978) Abrupt withdrawal from therapeutically administered diazepam. Arch. Gen. Psychiatry 35, 995–998.

Schopf, J. (1983) Withdrawal phenomena after long-term administration of benzodiazepines. A review of recent investigations. Pharmacopsychiat. 16, 1–8.

Squires, R. F. and Braestrup, C. (1977) Benzodiazepin receptors in rat brain. Nature 266, 732–734.

Tallman, J. F., Paul, S. M., Skolnick, P. and Gallagher, D. W. (1980) Receptors for the age of anxiety: pharmacology of the benzodiazepines. Science 207, 274–281.

Taylor, D. P., Riblet, I. A., Stanton, H. C., Eison, A. S., Eison, M. S. and Temple, D. P. (1982) Dopamine and antianxiety activity. Pharmac. Biochem. Behav. 17 (Suppl.1), 25–35.

Thompson, W. L., Johnson, A. D., Maddrey, W. L. and Osler Housestaff. (1975) Diazepam and paraldehyde for treatment of severe delirium tremens. Ann. Int. Med. 82, 175–180.

Wilensky, A. J., Ojemann, L. M. Temkin, N. R., Troupin, A. S. and Dodrill, C. B. (1981) Clorazepate and phenobarbital as antiepileptic drugs: a double-blind study. Neurology 31, 1271–1276.

Wilson, J. and Ellis, F. R. (1973) Oral premedication with lorazepam (Ativan): a comparison with heptobarbitone (Medomin) and diazepam (Valium). Br. J. Anaesthesia 45, 738–744.

Winstead, D. K., Anderson, A., Eilers, M. K., Blackwell, B. and Zeremba, A. L. (1974) Diazepam on demand: drug-seeking behavior in psychiatric inpatients. Arch. Gen. Psychiatry 30, 349–351.

Wu, P. H., Phillis, J. W. and Bender, A. S. (1981) Do benzodiazepines bind at adenosine uptake sites in CNS? Life Sci. 28, 1023–1031.

Burrows/Norman/Davies (eds) Antianxiety agents
© *Elsevier Science Publishers B.V., 1984*

Chapter 9

Tolerance, dependence and abuse in relation to antianxiety drugs

MALCOLM LADER

and

HANNES PETURSSON

Department of Pharmacology, Institute of Psychiatry, University of London, Decrespigny Park, London SE5 8AF, U.K.

INTRODUCTION

The benzodiazepines are among the most widely used of all prescribed drugs. They have largely replaced the barbiturates in clinical practice because of the following advantages: 1) they are more effective in alleviating anxiety and stress responses although possibly less powerful as hypnotics: 2) they have fewer and less severe side effects: 3) they are much safer in overdosage: 4) they induce liver microsomal enzymes much less and so do not interact to any clinically relevant extent with other drugs; and finally, 5) they are generally believed to be less liable to induce dependence. However, this last belief has been entertained before with respect to the bromides, paraldehyde, chloral, barbiturates and meprobamate. Introduced as safe sedatives, the dependence liability was only apparent later, sometimes after decades of use. Escalation of dosage was noted with concern, tell-tale signs of drug-seeking behaviour were detected, and a characteristic withdrawal syndrome was eventually described.

This review outlines the evidence concerning the dependence-inducing properties of the benzodiazepines, focussing in particular on the clinical therapeutic situation. On the basis of the reviewed topics, the clinician must then decide in each case whether benzodiazepine treatment is warranted.

The topic of definitions of dependence has always been a thorny problem (WHO, 1974). However, for practical, clinical purposes, the prescriber is concerned to know:

1) How assiduously the patient seeks the drug in question;
2) whether tolerance has developed as evidence by escalation of dosage; and
3) whether a definable withdrawal syndrome supervenes when the drug is stopped.

CLINICAL EFFECTS OF BENZODIAZEPINES

The benzodiazepines relieve anxiety in doses which do not produce sedation, although higher doses cause drowsiness and lethargy. They are also effective as hypnotics without the 'knock-out' action of the barbiturates, although some benzodiazepines such as nitrazepam and flurazepam may subsequently cause subjective 'hangover' symptoms. Amnesia has been reported following the intravenous administration of lorazepam (Heisterkamp and Cohen, 1975). Other clinical indications include: 1) muscle spasm, especially that secondary to musculo-skeletal lesions; 2) status epilepticus; 3) intravenous administration of diazepam or lorazepam is widely used preoperatively and as a soporific during dental and endoscopic procedures. Diazepam can substitute for alcohol during withdrawal and, unfortunately, during the self-induction of intoxication. Effects on mood, sex, aggression, and sociability are complex and are probably influenced by expectation. In general, benzodiazepines decrease rather than increase hostility and aggression, but aggression can be released. This is probably influenced by sex, route of administration and the social setting (Valzelli, 1967; Bond and Lader, 1979).

Drug addicts who take large doses of diazepam, either alone or with narcotics, experience a pleasant, relaxed sensation which they describe as a 'high' (Woody et al., 1975). Large doses produce drowsiness, sleep, incoordination, muscle weakness, ataxia and dysarthria. Our study patients have described a 'rush' effect in response to 10 mg intravenous diazepam, with euphoria, flight of ideas, pressure of speech, enhanced self-confidence, pleasant relaxation and calmness, followed by increasing drowsiness.

In recent years concern has been increasing about possible long-term effects on cognitive performance of chronic drug intake (Edwards and Medlicott, 1980). The evidence mainly involves poly-drug abusers (Grant and Judd, 1976; Grant et al., 1978), but many such individuals also take benzodiazepines chronically. More importantly, intellectual functioning declines in patients taking prescribed benzodiazepines in therapeutic doses (Maruta, 1978). Although the intellectual deficit is fairly readily reversible, the problem requires urgent investigation because of the large numbers of long-term benzodiazepine users.

Patterns of usage

Of over 2,500 persons aged 18–74 surveyed in the U.S.A., 13% of men and 29% of women had taken prescribed psychotropic drugs at some time during the previous year (Parry et al., 1973). An extension of this study to Europe (Balter et al., 1974), focussing on tranquillizers, revealed that the drug-use rates during the year before interview ranged from 10% in Spain to 17% in Belgium and France, with the U.K. and Germany falling at the median of 14%. Parallel data from the U.S.A. resembled those from the U.K. Male rates were lower than the female rates in every country and more of those over 35 tended to use the drugs than younger individuals. Regular daily usage for one month or more showed somewhat different patterns. The U.K., Denmark, The Netherlands and Belgium, had the highest usage with about 8% of adults using sedatives; Spain and Italy were at the bottom with less than half that figure. Again, female chronic usage was about twice the male rates. In general, respondents thought that tranquillizers did more good than harm; those who had used them had a more favourable attitude than those who had not, suggesting a high degree of consumer satisfaction.

A replication of this study in the U.S.A. involved an interview with a rigorous cross-section sample of the population, totalling 3,161 persons. In all 7.5% of men and 14.1% of women had used antianxiety agents (mainly benzodiazepines) at some time during the previous year. Also 2.1% of men and 3.0% of women had taken sleeping tablets. Tranquillizer use increased with age until the 50–64 age group and then decreased, especially in women. Most respondents had used tranquillizers for short-term treatment but 1.4% of the total sample had used the drugs for between 1 and 4 months, 0.6% between 4 and 12 months, and 1.6% (i.e. 15% of the users) had taken their tranquillizers during the entire previous year (Mellinger and Balter, 1981).

A survey of prescribing in general practice showed that during one year 10% of adult males and 21% of adult females received a prescription for at least one psychotropic drug. Until recently, diazepam alone accounted for almost 5% of all general practice prescriptions (Skegg et al., 1977). In addition, benzodiazepines are common constituents of mixtures formulated for stress-related conditions such as peptic ulcers. Tranquillizers also head the list for repeat prescriptions. In the U.K. the number of prescriptions for benzodiazepine tranquillizers has risen steadily until the last few years.

Extent of anxiety

The prescribing of tranquillizers is obviously very extensive. The prescriber must then ask whether this reflects genuine symptomatic distress in the recipients, whether tranquillizers are prescribed indiscriminately, or whether chronic usage reflects an insidious development of dependence.

One large scale study 20 years ago suggested that about 30% of a sample of adults suffered from 'nerves', depression, insomnia or undue irritability (Taylor and Cave, 1964). This prevalence was the same in a planned New Town, a dormitory computer suburb or a decaying inner city region. The percentage of females reporting such symptoms was twice that of males. Older and poorer people also reported symptoms more frequently. These high prevalence rates were confirmed by Salkind (1973) using a standardised self-rating scale for anxiety: a third of people scored in the clinically anxious range. Data from the U.S.A. are very similar (Mellinger et al., 1978).

Uhlenhuth and his colleagues (1978) have directly examined the relationship between tranquillizer usage, psychological distress and situational stresses using a sample of subjects in Oakland, California. Drug usage was related more to the psychological state of the individual, essentially whether they were anxious or not, rather than to whether situational stresses were experienced. However, the survey was retrospective which might bias the data towards continuing deepseated psychological problems and away from transient situational difficulties. The authors conclude that the use of tranquillizers does comply "with a rational medical model in relation to both the type and amount of disturbance experienced".

DEPENDENCE ON BENZODIAZEPINES

Tolerance

Tolerance to the sedative effects of benzodiazepines can be demonstrated in animals as the depression of exploratory and general motor activity induced by these drugs wanes after a few days (File, 1981). Most patients reporting initial drowsiness find it disappears after a few days (Kaplan et al., 1973; Hillstad et al., 1974; Gamble et al., 1976; Eatman et al., 1977). It is possible that tolerance to the anxiolytic effects of the benzodiazepines may develop less readily although this has not been reliably documented within the clinical situation.

Further support for a non-pharmacokinetic tolerance comes from case studies of acute overdosage where plasma levels wane slowly whereas the soporific effects last only a short time (Greenblatt et al., 1978). Finally, there is cross-tolerance between the benzodiazepines and barbiturates and alcohol (Greenblatt and Shader, 1974, 1975). Patients with histories of drug abuse of the alcohol/sedative type tend to use benzodiazepines if the opportunity arises but still prefer barbiturates or alcohol.

Most patients maintain themselves on a fairly constant dose of benzodiazepine while others steadily escalate their dosage (Winstead et al., 1974). Clinical observations suggest that increased problems and stresses are associated with increase in dose. When these resolve, the dosage is reduced in most patients (Allgulander, 1978). Some patients, however, seem to become rapidly tolerant to the anxiolytic effects and do not reduce their dosage when the stress is alleviated. Thus, a relevant question may concern the factors which govern variations in the rate of acquiring tolerance.

The practical implications of these various studies and observations mainly concern patients with previous histories of drug abuse or alcoholism. Such patients are more likely than others to become tolerant to benzodiazepines and to push up the dose. Other methods of management and alternative medications should be considered.

Animal studies

Animal models of withdrawal show that a definite withdrawal syndrome can be recognized on discontinuation of benzodiazepines. They can also be cross-substituted in animals previously rendered dependent on other drugs (Deneau and Weiss, 1968). However, drug-seeking or maintaining behaviour is not easily induced by the benzodiazepines.

Human studies

Attempts have been made in the past to induce dependence in humans. In the most vigorously pursued study (Hollister et al., 1961), psychiatric patients in hospital were treated with chlordiazepoxide, 100–600 mg daily for 1–7 months, most patients for over 3 months. Ten of 11 patients abruptly switched to placebo reported new symptoms or developed new signs. Psychoses were aggravated in 5 patients, insomnia and agitation supervened in 5, and 4 lost their appetite. Two patients had major epileptiform convulsions on the seventh and eighth day following discontinuation. Symptoms following benzodiazepine withdrawal were more delayed and less severe than those following withdrawal of barbiturate or meprobamate but were of the same type.

Another approach is to make available to volunteer human subjects with documented histories of drug abuse various psychotropic drugs. Such subjects would undertake physical work in exchange for doses of alcohol, sodium pentobarbital or diazepam. Both dose and minimum interingestion interval were important controlling parameters of drug ingestion (Griffiths et al., 1976). By contrast, chlorpromazine did not maintain self-administration (Griffiths et al., 1979). However, given the choice of the barbiturate or diazepam, most erstwhile drug abusers preferred pentobarbital (Griffiths et al., 1980).

Several hundred papers are extant reporting cases of dependence on the benzodiazepines. This literature has been comprehensively reviewed by Marks (1978), and by Greenblatt and Shader (1978), Palmer (1978), Jepsen and Haastrup (1979), and Petursson and Lader (1981). Maletzky and Klotter (1976) have reviewed the literature on the dependence potential of diazepam. Marks (1978) found that only

118 of these publications contained fully verified cases of physical dependence with a definite withdrawal syndrome or carefully documented cases of psychological dependence. The cases collected by Marks fell into two categories: 1) those occurring in a therapeutic situation, and 2) Those arising within the context of the 'drug scene' with evidence of multiple drug abuse or alcoholism. He listed 151 cases worldwide of benzodiazepine dependence within the framework of multiple drug abuse or alcoholism, plus 250 less definite cases. As he points out, it is difficult to assign individual cases to the 'abuse' or the 'therapeutic' group, the main criterion being whether the supplies of benzodiazepines come via a prescription or from illicit sources.

Cases of benzodiazepine dependence reported to have occurred solely within the therapeutic situation, and in which other forms of drug dependence do not seem to have played a major contributory role, constitute a minority of the several hundred cases reported in the literature. Many clinically reported cases of dependence arising within the therapeutic context described patients who had usually taken 2–5 times the normal therapeutic doses of the various benzodiazepines. Several reports indicate that on such *high doses* physical dependence can develop within 2–3 weeks (Relkin, 1966; Woody et al., 1975), and certainly within 4 months (Hayashki et al., 1974). In the majority of cases, however, the drugs have been taken for much longer, usually a few years (Aivazian, 1964; Kryspin-Exner, 1966; Slater, 1966; Gordon, 1967; Badura, 1972; von Mader, 1972; Venzlaff, 1972; Misra, 1975; Preskorn and Denner, 1977; Allgulander and Borg, 1978; Bliding, 1978; Acuda and Muhangi, 1979; Laux, 1979; Miller and Nulsen, 1979; Bismuth et al., 1980; Le Bellec et al., 1980).

There are few systematic studies of benzodiazepine withdrawal following ingestion of *therapeutic doses*. Covi et al. (1969, 1973) investigated the effect of abrupt discontinuation of chlordiazepoxide treatment, 45 mg daily for 20 weeks. They found a mild abstinence syndrome, consisting mainly of subjective feelings of anxiety and tension as well as minor symptoms, such as trembling, poor appetite, and faintness or dizziness. A recent study by Tyrer and colleagues (1980, 1981) investigated benzodiazepine dependence in patients seen in general practice and psychiatric out-patient clinics. Eighty-six patients satisfied the inclusion criteria, namely that they had taken either diazepam or lorazepam regularly for 4 months or longer, were not on any other psychotropic drugs, and were not considered to need the drug on clinical grounds. Only 40 agreed to be withdrawn, of whom 18 dropped out and returned to taking their benzodiazepine again. Of the 40 patients a substantial minority, 27–45% depending on the criteria used, suffered a withdrawal syndrome when their medication was abruptly stopped.

During the last 3 years we have withdrawn, under double-blind, placebo-controlled conditions, over 40 patients who had all received benzodiazepines in therapeutic doses for at least one year (range: 1–20 years). All experienced some form of withdrawal reaction, but more importantly, the changes on withdrawal of normal doses have in most cases been indistinguishable from those on withdrawal of high doses in other patients (Hallstrom and Lader, 1981), either in quality or quantity. The withdrawal reaction has ranged from anxiety and dysphoria to severe affective and perceptual changes. Anxiety ratings rose as the drugs were discontinued but usually subsided to pre-withdrawal levels over the next 2–4 weeks. This in itself suggests that the symptoms represented a true withdrawal syndrome and not a revival of the original anxiety symptoms. Furthermore, some of the symptoms were untypical of anxiety. The dysphoria was an amalgam of anxiety, depression, nausea, malaise and depersonalisation. Perceptual changes were common; patients noted intolerance to loud noises, bright lights and touch, and complained of numbness, paresthesia, unsteadiness and a feeling of motion. Some patients have reported strange smells and a metallic taste.

Several papers are extant reporting cases of physical withdrawal reactions from short-term (weeks–months) (Fruensgaard and Vaag, 1975; Haskell, 1975; Woody et al., 1975; Fruensgaard, 1976; Rifkin et al., 1976; de la Fuente et al., 1980; Haselrud and Heskestad, 1981), and long-term (years) (Peters and Boeters, 1970; Darcy, 1972; Bant, 1975; Vyas and Carney, 1975; Floyd and Murphy, 1976; Fruensgaard, 1976; Dysken and Carlyle, 1977; Bliding, 1978; Pevnick et al., 1978; Bismuth et al., 1980; Howe, 1980; Khan et al., 1980; Le Bellec, 1980; Stewart et al., 1980; Winokur et al., 1980; Haselrud and Heskestad, 1981; Tyrer et al., 1981), low-dosage benzodiazepine treatment. In most instances these abstinence phenomena qualitatively and quantitatively resembled those on withdrawal from high-doses of benzodiazepines.

Benzodiazepines vary among themselves in their duration of action. Diazepam, chlordiazepoxide, clorazepate and clobazam have long plasma half-lives (or have long-acting metabolites); lorazepam, oxazepam, temazepam and triazolam are short-acting. These pharmacokinetic differences may also be important as regards benzodiazepine dependence. Tyrer et al. (1981) have found that withdrawal phenomena were more troublesome in patients dependent on lorazepam than in those discontinuing diazepam. They suggest that if the drugs are reduced very gradually, the withdrawal symptoms may even be avoided so they advocate the use of a benzodiazepine with a long duration of action for effecting withdrawal since it is more difficult to achieve a smooth fall in plasma levels with short-acting benzodiazepines. Walters and Nel (1981) have also demonstrated that a withdrawal syndrome occurs more frequently with the use of a short-acting benzodiazepine such as oxazepam, compared to chlordiazepoxide.

Incidence of dependence

The peak of reporting of cases of possible benzodiazepine dependence was in 1969–73, that is, about 10 years after the introduction of the first benzodiazepine. Since then and until recently, the number has been few despite increasing use of

134

the drugs. This can be construed as lack of concern among the medical profession rather than paucity of cases.

Two reviews of pre-1965 studies of chlordiazepoxide (Svenson and Hamilton, 1966), and diazepam (Maletzky and Klotter, 1976), detected no cases of dependence. The latter authors concluded, however, from their review of 27 articles in which diazepam was claimed to be free of addicting properties, that none had used adequate methods: withdrawal was not systematic, and in some, no data regarding tolerance were collected. Some survey data have suggested little concern. In the Boston Collaborative Drug Surveillance Porgram, trained nurses monitored data on medical patients in nine hospitals in North America, New Zealand and Israel. Of 25,000 interviewed, 4,500 patients were taking benzodiazepine but no signs of dependence were detected (Boston Collaborative Drug Surveillance Program, 1973; Miller, 1973). Two other large-scale surveys of patients have only reported 2–3 cases of benzodiazepine dependence (Grant, 1969; Miller, 1974).

Greenblatt and Shader (1978) opine that the hazards of benzodiazepine addiction and habituation have probably been greatly exaggerated. Jepsen and Haastrup (1979) maintain that severe withdrawal reactions can occur, but apparently very rarely, although they admit these may be underreported. On the other hand, they believe that milder abstinence syndromes are quite frequent. Leading medical journals on both sides of the Atlantic have recently published editorials on benzodiazepine withdrawal and dependence. The Lancet (Editorial, 1979) states that 'in view of the extensive world-wide usage of the benzodiazepines, serious physical dependence on benzodiazepines must be uncommon, the risk being much lower than with barbiturates and meprobamate.'

The Journal of the American Medical Association (Ayd, 1979) refers to the views of Marks (1978), Hollister (1977) and Covi et al. (1973), and states that 'while psychological and physical dependence on benzodiazepines may occur, this is rare and is not cause for alarm.' In addition to daily dosage, benzodiazepine dependence and withdrawal is a consequence of time 'which is the more important variable when small amounts of the benzodiazepine are consumed'. Ayd (1979) concludes that the risk of serious physical dependence on benzodiazepines is low, even with high doses, and that the risk of dependence with normal dosage is even lower.

It is difficult to reconcile these views with the more recent reports which appear to show that a sizeable proportion of patients taking benzodiazepines will develop some form of dependence.

Assessing the addiction potential of diazepam, Maletzky and Klotter (1976) interviewed 50 subjects referred from medical, surgical, and psychiatric clinics. They found substantial evidence for "diazepam's capacity to elicit tolerance and withdrawal", but that psychiatric patients were no more 'addiction-prone' in this regard than patients given diazepam for medical reasons. Of 24 patients who had attempted to stop diazepam abruptly at some time, 17 (79%) experienced withdrawal symptoms of moderate to extreme severity.

Kemper et al. (1980) reviewed the case-notes of all in-patients at the Psychiatric Clinic, Göttingen, for a 3-year period (1977–80). For this short period alone, many more patients had been admitted to their clinic because of benzodiazepine dependence than Marks (1978) found for the years 1961–77 for the whole of the Federal Republic of Germany. The most common admission diagnoses to the clinic were alcoholism and other forms of drug dependency. Whereas only a few years ago bromureides and/or barbiturates were the most commonly abused agents, the benzodiazepines now topped the list of agents leading to drug dependence and subsequent admission. While in previous years secondary benzodiazepine dependence ('switchers from bottle to pill') was most frequent, among the admissions in recent years a growing number of patients had never before taken addictive agents other than benzodiazepines (primary dependence).

A further confirmation that the dependence potential of benzodiazepines is greater than previously assumed, comes from the recent study by Tyrer et al. (1981) and from our own observations in over 40 patients studied to date. It appears that many patients who have taken benzodiazepines in therapeutic dosage for several years will develop recognisable withdrawal symptoms if their medication is stopped.

The British Committee on the Review of Medicines (1980) concluded that, although benzodiazepines are safe and effective in the short-term treatment of anxiety and insomnia, their long-term use should be avoided where possible because of unwanted effects and the risk of dependence.

WITHDRAWING PATIENTS FROM BENZODIAZEPINES

In each case, the first thing to consider is whether withdrawal is indicated or not. If the patients firmly believe they cannot stop their benzodiazepines because every time they attempt to do so they develop distressing abstinence symptoms which lead them to resume taking benzodiazepines for relief, then withdrawal is usually indicated. Normal-dosage dependence should be suspected when a patient repeatedly tries to wean himself from his medication and restarts the drug because of dysphoria, headache, perceptual hypersensitivity, or other symptoms unrelated to the anxiety syndrome for which the tranquillizers were given initially. The same applies to any signs of active drug-seeking behaviour, such as insistent statements like: 'I must have the tablets,' or hoarding, future planning to ensure an uninterrupted supply of benzodiazepines, using the drugs 'to freshen up', conspicuous pleading and whining in response to attempts to stop or to curtail the prescriptions. Equally any signs of development of tolerance and/or increase in dosage should alert the physician to the possibility that dependence is developing. Because of the unpredictable and often remitting course of anxiety states, a trial of withdrawal is often justified in cases of prolonged benzodiazepine use, even in the absence of any signs of potential dependence. If laboratory assays are available these can often help in doubtful cases. Signs which should arouse suspicion include high plasma benzodiazepine levels (over 1000 ng/ml of diazepam or equivalent) without correspondingly marked signs of intoxication, higher than expected plasma concentrations during intake of apparently therapeutic doses, and a marked discrepancy between reported dose and frequency of intake, and plasma drug concentrations.

The second question is whether the withdrawal is feasible on an out-patient basis, or whether admission to hospital is needed. Patients who have taken high-doses for a long time or who have previously experienced severe withdrawal reactions, such as psychosis or seizures, should be admitted to hospital for safe and successful withdrawal. Other factors to be considered are the patient's tolerance for subjective distress and his methods of coping with this, e.g. self-medication with sedatives or misuse of alcohol. Adequate social support is important, and compliance is also affected by the physician's attitudes, whether he attains full cooperation of the patient and his family, explains the possibility of withdrawal effects, and so on.

In our experience out-patient withdrawal is safe in most patients who have been on normal doses, even in cases of prolonged treatment, although frequent medical supervision is needed. Dosage can usually be reduced gradually over a period of 4 weeks. The severity of withdrawal symptoms may be related to the rate at which circulating benzodiazepines and their active metabolites are metabolised and excreted (Tyrer et al., 1981). Thus, these authors claim that if the drugs are reduced very gradually, for example over 4–8 weeks, the withdrawal symptoms may even be avoided. Hence, the merits of using a benzodiazepine with a long half-life for effecting withdrawal in order to achieve a smoother fall in the bodily concentrations. However, our own data suggest that once the patient has become physically dependent, he will inevitably experience some withdrawal symptoms although prolonged withdrawal will probably reduce its severity to tolerable levels. Most of our patients have also appreciated the placebo substitution procedure which reduces their apprehension about the date when the drug withdrawal has been completed.

At one-year follow-up, about one-third of our patients are doing well with few or no problems since completing the withdrawal. Another third of our patients experience occasional episodes of anxiety and tension but are gratified to find that they can manage without chronic sedative medication. The last third of our patients are more or less chronically anxious and find it very difficult to stay off their drugs. In fact, most of them have recommenced some form of anxiolytic medication. During the months following the withdrawal we have utilised general out-patient support and relaxation training, and two patients have started in formal analytical psychotherapy. A further two patients have been treated with anti-depressives.

Preventive measures

The benzodiazepines are safe and effective in the short-term management of anxiety and insomnia. Because of unwanted effects and risk of dependence, long-term usage should be avoided wherever possible. Prolonged benzodiazepine treatment should never be stopped abruptly because of the danger of withdrawal symptoms including fits. Short-acting benzodiazepines are preferable in the treatment of insomnia which is not accompanied by daytime anxiety. There is no good scientific evidence that the anxiolytic effect of the drugs last longer than 4 months although clinical experience would suggest that some chronically anxious patients are helped. Prescriptions should be reserved for valid clinical indications, the lowest possible doses prescribed, and repeat prescriptions should be limited. The patient's circumstances need to be carefully assessed before prescribing a benzodiazepine and adverse influences removed wherever possible, and subsequently his condition should be regularly monitored, especially in cases with previous histories of alcohol or drug abuse.

We are not urging that benzodiazepines should be phased out. But the recent demonstration of a dependence risk on longterm use should be kept in mind when deciding whether to prescribe tranquillizers. The benefits must always outweigh the risks and it is doubtful if benzodiazepines are justified in patients reacting to life-stresses with minor transient anxiety symptoms.

CONCLUSIONS

The contradictions and opposing views expressed in the literature could suggest that the problem of benzodiazepine dependence is either extremely rare, or is very rarely recognised by doctors. One reason why signs of benzodiazepine dependence may be missed or misdiagnosed is that anxiety is the cardinal symptom of the benzodiazepine withdrawal syndrome. Furthermore, the temporal relationships of the respective syndromes are quite different because of pharmacokinetic differences. Also the wide availability of the drugs would suppress any obvious signs of drug-seeking behaviour. Nevertheless, published reports cannot be relied on as an accurate or even approximate estimate since many cases will not be reported. Furthermore, the best evidence for dependence-inducing properties is obtained by careful observation of withdrawal symptoms, and many patients may be reluctant to have their medication withdrawn. Most of the recent studies and reviews seem to agree that withdrawal symptoms may occur with therapeutic doses of benzodiazepines, especially if the treatment has been prolonged. This is the crux of the matter. Although the extent of such normal-dosage dependence is unknown, and even if it only supervened to a minor degree, the extensive and chronic usage of these drugs could mean that thousands of patients are at risk. Careful withdrawal is necessary using the principles we have enunciated earlier.

138

REFERENCES

Acuda, S. W. and Muhangi, J. (1979) Diazepam addiction in Kenya. East Afr. Med. J. 56, 76–79.

Aivazian, G. H. (1964) Clinical evaluation of diazepam. Dis. Nerv. Syst. 25, 491–496.

Allgulander, C. (1978) Dependence on sedative and hypnotic drugs. A comparative clinical and social study. Acta Psychiatr. Scand., Suppl. 270.

Allgulander, C. and Borg, S. (1978) Case report: a delirious abstinence syndrome associated with clorazepate (Tranxilen). Br. J. Addict. 73, 175–177.

Ayd, F. J. (1979) Benzodiazepines: dependence and withdrawal. J. Am. Med. Assoc. 242, 1401–1402.

Badura, H. O. (1972) Valiumsucht. Internist Prax. 12, 352.

Balter, M. B., Levine, J. and Manheimer, D. I. (1974) Cross-national study of the extent of anti-anxiety/sedative drug use. N. Engl. J. Med. 290, 769–774.

Bant, W. (1975) Diazepam withdrawal symptoms. Br. Med. J. 4, 285.

Bismuth, C., Le Bellec, M., Dally, S. and Lagier, G. (1980) Dépendence physique aux benzodia-zépines. Nouv. Presse Med. 9, 1941–1945.

Bliding, Å. (1978). The abuse potential of benzodiazepines with special reference to oxazepam. Acta Psychiatr. Scand. Suppl. 274, 111–116.

Bond, A. J. and Lader, M. H. (1979) Benzodiazepines and aggression. In: M. Sandler (Ed.), Psychopharmacology of Aggression. Raven Press, New York, pp. 173–182.

Boston Collaborative Drug Surveillance Program (1978) Clinical depression of the central nervous system due to diazepam and chlordiazepoxide in relation to cigarette smoking and age. N. Engl. J. Med. 288, 277–280.

Committee on the Review of Medicines (1980) Systematic review of the benzodiazepines. Br. Med. J. 2, 719–720.

Covi, L., Park, L. C., Lipman, R. S., Uhlenhuth. E. H. and Rickels, K. (1969) Factors affecting withdrawal response to certain minor tranquillizers. In: J. O. Cole and J. R. Wittenborn (Eds.), Drug Abuse: Social and Psychopharmacological Aspects. Thomas, Springfield, Ill., pp. 93–108.

Covi, L., Lipman, R. S., Pattison, J. H., Derogatis, L. R. and Uhlenhuth, E. H. (1973) Length of treatment with anxiolytic sedatives and response to their sudden withdrawal. Acta Psychiatr. Scand. 49, 51–64.

Darcy, L. (1972) Delirium tremens following withdrawal of nitrazepam. Med. J. Aust. 2, 450.

De la Fuente, J. R., Rosenbaum, A. H., Martin, H. R. and Niven, R. G. (1980) Lorazepam-related withdrawal seizures. Mayo Clin. Proc. 55, 190–192.

Deneau, G. A. and Weiss, S. (1968) A substitution technique for determining barbiturate-like physiological dependence capacity in the dog. Pharmacopsychiatr. Neuro-Psychopharmakol. 1, 270–275.

Dysken, M. W. and Carlyle, H. C. (1977) Diazepam withdrawal psychosis: a case report. Am. J. Psychiatry 134, 573.

Eatman, F. B., Colburn, W. A., Boxenbaum, H. G., Postmanter, H. H., Weinfeld, R. W., Ronfeld, R., Weissman, L., Moore, J. D., Gibaldi, M. and Kaplan, S. A. (1977) Pharmacokinetics of diazepam following multiple-dose oral administration to healthy human subjects. J. Pharmacokinet. Biopharmacol. 5, 481–495.

Editorial (1979) Benzodiazepine withdrawal. Lancet 1, 196.

Edwards, R. A. and Medlicott, R. W. (1980) Advantages and disadvantages of benzodiazepine prescription, N. Z. Med. J. 92, 357–359.

File, S. E. (1981) Rapid development of tolerance to the sedative effects of lorazepam and triazolam in rats. Psychopharmacology 73, 240–245.

Floyd, J. B. and Murphy, M. (1976) Hallucinations following withdrawal of valium. J. Kentucky Med. Assoc. 74, 549–550.

Fruensgaard, K. (1976) Withdrawal psychosis: a study of 30 consecutive cases. Acta Psychiatr. Scand. 53, 105–118.

Fruensgaard, K. and Vaag, U. H. (1975) Abstinenspsykose efter nitrazepam. Ugeskr. Læg. 137, 633–634.

Gamble, G. A. S., Dundee, G. W. and Gray, R. C. (1976) Plasma diazepam concentrations following prolonged administration. Br. J. Anaesth. 48, 1087–1090.

Gordon, E. B. (1967) Addiction to diazepam (Valium). Br. Med. J. 1, 112.

Grant, I. (1969) Drug habituation in an urban general practice. Practitioner 202, 428–430.

Grant, I. and Judd, L. L. (1976) Neuropsychological and EEG disturbances in polydrug users. Am. J. Psychiatry 133, 1039–1042.

Grant, I. N., Adams, K. M., Carlin, A. S., Rennick, P. M., Judd, L. L., Schooff, K. and Reed, R. (1978) Organic impairment in polydrug users: risk factors. Am. J. Psychiatry 135, 178–184.

Greenblatt, D. J. and Shader, R. I. (1974) Benzodiazepines in Clinical Practice. Raven Press, New York.

Greenblatt D. J. and Shader, R. I. (1975) Treatment of the alcohol withdrawal syndrome. In: Shader (Ed.), Manual of Psychiatric Therapeutics. Little Brown, Boston, pp. 211–235.

Greenblatt, D. J. and Shader, R. I. (1978) Dependence, tolerance and addiction to benzodiazepines: clinical and pharmacokinetic considerations. Drug Metab. Rev. 8, 13–28.

Greenblatt, D. J., Woo, E., Allen, M. D., Orsulak, P. J. and Shader, R. I. (1978) Rapid recovery from massive diazepam overdose. J. Am. Med. Assoc. 240, 1872–1874.

Griffiths, R. R., Bigelow, G. E. and Liebson, I. (1976) Human sedative self-administration: effects of interingestion interval and dose. J. Pharmacol. Exp. Ther. 197, 488–494.

Griffiths, R. R., Bigelow, G. E. and Liebson, I. (1979) Human drug self-administration: double-blind comparison of pentobarbital, diazepam, chlorpromazine and placebo. J. Pharmacol. Exp. Ther. 210, 301–310.

Griffiths, R. R., Bigelow, G. G., Liebson, I. and Kaliszak, J. E. (1980) Drug preference in humans: double-blind choice comparison of pentobarbital, diazepam and placebo. J. Pharmacol. Exp. Ther. 215, 649–661.

Hallstrom, C. and Lader, M. H. (1981) Withdrawal phenomena in patients on high and normal doses of diazepam. Int. Pharmacopsychiatr. 16, 235–244.

Haselrud, J. and Heskestad, S. (1981) Abstinens og forvirringsreaksjoner etter Rohypnol-bruk. Tidsskr. Nor. Lægeforen. 101, 112.

Haskell, D. (1975) Withdrawal of diazepam, J. Am. Med. Assoc. 233, 135.

Hayashki, T., Higashki, T. and Kadota, K. (1974) 3 cases of chronic chlordiazepoxide intoxication and their withdrawal symptoms. Clin. Psychiatr. 16, 77–83.

Heisterkamp, D. V. and Cohen, P. J. (1975) Effect of intravenous premedication with lorazepam, pentobarbitone or diazepam on recall. Br. J. Anaest. 47, 79.

Hillstad, L., Hansen, T. and Melsom, H. (1974) Diazepam metabolism in normal man. II. Serum concentrations and clinical effect after oral administration and cumulation. Clin. Pharmacol. Ther. 16, 495–489.

Hollister, L. E. (Ed.) (1977) Valium: a discussion of current issues. Psychosomatics 18, 1–15.

Hollister, L. E., Motzenbecker, F. P. and Degan, R. O. (1961) Withdrawal reactions from chlordiazepoxide ('Librium'). Psychopharmacologia, 2, 63–68.

Howe, J. G. (1980) Lorazepam withdrawal seizures. Br. Med. J. I, 1163–1164.

Jepsen, P. W. and Haastrup, S. (1969) Abstinensreaktioner efter benzodiazepiner. Ugeskr. Læg. 141, 1121–1125.

Kaplan, S. A., Jack, M. L., Alexander, K. and Winfeld, R. E. (1973) Pharmacokinetic profile of diazepam in man following single intravenous and oral and chronic oral administration. J. Pharmacol. Sci. 62, 1789–1796.

Kemper, N., Poser, W. and Poser S. (1980) Benzodiazepin-Abhängigkeit. D. Med. Wochenschr. 105, 1707–1712.

Khan, A., Joyce, P. and Jones, A. V. (1980) Benzodiazepine withdrawal syndromes. N. Z. Med. J. 92, 94–96.

Kryspin-Exner, K. (1966) Missbrauch von Benzodiazepin-derivaten bei Alkoholkranken. Br. J. Addict. 61, 283–290.

Laux, G. (1979) Ein Fall von Lexotanil-Abhängigkeit. Nervenarzt 50, 326–327.

Le Bellec, M., Bismuth, C., Lagier, G. and Dally, S. (1980) Syndrome de sevrage sévère apres arrêt des benzodiazepines. Thérapie 35, 113–118.

Maletzky, B. M. and Klotter, J. (1976) Addiction to diazepam. Int. J. Addict. 11, 95–115.

Marks, J. (1978) The Benzodiazepines. Use, Overuse, Misuse, Abuse. MTP Press, Lancaster.

Maruta, T. (1978) Prescription drug-induced organic brain syndrome. Am. J. Psychiatry 135, 378–377.

Mellinger, G. D. and Balter, M. B. (1981) Prevalence and patterns of use of psychotherapeutic drugs: results from a 1979 national survey of American adults. In: G. Tognoni et al. (Eds.) Epidemiological Impact of Psychotropic Drugs. Elsevier, Amsterdam, pp. 117–136.

Mellinger, G. D., Balter, M. B., Manheimer, D. I., Cisin, I. H. and Parry, H. J. (1978) Psychic distress, life crisis and use of psychotherapeutic medications. National Household Survey Data. Arch. Gen. Psychiatry 25, 1045–1052.

Miller, F. and Nulsen, J. (1979) Diazepam (Valium) detoxification. J. Nerv. Ment. Dis. 167, 637–638.

Miller, R. R. (1973) Drug surveillance utilizing epidemiologic methods. Am. J. Hosp. Pharm. 30, 584–592.

Miller, R. R. (1974) Hospital admissions due to adverse drug reactions. Arch. Int. Med. 134, 219–223.

Misra, P. C. (1975) Nitrazepam (Mogadon) dependence. Br. J. Psychiatry 126, 81–82.

Palmer, G. C. (1978) Use, overuse, misuse, and abuse of benzodiazepines. Alabama J. Med. Sci. 15, 383–392.

Parry, H. J., Balter, M. B., Mellinger, G. D., Cisin, I. H. and Manheimer, D. I. (1973) National patterns of psychotherapeutic drug use. Arch. Gen. Psychiatry 28, 769–783.

Peters, U. H. and Boeters, U. (1970) Valium-Sucht. Eine Analyse anhand von 8 Fällen. Pharmacopsychiatrie, Neuropsychopharmacol. 3, 339–348.

Petursson, H. and Lader, M. H. (1981) Benzodiazepine dependence. Br. J. Addict. 76, 133–145.

Pevnick, J. S., Jasinski, D. R. and Haertyen, C. A. (1978) Abrupt withdrawal from therapeutically administered diazepam. Arch. Gen. Psychiatry 35, 995–998.

Preskorn, H. and Denner, J. (1977) Benzodiazepines and withdrawal psychosis. Report of three cases. J. Am. Med. Assoc. 237, 36–38.

Relkin, R. (1966) Death following withdrawal of diazepam. N.Y. State J. Med. 66, 1770–1772.

Rifkin, A., Quitkin, F. and Klein, D. F. (1976) Withdrawal reaction to diazepam. J. Am. Med. Assoc. 236, 2172–2173.

Salkind, M. R. (1973) The construction and validation of a self-rating anxiety inventory, Ph.D. Thesis. University of London.

Skegg, D. C. G., Doll, R. and Perry, J. (1977) Use of medicines in general practice. Br. Med. J. 2, 1561–1563.

Slater, J. (1966) Suspected dependence on chlordiazepoxide hydrochloride (Librium). Can. Med. Assoc. J. 95, 416.

Stewart, R. B., Salem, R. B. and Springer, P. K. (1980) A case report of lorazepam withdrawal. Am. J. Psychiatry 137, 1113–1114.

Svenson, S. E. and Hamilton, R. G. (1966) A critique of overemphasis on side-effects with the psychotropic drugs: an analysis of 18000 chlordiazepoxide-treated cases. Curr. Ther. Res. 8, 455–464.

Taylor, Lord and Chave, S. (1964) Mental Health and Environment. Longmans, London.

Tyrer, P. J. (1980) Benzodiazepine dependence and propranolol. Pharmaceut. J. 225, 158–160.

Tyrer, P. J., Rutherford, D. and Huggett, T. (1981) Benzodiazepine withdrawal symptoms and propranolol. Lancet i, 520–522.

Uhlenhuth, E. H., Balter, M. B. and Lipman, R. S. (1978) Minor tranquillizers. Clinical correlates of use in an urban population. Arch. Gen. Psychiatry 35, 650–655.

Valzelli, L. (1967) In: S. Garattini and P. A. Shore (Eds.), Advances in Pharmacology. Academic Press, New York, pp. 79–108.

Venzlaff, V. (1972) Valiumsucht. Internist Prax. 12, 349.

Von Mader, R. (1972) Primäre Valiumhängigkeit bei einem Jugendlichen. Wiener Med. Wochenschr. 122, 699–700.

Vyas, I. and Carney, M. W. P. (1975) Diazepam withdrawal fits. Br. Med. J. 4, 44.

Walters, L. and Nel, P. (1981) Die afhanklikheidspotensiaal van die bensodiasepine. South Afr. Med. J. 54, 115–116.

WHO Expert Committee on Drug Dependence (1974) Twentieth report. WHO technical report series, no. 551.

Winokur, A., Rickels, K., Greenblatt, D. J. Snyder, P.J. and Schatz, N. J. (1980) Withdrawal reaction from long-term low-dosage administration of diazepam. Arch. Gen. Psychiatry 37, 101–195.

Winstead, D. K., Anderson, A., Eilers, M. K., Blackwell, B. and Zaremba, A. L. (1974) Diazepam on demand. Drug-seeking behaviour in psychiatric inpatients. Arch. Gen. Psychiatry 30, 349–351.

Woody, G. E., O'Brien, C. P. and Greenstein, R. (1975) Misuse and abuse of diazepam: an increasingly common medical problem. Int. J. Addict. 10, 843–848.

Burrows/Norman/Davies (eds) Antianxiety agents
© *Elsevier Science Publishers B.V., 1984*

Chapter 10

Antianxiety drugs in the aged

WILLIAM M. PETRIE

and

THOMAS A. BAN

Tennessee Neuropsychiatric Institute and Vanderbilt University, Nashville, Tennessee, U.S.A.

INTRODUCTION

The prevalence of neuroses ranges from 9 to 30% in various surveys, and anxiety disorders are particularly widespread in the elderly (Shepherd and Gruenberg, 1957; Ernst, 1959; Neilsen, 1963; Kay et al., 1964; Balier, 1968; Busse and Pfeiffer, 1973). For some time they were attributed to hidden character traits, brought to the forefront by the increased frequency of life crises and physical illness in this age group (Bergman, 1971). More recently, however, the possibility has been raised that anxiety disorders in the elderly are related to biochemical changes, such as the decrease in glutamic decarboxylase activity, the enzyme responsible for γ-aminobutyric acid (GABA) formation (McGeer and McGeer, 1976).

The prevailing manifestations of anxiety in the aged are somatic. They include autonomic signs, agitation, insomnia, aches and pains. Because of this, elderly anxious patients consult physicians more often than young anxious patients. Considering that anxiety in the elderly may be symptomatic of depression (Gurland, 1972), incipient dementia (Post, 1975) or a wide variety of somatic illness, psychiatric examination – including family history and an evaluation of premorbid personality – should be supplemented with careful physical examination and laboratory studies in all anxious patients in this age group.

ANXIOLYTIC SEDATIVES

The most frequently employed treatment of anxiety disorders is with anxiolytic sedative drugs. They include substances which reduce pathologic anxiety, tension and agitation without adverse effects on cognitive and perceptual processes (WHO, 1967; Lehmann and Ban, 1970). Alcohol, chloral derivatives, and cyclic ethers are among the oldest anxiolytic sedative substances. During the first half of the century they were gradually replaced by barbiturates. During the 1950s the propanediols and diphenylmethanes were widely used. Since 1960 the benzodiazepines have gained an overwhelming popularity for the treatment of anxiety (Ban, 1980).

Alcohol

It is a common contention that alcohol alleviates anxiety (Renshaw, 1973); there are indications that both wine and beer reduce a number of behavioural symptoms of fear, increase social interaction and decrease the need for hypnotics in the aged (Kastenbaum, 1965; Chien et al., 1973; Stotsky, 1975). In a comparative clinical study carried out at a nursing-home, Chien (1971) found more favourable changes with a combination of beer and sociotherapy than with the neuroleptic thioridazine, a piperazine phenothiazine.

In spite of the favourable changes with small amounts of alcohol over a short period of time, alcohol consumption over extended periods is undesirable in this age group. Amnesic syndromes – assumedly the result of an inborn abnormality of transketolase, a thiamine regulating enzyme – may occur considerably sooner in old than in young patients (Blass and Gibson, 1977). One possible reason for this is that chronic alcohol-induced thiamine deficiency is frequently coupled with lowered thiamine intake in the elderly (Ban, 1980).

Cyclic ethers

Paraldehyde is the only cyclic ether with anxiolytic sedative properties. It has been employed in the treatment of anxiety, agitation and insomnia in the elderly.

Paraldehyde is a rapidly acting substance that can be administered orally, rectally or parenterally; sleep ensues within 10 to 15 min. when taken by mouth (Ban, 1969). In high concentrations, however, by reducing acetylcholine liberation, it depresses cholinergic transmission in ganglionic and neuromuscular junctions. Because of this, and its unpleasant odour, the use of paraldehyde has been abandoned.

Chloral derivatives

Chloral hydrate was the first chloral derivative employed in the treatment of anxiety. It is an anticholinesterase that transforms into trichloroethanol, a basal anaesthetic. Since inactivation of trichlorethanol takes place in the liver, chloral hydrate should be prescribed cautiously for elderly patients with hepatic damage.

Barbiturates

While some believe that barbiturates are contraindicated in aged patients due to serious adverse effects (Dawson-Butterworth, 1970), a 4-week double-blind clinical study carried out by Stotsky and Borozne revealed that the therapeutic effects of butabarbital (in the daily dosage of 58 mg) was superior to chlordiazepoxide, within the first 2 weeks of treatment, and equal or superior to chlordiazepoxide (CDZ) during the rest of the investigational period. Another longer acting barbiturate preparation, phenobarbital (in the daily dosage of 64 mg) was found to be equal to the piperazine phenothiazine (80 mg/day), in reducing anxiety and tension associated with angina pectoris and hypertension (Welborn, 1961).

When prescribing a barbiturate to elderly patients, consideration should be given to the narrow therapeutic ratio of these drugs. Not only are excessive drowsiness and hangover frequent (Exton-Smith et al., 1963), but respiratory depression may also occur. Furthermore, even in low doses barbiturates may produce a paradoxical excitement and/or confusion in patients with organic brain disease. Because of this, it is generally agreed that barbiturates should not be given to patients with multi-infarct dementia (Bender, 1964; Gibson, 1966).

Propanediols

There are at least two propanediol preparations with proven therapeutic efficacy in the elderly: meprobamate and tybamate. Both were found to be superior to inactive placebo in elderly psychiatric patients (Chesrow et al., 1965a; Chesrow and Kaplitz, 1970). In one clinical study, tybamate (1250–1500 mg per day) was found to be superior in its therapeutic effects to its parent substance, meprobamate (1000-1200 mg per day). Since tybamate is less soporific than meprobamate, and has a lower potential for abuse – possibly because of its shorter half-life – it is probably the more suitable preparation for elderly patients (Stern, 1964; Shelton and Hollister, 1967).

Diphenylmethane

Hydroxyzine is the only diphenylmethane preparation with psychogeriatric significance. It is an antihistamine with both anxiolytic and muscle relaxant properties that has been successfully employed in the treatment of agitation, anxiety and insomnia in the aged (Negri, 1957). Hydroxyzine might be a particularly suitable substance for aged psychiatric patients, because it produces coronary dilation (Burrell et al., 1958). There has been no tolerance or dependence associated with the administration of this drug, so that it is useful in the treatment of dependence-prone patients.

Benzodiazepines

Benzodiazepines are the most extensively employed antianxiety drugs; as many as one-third of elderly patients hospitalized for medical illness are administered a benzodiazepine – most frequently diazepam – to alleviate their anxiety (Shaw and Opit, 1976).

In spite of their wide use, the action mechanism of benzodiazepines has not been fully elucidated. Recent studies suggest that selective enhancement of gabaminergic neurotransmission may account for their action (Mohler and Okada, 1977; Hoehn-Saric, 1981). Relative affinities of pharmacologically active benzodiazepines for benzodiazepine receptors correlate well with their ability to antagonize GABA-modulin, the endogenous GABA receptor in vitro and with their ability to potentiate GABA-mediated electrically evoked cortical inhibition in vivo. Furthermore, benzodiazepines displace ^{3}H-diazepam from receptor binding sites in rat brain membranes with a potency which shows a significant correlation with the scores of these drugs on in vivo pharmacological tests which predict anxiolytic activity in man (Nestoros, 1981).

Pharmacokinetics

Considering incomplete drug absorption, a lowered serum albumin fraction, slowed circulation, reduced renal clearance and decreases in neuronal tissue in the aged, an understanding of the pharmacokinetics of benzodiazepines is essential for their proper use.

Of the two most frequently employed benzodiazepine preparations, chlordiazepoxide (CPZ) shows an age-related increase in elimination half-life from 6 hours in a 20-year old to 36 hours in an 80-year old, and diazepam increases from 20 hours to 90 hours, respectively (Wilkinson, 1978). In the case of CDZ, this is due in part to the reduction in plasma clearance with aging, while in the case of diazepam, to an increased volume of distribution rather than decreased clearance of the drug (Triggs et al., 1975).

Diazepam has two active metabolites: *N*-desmethyldiazepam and oxazepam. *N*-desmethyldiazepam is commercially available in the form of this dipotassium acetate salt (chlorazepate), a 'pro-drug' which must be hydrolysed to regenerate the parent compound. Since this hydrolysis occurs in the acid medium of the stomach, the pro-drug may not become active in the presence of achlorhydria or excessive use of antacids, both frequently encountered in the aged (Hollister, 1981).

Oxazepam, the other active metabolite of diazepam, is marketed as a separate drug and has a considerably shorter half-life than diazepam or desmethyldiazepam. From a psychogeriatric point of view, oxazepam's value is that it shows no age-related changes in either elimination half-life or clearance (Shull et al., 1976). The same applies to lorazepam and temazepam, another short half-life benzodiazepine which has shown only slight age-dependent changes in pharmacokinetic parameters (Kraus, et al., 1978; Schwarz, 1979; Greenblatt, 1980).

Among the other benzodiazepines, flurazepam has a long half-life and several active metabolites. Its monodesmethylated metabolite has an elimination half-life of 51–100 hours, and there are indications that it shows accumulation during chronic oral administration in the aged (Greenblatt et al., 1975).

Nitrazepam, another benzodiazepine, has produced similar plasma concentrations, with an apparently equal elimination half-life, in both young and old volunteers (Castleden et al., 1977). However, it has a prolonged half-life in hospitalized geriatric patients (Kangas et al., 1979).

Clinical use

Chlordiazepoxide. In open clinical trials, CDZ has shown favourable changes in the control of anxiety and tension in the elderly (Jones, 1962); in double-blind clinical studies in the dosage range of 20–40 mg per day, it has been found to be superior in its therapeutic effects to an inactive placebo and equal in its therapeutic effect to the propanediol, tybamate (Chesrow et al., 1965b) as well as the phenothiazine, thioridazine (Feigenbaum, 1971). On the other hand, in a comparative clinical study CDZ was found to be less effective than oxazepam, another benzodiazepine (Chesrow et al., 1965a).

Considering its pharmacokinetic properties, CDZ should be administered with caution in the elderly (Roberts et al., 1978). The incidence of excessive drowsiness is considerably greater in old than in young patients (Boston Collaborative Drug Surveillance Program, 1973) and there have been reports of ataxia, confusion and dysarthria with CDZ (Glasgow, 1969).

Diazepam. In open clinical trials, diazepam has shown favourable changes in the alleviation of anxiety, restlessness and somatic complaints in the elderly (Chesrow et al., 1962); it was found to be superior to an inactive placebo in the dosage range of 7.5–12.5 mg per day in the control of hyperactivity and insomnia (Cromwell, 1973; DeLamos et al., 1965). However, in at least two comparative clinical studies, diazepam (9–12 mg per day) was slightly less effective than the neuroleptic, thioridazine in the alleviation of anxiety (Kirven and Montero, 1973; Cerera, 1974). In symptomatic volunteers with anxious depression, only modest therapeutic effects were seen (Salzman and Shader, 1973; Salzman et al., 1975).

As with CDZ, diazepam also should be administered with caution in the elderly. The likelihood of developing fatigue and/or drowsiness is considerably greater in old than in young patients (Boston Collaborative Drug Surveillance Program, 1973) and dysmnesia with diazepam has been reported (Salzman et al., 1975). Female patients with organic brain syndrome are especially prone to confusion, impaired concentration and memory problems following diazepam treatment (Hall and Joffee, 1972).

Oxazepam. Because of its relatively short half-life and lack of active metabolite, oxazepam produces few cumulative and adverse effects. Another advantage of oxazepam in the elderly is that its major metabolic route of elimination is by conjugation, a function usually preserved in the aged even in cases of advanced liver disease.

In open clinical trials, oxazepam has shown favourable clinical effects in the elderly; in double-blind, clinical studies in the dosage range of 10–50 mg per day, it was found to be superior to an inactive placebo and equal to CDZ in reducing anxiety, tension, irritability, agitation and insomnia (Beber, 1965; Sanders, 1965; Holliday and Mihlayi, 1966). It was also superior to tybamate, haloperidol, chlorpromazine and thioridazine, in the treatment of restlessness in elderly, senile patients (Twefik et al., 1970). In a comparative clinical study of oxazepam and CDZ, the side effects of CDZ were significantly more severe; because of this, oxazepam was clearly the more clinically desirable drug (Chesrow et al., 1965b).

Lorazepam. Lorazepam, similar to oxazepam, has a short half-life without active metabolites. Possibly because of these advantages, lorazepam is frequently employed in the elderly. A possible disadvantage of lorazepam, however, is that it may produce amnesia and/or dysmnesia in the aged (Ban, 1980).

In open clinical trials, lorazepam has shown favourable therapeutic effects; it alleviated anxiety and attenuated restlessness in hospitalized psychogeriatric patients (Schrappe, 1971; Sizaret et al., 1974) and reduced the anxiety associated with medical illness in 90% of the reported cases (Amore et al., 1972; Metellus and Chappon, 1972). De Thibault et al. (1974) found that the dosage of analgesic medications in cancer patients could be reduced by adding lorazepam (4.5 mg per day) to the treatment regime. Banen and Resnick (1973) and Imlah (1973) used lorazepam as a hypnotic in aged patients with clinical success.

Flurazepam.   Flurazepam is one of the most frequently employed benzodiazepine hypnotics in elderly patients. In doses of 15–30 mg, it interferes less with the
normal sleep cycle than methaqualone, glutethimide or chloral hydrate (Raskind
and Eisdorfer, 1975). Possibly because of the extremely long elimination half-life
of its desmethylated metabolite, flurazepam administration results in oversedation and other adverse effects considerably more often in the old than in younger
patients. In one survey, a nightly dose of 30 mg produced oversedation in 39% of
the cases (Greenblatt et al., 1977), while in another survey, regular doses of flurazepam produced ataxia, confusion and/or hallucinations in 26% of nursing-home
patients. These adverse effects were encountered more frequently in patients over
75 and almost four times as often in females as in males (Martilla et al., 1977). On
the other hand, an advantage of flurazepam is that it causes less rebound insomnia, than some of the other benzodiazepines upon discontinuation of treatment
(Viukari et al., 1978).

Temazepam.   Like flurazepam, temazepam also is employed almost exclusively
as a hypnotic. In contradistinction to flurazepam, it has a short, approximately
10-hour half-life that is advantageous for the aged. Another advantage of temazepam is the lack of active metabolites. In at least one clinical trial temazepam was
found to be superior to chlormethiazole in its effects on the quality and duration of
sleep in psychogeriatric patients (Middleton, 1978).

Nitrazepam.   Nitrazepam is another benzodiazepine which is employed exclusively as a hypnotic. Possibly because of its long elimination half-life, however,
nitrazepam administration results in oversedation and other adverse effects considerably more often in old than in young adult patients (Linnoila and Viukari,
1976; Greenblatt and Shader, 1978). Impairment of psychomotor skills, confusion
and disorientation have been reported with the drug (Dawson-Butterworth, 1970;
Evans and Jarvis, 1972).

Miscellaneous.   Other benzodiazepines employed as anxiolytics and/or hypnotics in the aged include clobazam, prazepam and triazolam. One particular advantage of clobazam is that it has no effect on motor functions in doses sufficient for
successful tranquillization (Fielding and Hoffman, 1979). Triazolam, because of
its short half-life is considered to be a more desirable hypnotic than flurazepam in
elderly patients (Okawa, 1978). However, because of its shorter half-life, withdrawal insomnia is more frequent and severe with the drug (Linnoila et al.,
1980).

β-Adrenergic receptor blockers

The stimulation of β-adrenergic receptors results in the activation of hepatic phosphorylase and glycogenolysis with a subsequent rise in glucose and lactic acid levels. It also leads to the activation of a specific lipase which yields to increased mobilization of free fatty acids from peripheral tissues. Since these biochemical changes are frequently associated with the somatic manifestations of anxiety frequently seen in the aged, the possibility has been raised that the administration of β-adrenergic receptor blocking agents may have a particular role in the treatment of anxiety and possibly also agitation in elderly patients.

Propranolol. It has been suggested that peripheral autonomic symptoms may be more responsive to propranolol than psychological symptoms of anxiety (Lader, 1974). This profile of efficacy is particularly suitable to geriatric patients. Petrie and Ban (1981) have indicated that propranolol may be effective in the agitation and associated behavioural problems of demented geriatric patients, refractory to drug treatment with antipsychotic or benzodiazepine drugs. Another report suggests the efficacy of propranolol in agitated psychotic patients with organic deficits (Yudofsky et al., 1981). As a result of these reports, the use of propranolol is now being investigated in the aged.

Unlike the benzodiazepines, propranolol may improve performance on serial learning tasks; it also decreases free fatty acid levels in the serum (Eisdorfer and Raskind, 1970). However, propranolol may also cause bradycardia and hypotension, and depress myocardial function. Propranolol has also produced concentration difficulties and reversible confusional states (Kurland, 1979), and it should be avoided in patients with asthma, bronchitis and diabetes.

Oxprenolol. Unlike propranolol, oxprenolol, another β-adrenergic receptor blocker, does not seem to induce depressive symptoms (McClelland, 1973). In fact, Waal (1968) found that propranolol-induced depressive reactions remitted after the replacement of propranolol by oxprenolol. In addition, since oxprenolol has an intrinsic sympathomimetic action, it causes considerably less marked slowing of the heart rate at rest and carries less risk of inducing secondary heart failure. These distinct advantages are of a particular importance in elderly patients (Brunner et al., 1967; Naylor et al., 1969).

MONOAMINE OXIDASE INHIBITORS

In the treatment of severe anxiety, antidepressant drugs have been increasingly employed. There is sufficient evidence to believe that patients with agoraphobia respond favourably to imipramine, a tricyclic antidepressant and there are indications that phenelzine, the most commonly prescribed monoamine oxidase inhibitor (MAOI) antidepressant has markedly greater antianxiety effects than amitriptyline, the most frequently prescribed tricyclic antidepressant (Nies et al., 1981). Considering the age-related increase in brain and platelet MAO activity

(Robinson et al., 1978) one cannot ignore the possibility that MAOIs have a particular role in the treatment of anxiety in the elderly.

Irrespective of their therapeutic benefit, the hypotensive effect of MAOIs available for clinical use is a definite disadvantage in the elderly. Nevertheless, in a recent clinical study, Georgotas et al. (1981) found that the administration of MAOIs in conservative dosages is safe in depressed elderly patients. Even more, unlike amitriptyline, which within the therapeutic dose range increases the heart rate in an average of 20% of patients, phenelzine does not increase the heart rate. Because of this phenelzine might be a reasonable treatment for depressed patients with angina pectoris, coronary artery disease, or other cardiovascular disorders, for whom tricyclics would be contraindicated because of the tachycardia and blood pressure elevations they induce (Robinson et al., 1981).

CONCLUDING REMARKS

The presence of medical illness, e.g. liver disease and treatment with other non-psychotropic drugs are more frequently encountered problems in elderly than in young patients. They need to be carefully considered in the selection of the therapeutic agent in this age group.

Because of altered pharmacokinetics, regardless of the drug chosen, the dosage should always be low initially – approximately 1/3 of adult dose – in the elderly. This, however, can prevent serious adverse reactions only at an early stage of treatment, whereas with drug accumulation, even low doses may produce unwanted effects.

Antianxiety drugs may produce excessive sedation and/or confusion as a result of drug interaction when given to patients treated with analgesics or narcotics. The agitated elderly patient with milder or subclinical organic changes may be made worse by the CNS depressant effects of almost all of the antianxiety drugs.

REFERENCES

Amore, A., Delpiano, G., Mardente, S. and De Marchi, F. (1972) Clinical geriatric trials and bioavailability studies on a new benzodiazepine drug: lorazepam. Gazz. Med. Ital. 13, 608–621.
Balier, C. (1968) Les états neurotiques chez les personnes agées. Gaz. Med. Fr. 75, 3415–3416.
Ban, T. A. (1969) Psychopharmacology. Williams & Wilkins, Baltimore.
Ban, T. A. (1980) Psychopharmacology for the Aged. S. Karger, New York.
Banen, D. M. and Resnick, O. (1973) Lorazepam versus glutethimide as a sleep-inducing agent for the geriatric patient. J. Am. Geriat. Soc. 21, 507–511.
Beber, Ch. (1965) Management of behaviour in the institutionalized aged. Dis. Nerv. Syst. 26, 591–595.
Bender, A. D. (1964) Pharmacologic aspects of aging. A survey of the effect of increasing age on drug activity in adults. J. Am. Geriatr. Soc. 12, 114–134.
Bergman, K. (1971) The neuroses of old age. In: D. W. Kay and S. Walk (Eds.), Recent Developments in Geropsychiatrics. Br. J. Psychiatry 6 (spec. publ.) 39–49.

152

Blass, J. P. and Gibson, G. E. (1977) Abnormality of a thiamine-requiring enzyme in Korsakoff syndrome. N. Engl. J. Med. 2997, 1367–1370.

Boston Collaborative Drug Surveillance Program (1973) Clinical depression of the central nervous system due to diazepam and chlordiazepoxide in relation to cigarette smoking and age. N. Engl. J. Med. 288, 277–280.

Brunner, H., Hedwall, P. R. and Meier, M. (1967) Influence of adrenergic betareceptor blockage on the acute cardiovascular effects of hydralazone. Br. J. Pharmacol. 30, 123–133.

Burrell, Z. L., Gittinger, W. C. and Martinez, A. (1958) Treatment of cardiac arrhytmias with hydroxyzine. Am. J. Cardiol. 1, 624–628.

Busse, E. W. and Pfeiffer, E. (Ed.) (1973) Mental Illness in Later Life. Am. Psychiatr. Assoc., Washington.

Castleden, C. M., George, C. F., Marcer, P. and Hallett, C. (1977) Increased sensitivity to nitrazepam in old age. Br. Med. J. 1, 10–12.

Cerera, A. A. (1974) Psychoactive drug therapy in the senile patient. Controlled comparison of thioridazine and diazepam. Psychiatr. Digest 35, 16–21.

Chesrow, E. J. and Kaplitz, S. E. (1970) Sustained-release intherapy in hospitalized geriatric patients. J. Am. Geriatr. Soc. 18, 17–80.

Chesrow, E. J., Kaplitz, S. E. Breme, J. T., Musci, J. and Sabatini, R. (1962) Use of a new benzodiazepine derivative (Valium) in chronically ill and disburbed elderly patients. J. Am. Geriatr. Soc. 10, 667–670.

Chesrow, E. J., Kaplitz, S. E., Sabatini, R., Vetra, H. and Marquardt, G. H. (1965a) A new psychotherapeutic agent effective in the management of anxiety, depression and behavioural reactions. J. Am. Geriatr. Soc. 13, 449–454.

Chesrow, E. J., Kaplitz, S. E., Vetra, H., Breme, J. T. and Marquardt, G. H. (1965b) Double-blind study of oxazepam in the management of geriatric patients with behavioral problems. Clin. Med. 72, 1001–1005.

Chien, C. P. (1971) Psychiatric treatment for geriatric patients, 'pub' or 'drug'? Am. J. Psychiatry 127, 1070–1075.

Chien, C. P., Stotsky, B. A. and Cole, J. O. (1973) Psychiatric treatment for nursing home patients. Drug, alcohol and milieu. Am. J. Psychiatry 130, 543–548.

Cromwell, H. A. (1973) Management of anxiety – depression in geriatric patients. Med. Times N.Y. 101, 47–53.

Dawson-Butterworth, K. (1970) The chemopsychotherapeutics of geriatric sedation. J. Am. Geriatr. Soc. 18, 87–114.

DeLamos, G. P., Clements, W. R. and Nickels, E. (1965) Effect of diazepam suspension in geriatric patients hospitalized for psychiatric illness. J. Am. Geriatr. Soc. 13, 355–359.

DeThibault de Boesinghe, L. and Van Vaerenbergh, P. M. (1974) The use of lorazepam (Temesta) in cancer patients. Arch. Med. 29, 2481–2482.

Eisdorfer, C. and Raskind, M. A. (1970) Improvement in learning in the aged by modification of autonomic nervous system activity. Science 170, 1327–1329.

Ernst, K. (1959) Die Prognose der Neurosen. Springer-Verlag, Berlin.

Evans, J. G. and Jarvis, E. H. (1972) Nitrazepam in the elderly. Br. Med. J. iv, 487–489.

Exton-Smith, A. N., Hodkinson, H. M. and Crane, B. W. (1963) Controlled comparison for four sedative drugs in elderly patients. Br. Med. J. iv, 1037–1040.

Feigenbaum, E. M. (1971) Assessment of behavioral changes and emotional disturbance in a custodial geriatric facility. Read at the 124th Ann. Meet. of the Am. Psychiatr. Assoc., Washington.

Fielding, S. and Hoffman, I. (1979) Pharmacology of anti-anxiety drugs with special reference to clobazam. Br. J. Clin. Pharmacol. 7 (Suppl. 1), 7–16.

Georgotas, A., Ferris, S., Friedman, E., Reisberg, B. and Gershon, S. (1981) Clinical efficacy and safety of monoamine oxidase inhibitors in depressed elderly. Read at the Am. Psychiatr. Assoc. Meet., New Orleans.

Gibson, I. (1966) Barbiturate delirium. Practitioner 197, 345–347.

Glasgow, J. F. T. (1969) A neurological disorder associated with chlordiazepoxide therapy. Clin. Toxicol. 2, 456–462.

Greenblatt, D. J. (1980) Pharmacokinetic comparisons. Psychosomatics 21 (Suppl.), 98–140.

Greenblatt, D. J. and Shader, R. I. (1978) Pharmacotherapy of anxiety with benzodiazepines and β-adrenergic blockers. In: M. Lipton, A. DiMascio and K.T. Killam (Eds.), Psychopharmacology. A Generation of Progress. Raven Press, New York, pp. 1381–1390.

Greenblatt, D. J. Shader, R.I. and Koch-Weser, I. (1975) Flurazepam hydrochloride. Clin. Pharmacol. Ther. 17, 1–14.

Greenblatt, D. J., Allen, M. D. and Shader, R. I. (1977) Toxicity of high-dose of flurazepam in the elderly. Clin. Pharmacol. Ther. 21, 355–361.

Greenblatt, D. J., Allen, M. D., Locniskar, A., Harmatz, J. S. and Shader, R. I. (1980) Lorazepam kinetics in the elderly. Clin. Pharmacol. Ther. 26, 103–113.

Gurland, B. J. (1972) Age differentiation in depression: diagnostic and descriptive aspects. Read at the Gerontological Society Meet., Puerto Rico.

Hall, R. W. C. and Joffee, J. R. (1972) Aberrant response to diazepam: a new syndrome. Am. J. Psychiatry 126, 738–742.

Hoehn-Saric, R. (1981) Neurotransmitters in anxiety. Scientific Proceedings, American Psychiatric Assoc. Meeting, New Orleans.

Holliday, A. R. and Mihlayi, E. (1966) A controlled evaluation of two dose levels of oxazepam compared to placebo. J. New Drugs 6, 124.

Hollister, L. E. (1981) Pharmacokinetics of benzodiazepines. Scientific Proceedings, American Psychiatric Assoc. Meeting, New Orleans.

Imlah, N. W. (1973) Clinical experience with lorazepam in hospital patients. Curr. Med. Res. Opin. 1, 276–281.

Jones, T. H. (1962) Chlordiazepoxide (librium) and the geriatric patient. J. Am. Geriatr. Soc. 10, 259–263.

Kangas, L., Iisala, E., Kanto, J., Lehtinen, V., Pynnonen, S., Ruikka, I., Salminen, J., Sillapaa, M. and Syvalahti, E. (1979) Human pharmacokinetics of nitrazepam: effect of age and diseases. Eur. J. Clin. Pharmacol. 15, 163–170.

Kastenbaum, R. (1965) Wine and fellowship in aging. An exploratory action program. J. Hum. Relat. 13, 266–275.

Kay, D. W. K., Beamish. O. and Roth, M. (1964) Old age mental disorders in Newcastle upon Tyne. Part I. A study of prevalence. Br. J. Psychiatry 110, 146–158.

Kirven, L. E. and Montero, E. F. (1973) Comparison of thioridazine and diazepam in the control of nonpsychotic symptoms associated with senility. Double-blind study. J. Am. Geriatr. Soc. 21, 546–551.

Kraus, J. W., Desmond, P. V., Marshall, J. P., Johnson, R. E., Schenter, S. and Wilkinson, G. R. (1978) Effects of aging and liver disease on disposition of lorazepam. Clin. Pharmacol. Ther. 24, 411–414.

Kurland, M. (1979) Organic brain syndrome with propranolol. N. Engl. J. Med. 300, 366.

Lader, M. (1974) The peripheral and central role of the catecholamines in the mechanism of anxiety. Int. Pharmacopsychiatry 9, 125–137.

Lehmann, H. E. and Ban, T. A. (1970) Pharmacological load tests as predictors of pharmacotherapeutic response in geriatric patients. In: R. Wittenborn, S. M. Goldberg and P. R. A. May (Eds.), Psychopharmacology and the Individual Patient. Raven Press, New York, pp. 32–54.

Linnoila, M. and Viukari, M. (1976) Efficacy and side effects of nitrazepam and thioridazine as sleeping aids in psychogeriatric inpatients. Br. J. Psychiatry 128, 566–596.

Linnoila, M., Viukari, M., Lamminsivu, U. and Auvinen, J. (1980) Efficacy and side effects of lorazepam, oxazepam and temazepam as sleeping aids in psychogeriatric inpatients. Int. Pharmacopsychiatry 15, 129–135.

154

Martilla, J. K., Hammel, R. J., Alexander, B. and Zustiak, R.   (1977)   Potential unwanted effects of long-term use of flurazepam in geriatric patients. J. Am. Pharmaceut. Assoc. 17, 11, 692–695.

McClelland, H. A.   (1973)   Psychiatric complication of drug therapy. Adv. Drug React. Bull. 40, 128–129.

McGeer, R. and McGeer, P.L.   (1976)   Genesis and treatment of psychologic disorders in the elderly. In: R. D. Terry and S. Gershon (Eds.), Aging, Vol. 3. Raven Press, New York.

Metellus, P. and Chappon, C.   (1972)   Study of lorazepam in a neurological clinic. Gaz. Med. Fr. 79, 354–356.

Middleton, R. W. W.   (1978)   Temazepam (Euhypnos) and chlormethiazole. A comparative study in geriatric patients. J. Int. Med. Res. 6, 121–125.

Möhler, H. and Okada, T.   (1977)   Benzodiazepine receptors in the central nervous system. Science 198, 849–851.

Naylor, W. G., Chipperfield, D. and Lowe, T. E.   (1969)   The negative inotropic effect of adrenergic betareceptor blocking drugs on human ear muscle. Cardiovasc. Res. 3, 30–36.

Negri, F.   (1957)   The neuroleptic agents in the management of certain psychic disorders particular to old age. Minerva Med. 48, 607–611.

Neilsen, J.   (1963)   Geronto-psychiatric period prevalence investigation in a geographically delimited population. Acta Psychiatr. Scand. 38, 307–330.

Nesteros, J. N.   (1981)   Mechanisms and anxiety. Scientific Proceedings, American Psychiatric Assoc. Meet., New Orleans.

Nies, A., Robinson, D. S., Corcella, J., Bartlett, D. and Cooper, T. B.   (1981)   Read at the American Society for Clinical Pharmacology and Therapeutics, New Orleans.

Okawa, K. K.   (1978)   Comparison of triazolam 0.25 mg and flurazepam 15 mg in treating geriatric insomniacs. Curr. Ther. Res. 23, 381–387.

Petrie, W. M. and Ban, T. A.   (1981)   Propranolol in organic agitation. Lancet I (8215), 324.

Post, F.   (1975)   Dementia, depression and pseudo-dementia. In: D.F. Benson and D. Blumer (Eds.), Psychiatric Aspects of Neurological Disease. Grune and Stratton, New York.

Raskind, M. A. and Eisdorfer, C.   (1975)   Psychopharmacology of the aged. In: P. Simpson (Ed.), Drug Treatment of Mental Disorders. Raven Press, New York.

Renshaw, D. C.   (1973)   Management of the elderly patient. Chicago Med. 76, 229–233.

Roberts, R. K., Wilkinson, G. R., Branch, R. A. and Schenker, S.   (1978)   Effect of age and parenchymal liver disease on the dispositon and elimination of chlordiazepoxide (librium). Gastroenterology 75, 479–485.

Robinson, D. S., Nies, A., Ravaris, C. L., Ives, J. O. and Bartlett, D.   (1978)   Clinical psychopharmacology of phenelzine: MAO activity and clinical response. In: L. A. Lipton, A. DiMascio and K. F. Killam (Eds.), Psychopharmacology. A Generation of Progress. Raven Press, New York, pp. 961–974.

Robinson, D. S., Corcella, J., Nies, A., Cooper, T. B., Jounson, G. A. and Keefevor, R.   (1981)   Monoamine oxidase inhibitors. Paper read at American Society for Clinical and Therapeutics, New Orleans.

Salzman, C. and Shader, R. I.   (1973)   Responses to psychotropic drugs in normal elderly. In: W. E. Fann and C. Eisdorfer (Eds.), Psychopharmacology and Aging. Plenum Publishing, New York.

Salzman, C., Shader, R. I., Hormatz, J. and Robertson. L.   (1975)   Psychopharmacologic investigations in elderly volunteers. Diazepam in males. J. Am. Geriatr. Soc. 23, 451–457.

Sanders, J. F.   (1965)   Evaluation of oxazepam and placebo in emotionally disturbed aged patients. Geriatrics 20, 739–746.

Schrappe, O.   (1971)   Clinical study on WY-4036 (lorazepam), a new tranquillizer. Arzneim. Forsch. 21, 1079–1082.

Schwarz, H. J.   (1979)   Pharmacokinetics and metabolism of temazepam in man and several animal species. Br. J. Clin. Pharmacol. 8, 235–295.

Shaw, S. M. and Opit, L. J.   (1976)   Need for supervision in the elderly receiving long-term prescribed medication. Br. Med. J. 1, 505–507.

Shelton, J. and Hollister, L. E.   (1967)   Stimulated abuse of tybamate in man. J. Am. Med. Assoc. 199, 338–340.

Shepherd, M. and Gruenberg, E. M.   (1957)   The age for neuroses. Milbank Mem. Fund. Q. 35, 258–265.

Shull, H. J., Wilkinson, G. R., Johnson, R. and Schenker, S.   (1976)   Normal disposition of oxazepam in acute viral hepatitis and cirrhosis. Ann. Intern. Med. 84, 420–425.

Sizaret, P., Versavel, M. C., Engel, G. and Vervisch, J. C.   (1974)   Clinical investigation of lorazepam. Psychol. Med. 6, 591–598.

Stern, F. H.   (1964)   A new drug (Tybamate) effective in the management of chronic brain syndrome. J. Am. Geriatr. Soc. 12, 1066–1072.

Stotsky, B. A.   (1975)   Psychoactive drugs for geriatric patients with psychiatric disorders. In: S. Gershon and A. Raskin (Eds.), Aging, Vol. 2. Raven Press, New York.

Triggs, E. J., Nation, R. L., Long, A. and Ashley, J. J.   (1975)   Pharmacokinetics in the elderly. Eur. J. Clin. Pharmacol, 8, 55–62.

Twefik, G. I., Jain, V. K., Harcup, M. and Magowan, S.   (1970)   Effectiveness of various tranquilizers in the management of senile restlessness. Gerontol. Clin. 12, 351–359.

Viukari, M., Linnoila, M. and Aalto, V.   (1978)   Efficacy and side effects of flurazepam, fosazepam, and nitrazepam as sleeping aids in psychogeriatric patients. Acta Psychiatr. Scand. 57, 27–35.

Waal, H. J.   (1968)   Hypotensive, antiarrhythmic and chronotropic action of Trasicor (CIBA 39 089-Ba). N.Z. Med. Z. 67, 291–295.

Welborn, W. S.   (1961)   A trial of new tranquilizing agents in geriatric patients. Psychosomatics 2, 45–452.

WHO   (1967)   Report of a Scientific Group on Research in Psychopharmacology. WHO Technical Report series No. 371, Geneva.

Wilkinson, G. R.   (1978)   The effects of liver desease and aging on the disposition of diazepam, chlordiazepoxide, oxazepam and lorazepam in men. Acta. Psychiatr. Scand., Suppl. 270, 56–74.

Yudofsky, S., Williams, D. and Gorman, J.   (1981)   Propranolol in the treatment of rage and violent behaviour in patients with chronic brain syndromes. Am. J. Psychiatry 138, 218–220.

Burrows/Norman/Davies (eds) Antianxiety agents
© *Elsevier Science Publishers B.V., 1984*

Chapter 11

Antianxiety agents – drug interactions

LAWRENCE PLON

Department of Psychiatry and Human Behavior, California College of Medicine, University of California at Irvine, Irvine, CA 92717, U.S.A. and Department of Pharmacy, University of California, Irvine Medical Center, Orange, CA 92668, U.S.A.

and

LOUIS A. GOTTSCHALK

Department of Psychiatry and Human Behavior, National Alcohol Research Center and University of California, Irvine Medical Center, Orange, CA 92668, U.S.A.

INTRODUCTION

One of the hallmarks of medicine's treatment of the entire spectrum of human disease has been the proliferation in the number and kinds of medications available. It is indeed rare today to find a patient who is receiving only one medication, yet it is seldom recognized that increasing the number of medications a patient receives multiplies the chances for a drug-to-drug interaction. It is fortunate that most interactions are mild and patients are seldom harmed. Indeed, many interactions are unnoticed by either the patient or the clinician. While few drug-to-drug interactions pose serious problems, certain ones have been classically noted to have the potential for inducing fatalities.

Most of the medications used in the psychiatric area have well known side-effects. Their potentials for interactions tend to be limited and fairly well recognized. Perhaps the most famous interaction is the one between a tricyclic antidepressant and a monoamine oxidase inhibitor. The clinician needs to be aware of

158

the potential for other interactions, for many of his patients are treated by other physicians for medical problems. These non-psychiatric medications can interact with psychiatric agents and may create some problems in certain patients.

Evaluation of drug interactions pose many problems. The first is the recognition of the drug-to-drug interaction. Many are neither looked for nor anticipated and, therefore, are not recognized. The second and perhaps most significant problem is the evaluation of the validity and the significance of the interaction. The third area of concern in this field is the question of whether the interaction is significant to a given patient. There may, indeed, be an interaction, yet clinically, its overall impact is minimal and the patient is not harmed in any way nor is the outcome of the therapy significantly affected. In this chapter, we have not attempted to include every drug interaction reported or suspected. It becomes impossible to give a complete, updated picture of these interactions, for new data and new medications arrive constantly. What we have attempted to do is list well documented or substantiated drug-to-drug interactions in an attempt to make the ones which are clinically significant more apparent to the reader. Most of the data is based on American literature and, therefore, we did not include some medications which are established in Europe at this time. In reviewing the literature one runs certain risks. The astute clinician is tempted to make generalizations. For example, if diazepam has a given drug interaction, then should not all other benzodiazepines? Perhaps and perhaps not. Many of the interactions with benzodiazepines are dependent upon active metabolites. A number of the newer products has no active metabolites, and so the drug-to-drug interaction is not valid. A similar situation exists with the proliferation of beta-adrenergic blocking agents. Because propranolol interacts with another medication in a certain way there is no indication that one of its cousins will, indeed, interact in the same fashion. However, because there are no data on a given drug, that does not mean that there is no potential for an interaction. It is perhaps, wise to be cautious in one's practice concerning adding a second medication to a patient's regimen, rather than ignoring a potential for problems. Good clinicians will find themselves reviewing the literature on an ongoing basis for drug-to-drug interactions. This is a difficult area to ignore and one that requires a constant sense of vigilance if we are to protect our patients from the very agents by which we seek to help them.

MECHANISMS

A basic familiarity with the two major kinds of drug-to-drug interactions is necessary. This familiarization enables the clinician to predict future interactions and to have a sense of understanding rather than rote memorization. In general, drug-to-drug interactions fall into one of the two following categories: pharmacokinetic or pharmacologic. The pharmacokinetic factors are those which influence the absorption, the distribution, the metabolism, and the excretion of a drug in a given patient. In viewing these factors one should always look for, not only decreased, but enhanced reactions. The pharmacologic interactions are those where there can be an additive, synergistic, or antagonistic effect upon the biologic system, and this interaction may or may not involve a specific receptor site. Most drug interactions will fall into one of the two categories that we have listed and are essentially variations upon one of these two themes, differing only in a quantitative fashion.

Drug absorption

Drug interactions may involve an alteration in the amount of the drug absorbed or an alteration in the rate of absorption. If the rate of absorption is decreased, one may not achieve a fully effective serum level. A patient may experience a rate of onset which is decreased or the effect of the medication may persist past a desired interval. This is exemplified by slowing the absorption of a barbiturate which may produce a 'morning hangover'. Changes in absorption may or may not be significant in a given patient. For example, food affects the rate of aspirin absorption and not the total amount absorbed. This might be a significant interaction to a patient who has taken aspirin to relieve his headache, yet not significant to a patient with severe rheumatoid arthritis who takes a large amount of aspirin throughout the day to achieve an overall effect. The interaction between tetracycline and foods is well known and can result in a decreased total absorption of the medication, lower serum levels, and perhaps decreased clinical effectiveness.

Drug distribution

Many drugs are highly localized in specific tissues. When a second drug is administered, one may find competition for available binding sites in the tissue resulting in a higher concentration with resulting toxic side-effects for the patient. Another factor affecting drug distribution is plasma protein binding. Most drugs are reversibly bound, to various extents, with proteins found in the plasma, usually albumin. There may be competition for available binding sites by two different medications. A patient can be at a steady state in regard to the amount of drug that is free to diffuse to the site of action. If a second drug is added which displaces an increased amount of the first drug, then there will be an increase in the amount of medication reaching the receptor site with a potential for increased side effects or drug action.

Drug metabolism

Medications are predominately metabolized and excreted by renal or biliary routes. Medications which stimulate enzyme induction, such as phenobarbital, by increasing the size and the content of the endoplasmic reticulum, may result in an increased rate of metabolism of many different drugs. The most profound example of this kind of interaction is the effect of barbiturates upon the metabolism of anticoagulants. The enhanced rate of metabolism requires an increased amount of the anticoagulant to achieve the desired effect. If the enzyme-inducer is removed from the patient's medication regimen and the level of anticoagulant is continued, its effect can increase into the toxic range. Enzyme-inducers can also decrease the effect of certain drugs, for example, griseofulvin.

Drug excretion

Drug-to-drug interactions that effect the renal excretion are clinically significant only when the drug or its active metabolites are excreted in an appreciable quantity by the renal route. Since medications are eliminated by urinary excretion through either glomerular filtration, tubular reabsorption, or active tubular secretion, drugs which affect any of these mechanisms may result in increased levels of an active compound. Perhaps the most famous constructive use of a drug-to-drug interaction is the well-known method of increasing serum levels of penicillin by the addition of probenecid. This interaction occurs because there is a competition between these drugs for tubular transportation, resulting in much higher plasma penicillin levels than would normally be achieved.

Pharmacologic interactions

Pharmacologic interactions may accur at the site of drug action. Medications may compete for receptor sites, they may alter a receptor site, alter other components at the site of action, or affect the total biological system in such a way as to add to or diminish the total biological response of the patient. An example of this kind of interaction is the classical reaction between alcohol and another sedative drug, such as a barbiturate. Both agents probably have different sites of action, but the total effect upon the organism is a synergism of the sedative effect.

Other factors

In assessing a patient for drug interactions, one must look at several areas. Often the age of the patient is overlooked in considering drug interactions. Elderly patients are more sensitive to side-effects, such as anticholinergic effects, than are younger patients. One must also consider disease states which may cause the patient to respond differently to a given medication. Diseases such as alterations in thyroid function, diabetes, alcoholism, and gastrointestinal disease may affect the absorption, metabolism, distribution, or elimination of a medication. In a patient with renal disease it is important to know whether the medication is removed in an active form via that route. Assessment of hepatic function is very important, since many drugs are metabolized by the liver. A decrease in hepatic function could lead to increased drug blood levels and enhance the possibility of adverse interactions.

SUMMARY

In summary, various drug-to-drug interactions can occur due to a wide variety of conditions in a given patient. Factors affecting absorption, transportation, metabolism, distribution, and excretion of medications either by other drugs or by patient disease states may affect the therapeutic outcome. Most drug interactions are relatively benign. However, some interactions have potential for significant problems. A high level of expertise with psychoactive drugs alone is no longer adequate for the psychiatrist because many patients receive non-psychoactive medications from specialists in other areas. This poses another challenge to the astute clinician to insure that his patient is helped rather than harmed by his pharmacological interventions.

BENZODIAZEPINES-PHENYTOIN

Mechanism. It is thought that benzodiazepines alter the metabolism of phenytoin. It is also speculated that phenytoin may enhance the metabolism of diazepines (Hepner et al., 1977).

Clinical significance. One study reported that patients receiving phenytoin with either diazepam or chlordiazepoxide had a higher phenytoin blood level than patients receiving just the phenytoin (Vajda et al., 1971). Other studies have also indicated that the benzodiazepines may result in a higher phenytoin level (Kutt and McDowell, 1968). However, several other studies have indicated that benzodiazepines may actually decrease serum phenytoin levels (Houghton and Richens, 1974; Siris et al., 1974). Thus the results are somewhat conflicting and not consistent. It is suggested that it is not necessary to avoid benzodiazepines in patients who are receiving phenytoin. One should be aware that phenytoin levels may be altered when a benzodiazepine is added or deleted.

CHLORDIAZEPOXIDE-ANTACIDS

Mechanism. Magnesium aluminium hydroxide appears to reduce the rate of absorption but not the total amount of chlordiazepoxide absorbed.

Clinical significance. The completeness of absorption of chlordiazepoxide was not reduced in one study (Greenblatt et al., 1976). It would seem that this particular interaction would have no overall effect on the clinical efficacy of the agent, except that it could lower the blood level achieved of the drug.

DIAZEPAM-ORAL ANTICOAGULANTS

Mechanism.   Not known.

Clinical significance.   There was one early case reported of an interaction between diazepam and dicoumarol (Taylor, 1967). Subsequent studies have shown no significant interaction between these two medications; therefore, no special precautions appear to be necessary in the co-administration of these agents (Whitfield et al., 1973; DeCarolis et al., 1975).

DIAZEPAM-DISULFIRAM

Mechanism.   Disulfiram inhibits a variety of enzymes, including the hepatic microsomal enzymes responsible for drug metabolism. It is thought that disulfiram via this mechanism inhibits the metabolism of diazepam and chlordiazepoxide.

Clinical significance.   There is a relationship between chlordiazepoxide or diazepam and disulfiram administration and increased sedation. Because of the inhibition of drug metabolism, higher plasma levels of these agents were found resulting in increased sedation. Oxazepam was not affected by disulfiram administration; its plasma levels and rate of excretion were unchanged in the presence of disulfiram. Clinically, both of these agents, the disulfiram and the benzodiazepines, are sedating. Hence, a combination of these agents can result in increased sedation, at least in the initial phases of clinical treatment (MacLeod et al., 1978).

DIAZEPAM-ETHANOL

Mechanism.   A combination of diazepam and ethanol causes an intensification of the central nervous system effects of each drug. The exact mechanism of the central nervous system action is not known. Studies on absorption, metabolism, and excretion of alcohol and the benzodiazepines show that these are unaffected by concurrent ingestion of both agents (Morselli et al., 1971; Morland et al., 1974). The interaction is generally thought to occur at the receptor site in the central nervous system (Morland et al., 1974).

Clinical significance.   There have been many studies investigating the effects of ethanol and benzodiazepines (Linnoila, 1973a, b; Linnoila and Hakkinen, 1974; Linnoila et al., 1974; Saario, 1976; MacLeod et al., 1977; Gottschalk, 1978; Gottschalk et al., 1980). While there is a variation in the data reported and conclusions drawn in some studies, it is generally accepted that benzodiazepine when taken in combination with alcohol may produce a greater impairment of a patient's ability

163

to perform motor tasks, such as driving an automobile and operating hazardous machinery, than when taken alone. Patients should be warned that the ingestion of alcohol along with a benzodiazepine can be detrimental, even fatal (Gottschalk et al., 1980). This reaction can occur 30 min after simultaneous ingestion or even if alcohol is ingested, 10 hours after the last dose of a benzodiazepine. This is a clinically significant interaction in that it may result in a sufficient impairment of psychomotor skills that the individual may be harmed in an accident. One may assume that a similar reaction occurs with other benzodiazepines, although the data may be conflicting. Any patient taking a benzodiazepine should be warned of the possibility of this interaction.

DIAZEPAM-FOOD

Mechanism.   An increase in serum diazepam following ingestion of food seems to be related to the secretion of the medication in gastric juice with subsequent reabsorption and/or entero-hepatic circulation (Linnoila et al., 1975; Korttila et al., 1976). Food does not alter the binding of the medication to plasma proteins (Klotz et al., 1977).

Clinical significance.   The ingestion of food results in a decreased rate of absorption of orally administered diazepam, but does not decrease the total amount absorbed. However, there may be an increase in plasma diazepam levels when the drug is administered intravenously after the ingestion of food due to changes in the entero-hepatic circulation (Greenblatt et al., 1978). There is no indication that ingestion of meals with oral diazepam will reduce steady state plasma concentrations, although individual doses are absorbed more slowly. The ingestion of food does seem to prolong, to some degree, the effect of oral diazepam, though no special precautions are necessary.

DIAZEPAM-LEVODOPA

Mechanism.   Not known at this time.

Clinical significance.   There is a description of one patient who was treated with levodopa who demonstrated a deterioration of the control of his Parkinsonism when diazepam was added to his therapeutic regimen (Hunter et al., 1970). Three other levodopa patients have also demonstrated a similar deterioration of the control of their disease (Wodak et al., 1972). There is sufficient evidence to warrant caution in the administration of diazepam to patients receiving levodopa.

DIAZEPAM-LITHIUM CARBONATE

Mechanism.   Not known at this time.

Clinical significance. One patient became hypothermic while taking lithium and diazepam who did not manifest this condition while receiving either medication alone (Naylor and McHarg, 1977). The combination of medications was thought to be responsible for the reaction. Whether this reaction was idiosyncratic or may be expected in other patients is difficult to determine. A clinician should be aware that this reaction may occur in patients receiving both diazepam and lithium.

DIAZEPAM-SKELETAL MUSCLE RELAXANTS (SURGICAL)

Mechanism. Not established. That diazepam may directly inhibit the contractile mechanism of skeletal muscles has been reported (Ludin and Dubach, 1971).

Clinical significance. Diazepam was initially reported to increase the duration of action of gallamine and decrease the duration of activity of succinylcholine (Feldman and Crawley, 1970). However, subsequent work did not verify these findings (Dretchen et al., 1971; Webb and Bradshaw, 1971). It now appears that diazepam, itself, does not significantly affect a patient's response to neuromuscular blocking agents. Some effects upon neuromuscular blockage have been reported when the injectable form of diazepam is given intra-arterially. This effect may be due to one of the preservatives or solvents in the medication. Based on current evidence special precautions do not appear to be necessary with concomitant use of these drugs; however, physicians should be aware of possible interactions between them.

MEPROBAMATE-ETHANOL

Mechanism. Acute ethanol intoxication may inhibit the metabolism of meprobamate (Rubin et al., 1970). However, meprobamate metabolism is increased when it is administered to a patient receiving chronic ethanol via enhanced hepatic microsomal enzymes (Misra et al., 1971).

Clinical significance. Acute ingestion of ethanol with meprobamate in low doses (200–300 mg) usually results in some increase in central nervous system depression though its significance is usually slight (Zirkle et al., 1960; Forney and Hughes, 1964; Reisby and Theilgaard, 1969). However, some patients may exhibit more impairment than others especially while engaged in activities such as driving a car. In general, patients should be advised to avoid the consumption of ethanol while receiving meprobamate.

MEPROBAMATE-WARFARIN

Mechanism.   Because meprobamate is capable of inducing hepatic microsomal enzymes, it may enhance the metabolism of warfarin (Conney, 1967).

Clinical significance.   Clinical evidence for this interaction is lacking and concomitant use of these medications need not be avoided (Udall, 1970; Gould et al., 1972).

PHENOBARBITAL-DEXAMETHASONE (BARBITURATES AND COR-TICOSTEROIDS)

Mechanism.   Barbiturates enhance the metabolism of corticosteroids probably by the induction of hepatic microsomal enzymes (Kuntzman et al., 1968; Southren et al., 1969).

Clinical significance.   This drug interaction is of clinical significance in those patients who are maintained on corticosteroids, such as, chronic asthmatics or patients with adrenal insufficiency (Brooks et al., 1972). When such patients are given barbiturates or phenobarbital they may experience a decrease in the effectiveness of the corticosteroids. This reaction appears to be dose-related and occurs in those patients who are receiving high doses of phenobarbital (120 mg/day) (Falliers, 1972).

PHENOBARBITAL-DIGITOXIN

Mechanism.   Hepatic enzyme systems convert a small fraction of digitoxin into digoxin. Digoxin has a significantly shorter half-life than digitoxin. With phenobarbital hepatic enzyme induction, the amount of digitoxin converted to digoxin is significantly increased (Brown et al., 1957; Jelliffe and Blankenhorn, 1966; Solomon and Abrams, 1972).

Clinical significance.   There is currently no significant support that there is a clinical effect as a result of this interaction. Patients receiving both of these medications should be observed for signs of a decreased digitoxin therapeutic effect. Digoxin could be substituted for digitoxin because it is not significantly hepatically metabolized.

PHENOBARBITAL-DOXYCYCLINE

Mechanism.   Barbiturate enhancement of hepatic microsomal enzyme systems lead to an increased rate of metabolism of the doxycycline.

Clinical significance. Several studies have demonstrated a significant decrease in the plasma half-life of doxycycline when it was administered to patients receiving chronic barbiturates (Neuvonen and Penttila, 1974). There may be a significant decrease in clinical response in patients receiving both of these medications concomitantly.

PHENOBARBITAL-OESTRADIOL

Mechanism. Enhanced metabolism of oestradiol into its metabolites (Levin et al., 1968; Welch et al., 1968; Janz and Schmidt, 1974).

Clinical significance. There have been reported cases of patients receiving antiepileptic medications and becoming pregnant while taking oral contraceptives. While the cause and effect aspects of this interaction have not been well documented it may be advisable to suggest additional or alternated methods of contraception (Conney, 1967; Roberton and Johnson, 1976).

PHENOBARBITAL-ETHANOL (BARBITURATES-ETHANOL)

Mechanism. Exact mechanism is unclear. Net clinical effect is an enhancement of central nervous system depression, with drowsiness, and motor impairment being the most common effect.

Clinical significance. Patients should be warned that taking both of these agents at the same time may result in a marked impairment of motor functions and decreased alertness. Consumption of 150 ml of 100-proof ethanol in combination with barbiturates may result in significant respiratory depression or death. This dose-related drug interaction is of high clinical significance (Jetter and McLean, 1943; Gruber, 1955; Forney and Hughes, 1968; Kielholz et al., 1969; Morselli et al., 1971; Gupta and Kofoed, 1972).

PHENOBARBITAL-GRISEOFULVIN

Mechanism. Uncertain at this time, but possibly by hepatic enzyme induction.

Clinical significance. Phenobarbital has been shown to cause a decrease in the serum levels of oral griseofulvin to ineffective levels in some patients (Busfield et al., 1963; Lorenc, 1967; Riegelman et al., 1970). Patients receiving both of these medications concurrently should be observed for signs of poor clinical response. Phenobarbital should be avoided in those patients taking griseofulvin. If both drugs must be used and there are indications that the griseofulvin is ineffective, then the dosage of griseofulvin may have to be increased.

PHENOBARBITAL-METHYLDOPA

Mechanism. It has been proposed that phenobarbital, as well as other barbiturates, will enhance the metabolism of methyldopa by hepatic enzyme induction.

Clinical significance. Several studies (Kristensen et al., 1973a,b) have failed to demonstrate that phenobarbital induces the specific enzyme responsible for methyldopa conjugation and, therefore, there seems to be no need for dosage adjustments in this case.

PHENOBARBITAL-QUINIDINE

Mechanism. Enhanced hepatic microsomal enzyme systems resulting in an increased metabolism of quinidine.

Clinical significance. It has been demonstrated that phenobarbital can enhance the metabolism of quinidine resulting in lower serum levels (Data et al., 1976). Adding or removing phenobarbital to a patient receiving quinidine may necessitate an adjustment in the quinidine dosage.

PHENOBARBITAL-WARFARIN   (BARBITURATES-ANTICOAGULANTS)

Mechanism. Phenobarbital, as well as other barbiturates, increases the hepatic microsomal enzyme systems resulting in an increased metabolism of warfarin and perhaps other anticoagulants. The result is a decrease in the anticoagulant effect (Dayton et al, 1961; Antlitz et al., 1968; Levy et al., 1970; Koch-Weser and Sellers, 1971).

Clinical significance. It is very likely that the administration of a barbiturate concurrently with warfarin or another anticoagulant will result in a decrease of the anticoagulation effect (Corn, 1966). The amount of decrease has been reported as high as 50% (Koch-Weser and Sellers, 1971). If the dosage of warfarin is adjusted upward to compensate and later the barbiturate is withdrawn, the warfarin level is high and the patient may be too anticoagulated and haemorrhage can result (MacDonald and Robinson, 1968). If a patient is already receiving a barbiturate and then receives warfarin, a higher dose of warfarin may be necessary to achieve the desired level of anticoagulation. If the barbiturate is then withdrawn, excessive anticoagulation can occur. Anticoagulation levels should be monitored closely even when no other drugs are given. If barbiturates are necessary in these patients, then extreme care must be used and anticoagulant levels watched very closely. Particular caution should be used when giving any drug to a patient receiving anticoagulants.

168

PROPRANOLOL-CHLORPROMAZINE

Mechanism. There is a likely chlorpromazine-induced inhibition of the hepatic metabolism of propranolol. Also, both of these agents have hypotensive effects which could be additive.

Clinical significance. Subjects who received chlorpromazine (50 mg t.i.d.) and propranolol demonstrated an elevation in plasma propranolol concentrations with an apparent increase in beta-adrenergic blockade. It is not known if chlorpromazine therapy dictates a decrease in propranolol dosage. Propranolol therapy may also be associated with marked elevations in plasma chlorpromazine concentrations (Vestal et al., 1979; Peet et al., 1981).

PROPRANOLOL-CIMETIDINE

Mechanism. Acute and chronic administration of cimetidine appears to significantly reduce hepatic blood flow and thereby decrease the clearance and elimination of propranolol.

Clinical significance. Two hours after administration of both of these agents, subjects demonstrated significantly lower pulse rates than when receiving propranolol alone (Feely et al., 1981). The addition of cimetidine to a patient who is receiving propranolol may require that the dosage of propranolol be decreased. There is a need for caution with the simultaneous administration of both of these medications.

PROPRANOLOL-CLONIDINE

Mechanism. During withdrawal of clonidine, adrenaline is released. If propranolol is also being administered, the beta (vasodilating) response is blocked and there can be an exaggerated alpha (vasoconstricting) response with hypertension.

Clinical significance. Several cases of hypertension have been reported in patients who were receiving both of these medications and in whom the clonidine was withdrawn (Harris, 1976; Strauss et al., 1977; Vernon and Sakula, 1979). A case involving timolol (another beta-blocker) has also been reported (Bailey and Neale, 1976). Clonidine should be very carefully withdrawn in the presence of beta-blockade. It has also been suggested that propranolol be carefully withdrawn before the clonidine is halted (Bruce et al., 1979; Warren et al., 1979). Beta-adrenergic blockade can then be reinstituted after the clonidine is completely withdrawn. This is a potentially very significant drug interaction.

PROPRANOLOL-ENZYME INDUCING AGENTS (BARBITURATES)

Mechanism. Enzyme inducing agents, such as phenobarbital, induce hepatic microsomal enzymes and seem to enhance the metabolism of orally administered drugs on their first pass through the liver (Alvan et al., 1977; Sotaniemi et al., 1979).

Clinical significance. It would be expected that lower propranolol plasma levels would be seen in patients taking an enzyme inducer and propranolol at the same time. Enzyme inducers have been noted to affect significantly the plasma levels of several other beta-blocking agents. (metoprolol and alprenolol) (Collste et al., 1979; Haglund et al., 1979). The therapeutic significance of the reduced plasma levels has not yet been evaluated.

PROPRANOLOL-ADRENALINE

Mechanism. Adrenaline possesses both alpha and beta properties which result in vasoconstriction and vasodilation/cardiac stimulation. In the presence of pro-pranolol, the beta effects of the adrenaline are blocked resulting in predominately alpha effects with hypertension and reflex vagal tone leading to bradycardia (Berchtold and Bessman, 1974).

Clinical significance. Several cases of hypertension have been reported with the above combination of medications (Kram et al., 1974; Varma et al., 1976). This reaction is clinically significant and caution should be exercised if a patient who is already receiving propranolol is given adrenaline. It is also possible that proprano-lol may enhance the effects of other sympathomimetics.

PROPRANOLOL-FUROSEMIDE

Mechanism. Not clearly established. That there is a decreased glomerular-filtration rate when these medications are administered simultaneously has been proposed (Tilstone et al., 1977).

Clinical significance. Subjects given propranolol (40 mg orally) and furosemide (25 mg orally) concomitantly demonstrated significantly higher blood levels of propranolol in the presence of furosemide (Chiariello et al., 1979). Increased beta-blockade accompanied the increased propranolol blood levels. It has not been determined whether the dose of propranolol should be decreased when taken with furosemide.

PROPRANOLOL-HYPOGLYCAEMICS, ORAL AND INSULIN

Mechanism. Glycogenolysis normally leads to decreased glucose utilization and propranolol has been shown to inhibit glycogenolysis (Salvador et al., 1967; Brown et al., 1968; Abramson and Arky, 1968). This inhibition may contribute indirectly to hypoglycaemia by permitting the continued peripheral utilization of glucose. Propranolol also interferes with insulin release by either blocking the beta-adrenergic receptors in the pancreatic beta-cells or enhancing the alpha-adrenergic suppression of insulin release by adrenaline (Porte, 1967; DeDivitiis et al., 1968; Blum et al., 1975).

Clinical significance. There have been many case reports of severe hypogly-caemia in patients receiving propranolol (Kotler et al., 1969; Wray and Sutcliffe, 1972; Podolsky and Pattavina, 1973). It has also been suggested that propranolol may cause hyperglycaemia. The situation is further complicated by propranolol's ability to block some of the warning symptoms of hypoglycaemia, such as palpitations or tachycardia. While there may be a few, selected uses of propranolol in certain patients with carbohydrate metabolism problems, in general, the use of propranolol in diabetic patients or in patients predisposed to diabetes may result in alterations of carbohydrate metabolism. If both insulin or an oral hypoglycaemic agent and propranolol must be given together, frequent serum glucose levels should be determined and medication dosages adjusted if necessary.

PROPRANOLOL-INDOMETHACIN

Mechanism. Possibly by prostaglandin inhibition.

Clinical significance. In several studies, the antihypertensive effect of propra-nolol was inhibited by indomethacin (100 mg/day) (Durao et al., 1977; Watkins et al., 1980). It is suggested that other prostaglandin inhibitors may also produce a similar inhibition. Patients receiving both of these agents should be monitored for inhibition of antihypertensive response.

PROPRANOLOL-LIDOCAINE

Mechanism. Currently thought to be the result of the effect of propranolol upon decreasing hepatic blood flow.

Clinical significance. Subjects receiving 240 mg/day of propranolol experi-enced a significant decrease in plasma clearance of constantly infused lidocaine resulting in a 30% increase in lidocaine steady-state serum levels (Ochs et al., 1980). This is a significant alteration in serum lidocaine levels and may require alteration of lidocaine dosage in patients receiving both of these medications. Several cases of lidocaine toxicity have been reported which may be the result of this interaction (Grahm et al., 1981).

PROPRANOLOL-PRAZOSIN

Mechanism.   Uncertain.

Clinical significance.   There appears to be an enhancement of the 'First dose hypotensive response' to prazosin when the patient also is receiving propranolol (Graham et al., 1976; Elliott et al., 1981). Patients receiving propranolol or other beta-blocking agents may be more susceptible to an initial episode of hypotension.

REFERENCES

Abramson, E. A. and Arky, R. A.   (1968)   Role of beta-adrenergic receptors in counterregulation to insulin-induced metabolic responses. Diabetes 17, 141–146.

Alvan, K. G., Piafsky, K., Lind, M. and von Bahr, C.   (1977)   Effect of phenobarbital on the disposition of alprenolol. Clin. Pharmacol. Ther. 22, 316–321.

Antlitz, A. M., Tolentino, M. and Kosai, M. F.   (1968)   Effect of butabarbital on orally administered anticoagulants. Curr. Ther. Res. 10, 70–73.

Bailey, R. R. and Neale, T. J.   (1976)   Rapid clonidine withdrawal with blood pressure overshoot exaggerated by beta blockade. Br. Med. J. 1, 942–943.

Berchtold, P. and Bessman, A. N.   (1974)   Propranolol (letter). Ann. Int. Med. 80, 110.

Blum, I., Doron, M., Laron, Z. and Atsmon, A.   (1975)   Prevention of hypoglycemic attacks by propranolol in a patient suffering from insulinoma. Diabetes 24, 535–537.

Brooks, A. M., Werk, E. E., Ackerman, J., Sullivan, I. and Thrasher, K.   (1972)   Adverse effects of phenobarbital on corticosteroid metabolism in patients with bronchial asthma. N. Engl. J. Med. 286, 1125–1128.

Brown, B. T., Wright, S. E. and Okita, G. T.   (1957)   C-12 hydroxylation of digitoxin. Nature 180, 607–608.

Brown, J. H., Riggilo, D. A. and Dungan, K. W.   (1968)   Oral effectiveness of beta-adrenergic antagonists in preventing epinephrine-induced metabolic responses. J. Pharmacol. Exp. Ther. 163, 25–35.

Bruce, D. L., Croley, T. F. and Lee, J. S.   (1979)   Preoperative clonidine withdrawal syndrome. Anesthesiology 51, 90–92.

Busfield, D., Child, K. J., Atkinson, R. M. and Tomich, E. G.   (1963)   An effect of phenobarbitone on blood-levels of griseofulvin in man. Lancet 2, 1042–1043.

Chiariello, M., Volpe, M., Rengo, F., Trimarco, B., Violini, R., Ricciardelli, B. and Condorelli, M.   (1979)   Effect of furosemide on plasma concentration and beta-blockade by propranolol. Clin. Pharmacol. Ther. 26, 433–436.

Collste, P., Seideman, P., Borg, K. O., Haglund, K. and von Bahr, C.   (1979)   Influence of pentobarbital on effect and plasma levels of alprenolol and 4-hydroxy-alprenolol. Clin. Pharmacol. Ther. 25, 423–427.

Conney, A. H.   (1967)   Pharmacological implications of microsomal enzyme induction. Pharmacol. Rev. 19, 317–366.

172

Corn, M. (1966) Effect of phenobarbital and glutethimide on biological half-life of warfarin. Thromb. Diath. Haemorrh. 16, 606.

Data, J. L., Wilkinson, G. R. and Nies, A. S. (1976) Interaction of quinidine with anticonvulsant drugs. N. Engl. J. Med. 294, 699–702.

Dayton, P. G., Tarcan, Y., Chenkin, T. and Weiner, M. (1961) The influence of barbiturates on coumarin plasma levels and prothrombin response. J. Clin. Invest. 40, 1797–1802.

DeCarolis, P. P. and Gelfand, M. L. (1975) Effect of tranquillizers on prothrombin time response to coumarin. J. Clin. Pharmacol. 15, 557.

DeDivitiis, O., Giordano, F., Gallo, B. and Jacono, A. (1968) Tolbutamide and propranolol. Lancet 1, 749.

Dretchen, K., Ghoneim, M. M. and Long, J. P. (1971) The interaction of diazepam with myoneural blocking agents. Anesthesiology 34, 463–468.

Durao, V., Martins-Prata, M. and Goncalves, L. M. P. (1977) Modifications of antihypertensive effect of beta-adrenoreceptor blocking agents by inhibition of endogenous prostaglandin synthesis. Lancet 2, 1005–1007.

Elliott, H. L., McLean, K., Sumner, D. J., Meredith, P. A. and Reid, J. L. (1981) Immediate cardiovascular responses to oral prazosin; effects of concurrent beta-blockers. Clin. Pharmacol. Ther. 29, 303–309.

Falliers, C. J. (1972) Corticosteroids and phenobarbital in asthma. N. Engl. J. Med. 287, 201.

Feely, J., Wilkinson, G. R. and Wood, A. J. J. (1981) Reduction of liver blood flow and propranolol metabolism by cimetidine. N. Engl. J. Med. 304, 692–695.

Feldman, S. A. and Crawley, B. E. (1970) Interaction of diazepam with the muscle relaxant drugs. Br. Med. J. 2, 336–338.

Forney, R. F. and Hughes, F. W. (Eds) (1968) Combined Effects of Alcohol and Other Drugs. Charles C. Thomas Publishers, Springfield, Ill., 48 pp.

Forney, R. F. and Hughes, F. W. (1964) Meprobamate, ethanol or meprobamate-ethanol combinations on performance of human subjects under delayed audiofeedback (DAF). J. Psychol. 57, 431–436.

Gould, L., Michael, A., Fisch, S. and Gomprecht, R.F. (1972) Prothrombin levels maintained with meprobamate and warfarin. J. Am. Med. Assoc. 220, 1460–1462.

Gottschalk, L. A. (1978) Pharmacokinetics of the minor tranquilizers and clinical response. In: M.A. Lipton, A. DiMascio and K. S. Killam (Eds), Psychopharmacology: A Generation of Progress. Raven Press, New York, pp. 975–986.

Gottschalk, L. A., McGuire, F. L., Heiser, J. F., Dinovo, E. C. and Birch, H. (1980) Drug Abuse Deaths in Nine Cities: A Survey Report. U.S. Government Printing Office, Institute on Drug Abuse, NIDA Research Monograph 29, Washington D.C. pp. 1–176.

Graham, R. M., Thornell, I. R., Gain, J. M., Bagnoli, C., Oates, H. F. and Stokes, G. F. (1976) Prazosin; the first dose phenomenon. Br. Med. J. 4, 1293–1294.

Grahhm, C. F., Turner, W. M. and Jones, J. K. (1981) Lidocaine-propranolol interactions (letter). N. Engl. J. Med. 304, 1301.

Greenblatt, D. J., Shader, R. I. and Harmatz, J. S. (1976) Influence of magnesium and aluminum hydroxide mixture on chlordiazepoxide absorption. Clin. Pharmacol. Ther. 19, 234–239.

Greenblatt, D. J., Allen, M. D., MacLaughlin, D. S. and Harmatz, J. S. (1978) Diazepam absorption; effect of antacids and food. Clin. Pharmacol. Ther. 24, 600–609.

Gruber, C. M. (1955) A theoretical consideration of additive and potentiated effects between drugs with a practical example using alcohol and barbiturates. Arch. Int. Pharmacodyn. Ther. 102, 17.

Gupta, R. C. and Kofoed, J. (1972) Toxicological statistics for barbiturates, other sedatives and tranquillizers in Ontario; a 10 year survey. Can. Med. Assoc. J. 94, 863.

Haglund, K., Seideman, P., Collste, P., Borg, K.O. and von Bahr, C. (1979) Influence of phenobarbital on metoprolol plasma levels. Clin. Pharmacol. Ther. 26, 326–329.

Harris, A. L. (1976) Clonidine withdrawal and blockade (letter). Lancet 1, 596.

Hepner, G. W., Vesell, E. S., Lipton, A., Harvey, H. A., Wilkinson, G. R. and Schenker, S. (1977) Disposition of aminopyrine, antipyrine, diazepam and indocyanine green in patients with liver disease or on anticonvulsant drug therapy; diazepam breath test and correlations in drug elimination. J. Lab. Clin. Med. 90, 440–456.

Houghton, G. W. and Richens, A. (1974) The effect of benzodiazepines and pheneturide on phenytoin metabolism in man. Br. J. Clin. Pharmacol. 1, 344.

Hunter, K. R., Stern, G. M. and Laurence, D. R. (1970) Use of levadopa with other drugs. Lancet 2, 1283–1285.

Janz, D. and Schmidt, D. (1974) Anti-epileptic drugs and failure of oral contraceptives. Lancet 1, 1113.

Jelliffe, R. W. and Blankenhorn, D. H. (1966) Effect of phenobarbital on digitoxin metabolism. Clin. Res. 14, 160.

Jetter, W. W. and McLean, R. (1943) Poisoning by the synergistic effect of phenobarbital and ethyl alcohol, an experimental study. Arch. Pathol. 36, 112.

Kielholz, P., Goldberg, L., Obersteg, J. I., Poldinger, W., Ramseyer, A. and Schmid, P. (1969) Fahrversuche zur frage der beeintrachtigung der verkehrstuchtigkeit durch alkohol, tranquilizer und hypnotika. Dtsch. Med. Wochenschr. 94, 301–306.

Klotz, U., Antonin, K. H. and Bieck, P. (1977) Food intake and plasma binding of diazepam (letter). Br. J. Clin. Pharmacol. 4, 85–86.

Koch-Weser, J. and Sellers, E.M. (1971) Drug interactions with coumarin anticoagulants. N. Engl. J. Med. 285, 547–558.

Korttila, K., Mattila, M. J. and Linnoila, M. (1976) Prolonged recovery after sedation; the influence of food, charcoal ingestion and injection rate on the effects of intravenous diazepam. Br. J. Anaesth. 48, 333–340.

Kotler, M. N., Berman, L. and Rubenstein, A. H. (1966) Hypoglycemia precipitated by propranolol. Lancet 2, 1389–1390.

Kram, J., Bourne, H. R., Melmon, K. L. and Maibach, H. (1974) Propranolol (letter). Ann. Intern. Med. 80, 282.

Kristensen, M., Jorgensen, M. and Hansen, T. (1973a) Plasma concentration of alfamethyldopa and its main metabolite, methyldopa-O-sulfate during long-term treatment with alfamethyl-dopa, with special reference to possible interaction with other drugs given simultaneously (abst.). Clin. Pharmacol. Ther. 14, 139–140.

Kristensen, M., Jorgensen, M. and Hansen, T. (1973b) Barbiturates and methyldopa metabolism (letter). Br. Med. J. 1, 49.

Kuntzman, R. M., Jacobson, M., Levin, W. and Conney, A. H. (1968) Stimulatory effect of N-phenylbarbital (phetharbital) on cortisol hydroxylation in man. Biochem. Pharmacol. 17, 565–571.

Kutt, H. and McDowell, F. (1968) Management of epilepsy with diphenylhydantoin sodium. J. Am. Med. Assoc. 203, 969.

Levin, W., Welch, R. M. and Conney, A. H. (1968) Effect of phenobarbital and other drugs on the metabolism and uterotropic action of estradiol-17B and estrone. J. Pharmacol. Exp. Ther. 159, 362–371.

Levy, G., O'Reilly, R. A., Aggeler, P. M. and Keech, G. M. (1970) Pharmacokinetic analysis of the effect of barbiturate on the anticoagulant action of warfarin in man. Clin. Pharmacol. Ther. 11, 372–377.

Linnoila, M. (1973a) Drug interaction on psychomotor skills related to driving; hypnotics and alcohol. Ann. Exp. Med. Biol. Fenn. 51, 118.

Linnoila, M. (1973b) Effects of diazepam, chlordiazepoxide, thioridazine, haloperidol, flupenthixole and alcohol on psychomotor skills related to driving. Ann. Exp. Med. Biol. Fenn. 51, 125.

Linnoila, M., Otterstrom, S. and Anttila, M.   (1974)   Serum chlordiazepoxide, diazepam and thioridazine concentration after the simultaneous ingestion of alcohol or placebo drink. Ann. Clin. Res. 6, 4–6.

Linnoila, M. and Hakkinen, S.   (1974)   Effects of diazepam and codeine, alone and in combination with alcohol, on simulated driving. Clin. Pharmacol. Ther. 15, 368–373.

Linnoila, M., Korttila, K. and Mattila, M. J.   (1975)   Effect of food and repeated injections on serum diazepam levels. Acta Pharmacol. Toxicol. 36, 181–186.

Lorenc, E.   (1967)   A new factor in griseofulvin treatment failures. Mo. Med. 64, 32–33.

Ludin, H. P. and Dubach, K.   (1971)   Action of diazepam on muscular contraction in man. Neurol. 199, 30–38.

MacDonald, M. G. and Robinson, D. S.   (1968)   Clinical observations of possible barbiturate interference with anticoagulation. J. Am. Med. Assoc. 204, 97.

MacLeod, S. M., Giles, H. G., Patzalek, J. J., Thiessen, J. J. and Sellers, E. M.   (1977)   Diazepam actions and plasma concentrations following ethanol ingestion. Eur. J. Clin. Pharmacol. 11, 345–349.

MacLeod, S. M., Sellers, E. M., Giles, H. G., Billings, B. J., Martin, P. R., Greenblatt, D. J. and Marshman, J. A.   (1978)   Interaction of disulfiram with benzodiazepines. Clin. Pharmacol. Ther. 24, 583–589.

Misra, P. S., Lefevre, A., Ishii, H., Rubin, E. and Lieber, C. S.   (1971)   Increase of ethanol, meprobamate and pentobarbital metabolism after chronic ethanol administration in man and in rats. Am. J. Med. 51, 346–351.

Morland, J., Setekleiv, J., Haffner, J. F. W., Stromsaether, C. E., Danielsen, A. and Holst Wethe, G.   (1974)   Combined effects of diazepam and ethanol on mental and psychomotor functions. Acta Pharmacol. Toxicol. 34, 5–15.

Morselli, P. L., Veneroni, E., Zaccala, M. and Bizzi, A.   (1971)   Further observations on the interaction between ethanol and psychotropic drugs. Arzneim. Forsch. 21, 20–23.

Naylor, G. J. and McHarg, A.   (1977)   Profound hypothermia on combined lithium carbonate and diazepam treatment. Br. Med. J. 2, 22.

Neuvonen, P. J. and Penttila, O.   (1974)   Interaction between doxycycline and barbiturates. Br. Med. J. 1, 535–536.

Ochs, H. R., Carstens, G. and Greenblatt, D. J.   (1980)   Reduction in lidocaine clearance during continuous infusion and by co-administration of propranolol. N. Engl. J. Med. 303. 373–377.

Peet, M., Middlemiss, D. N. and Yates, R. A.   (1981)   Pharmacokinetic interactions between propranolol and chlorpromazine in schizophrenic patients (letter) Lancet 2, 978.

Podolsky, S. and Pattavina, C. G.   (1973)   Coma: a complication of propranolol therapy. Metabolism 22, 685.

Porte, D   (1967)   A receptor mechanism for the inhibition of insulin release by epinephrine in man. J. Clin. Invest. 46, 86–94.

Reisby, N. and Theilgaard, A.   (1969)   The interaction of alcohol and meprobamate in man. Acta Psychiatr. Scand. 208 (Suppl. 5), 1–204.

Riegelman, S., Rowland, M. and Epstein, W.L.   (1970)   Griseofulvin-phenobarbital interaction in man. J. Am. Med. Assoc. 213, 426–431.

Roberton, Y. R. and Johnson, E. S.   (1976)   Interactions between oral contraceptives and other drugs; a review. Curr. Med. Res. Opin. 3, 647–661.

Rubin, E., Gang, H., Misra, P. and Lieber, C. S.   (1970)   Inhibition of drug metabolism by acute ethanol intoxication. Am. J. Med. 49, 801–806.

Saario, I.   (1976)   Psychomotor skills during subacute treatment with thioridazine and bromazepam, and their combined effect with alcohol. Ann. Clinic. Res. 8, 117–123.

Salvador, R. A., April, S. A. and Lemberger, L.   (1967)   Inhibition by butoxamine, propranolol and MJ 1999 of the glycogenolytic action of the catecholamines in the rat. Biochem. Pharmacol. 16, 2037.

175

Siris, J. H., Pippenger, C. E., Werner, W.L. and Masland, R. L. (1974) Anticonvulsant drug-serum levels in psychiatric patients with seizure disorders; effects of certain psychotropic drugs. N.Y. State J. Med. 74, 1554–1556.

Solomon, H. M. and Abrams, W. B. (1972) Interactions between digitoxin and other drugs in man. Am. Heart J. 83, 277–280.

Sotaniemi, E. A., Anttila, M., Pelkonen, O., Jarvensivu, P. and Sundquist, H. (1979) Plasma clearance of propranolol and sotalol and hepatic drug metabolizing enzyme activity. Clin. Pharmacol. Ther. 26, 153–161.

Southren, A. L., Gordon, G. G. and Tochimoto, S. (1969) Effect of N-phenylbarbital (phetharbital) on the metabolism of testosterone and cortisol in man. J. Clin. Endocrinol. Metab. 29, 251–256.

Strauss, F. G., Franklin, S. S. and Lewin, A. J. (1977) Withdrawal of antihypertensive therapy; hypertensive crisis in renovascular hypertension. J. Am. Med. Assoc. 238, 1734–1736.

Taylor, P. J. (1967) Hemorrhage while on anticoagulant therapy precipitated by drug interaction. Ariz. Med. 24, 697.

Tilstone, W. J., Semple, P. F., Lawson, D. H. and Boyle, J. A. (1977) Effects of furosemide on glomerular filtration rate and clearance of practolol, digoxin, cephaloridine, and gentamicin. Clin. Pharmacol. Ther. 22, 389–394.

Udall, J. A. (1970) Warfarin therapy not influenced by meprobamate; a controlled study in nine men. Curr. Ther. Res. 12, 724–728.

Vajda, F. J. E., Prineas, R. J. and Lovell, R. R. H. (1971) Interaction between phenytoin and the benzodiazepines (letter). Br. Med. J. 1, 346.

VanHerwaarden, C. L. A., Binkhorst, R. A., Fennis, J. M. and van 't Laar, A. (1977) Effects of adrenalin during treatment with propranolol and metoprolol (letter). Br. Med. J. 1, 1029.

Varma, D. R., Sharma, K. K. and Arora, R. C. (1976) Response to adrenaline and propranolol in hyperthyroidism (letter). Lancet 1, 260.

Vernon, C. and Sakula, A. (1979) Fatal rebound hypertension after abrupt withdrawal of clonidine and propranolol. Br. J. Clin. Pract. 33, 112–121.

Vestal, R. E., Kornhauser, D. M., Hollifield, J. W. and Shand, D. G. (1979) Inhibition of propranolol metabolism by chlorpromazine. Clin. Pharmacol. Ther. 25, 19–24.

Warren, S. E., Ebert, E., Swerdlin, R. E., Steinberg, S. M. and Stone, R. (1979) Clonidine and propranolol paradoxical hypertension (letter) Arch. Intern. Med. 139, 253.

Watkins, J., Abbott, E. C., Hensby, C. N., Webster, J. and Dollery, C. T. (1980) Attenuation of hypotensive effect of propranolol and thiazide diuretics by indomethacin. Br. Med. J. 281, 702–705.

Webb, S. N. and Bradshaw, E. G. (1971) Diazepam and neuromuscular blocking drugs (letter). Br. Med. J. 3, 640.

Welch, R. M., Levin, R. and Conney, A. H. (1968) Stimulatory effect of phenobarbital on the metabolism in vivo of estradiol-17β and estrone in the rat. J. Pharmacol. Exp. Ther. 160, 171–178.

Whitfield, J. B., Moss, D. W., Neale, G., Orme, M. and Breckenridge, A. (1973) Changes in plasma γ-glutamyl transpeptidase activity associated with alterations in drug metabolism in man. Br. Med. J. 1, 316–318.

Wodak, J., Gilligan, B. S., Veale, J. L. and Dowty, B. J. (1972) Review of 12 months treatment with L-DOPA in Parkinson's disease, with remarks on unusual side effects. Med. J. Aust. 2, 1277–1282.

Wray, R. and Sutcliffe, S. B. J. (1972) Propranolol-induced hypoglycemia and myocardial infarction (letter). Br. Med. J. 2, 592.

Zirkle, G. A.., McAtee, O. B., King, P. D. and VanDyke, R. (1960) Meprobamate and small amounts of alcohol; effects on human ability, coordination, and judgment. J. Am. Med. Assoc. 173, 1823–1825.

Burrows/Norman/Davies (eds) Antianxiety agents
© *Elsevier Science Publishers B.V., 1984*

Chapter 12

Adverse reactions, cardiotoxicity, and management of overdose

RICHARD J. MOLDAWSKY

and

LOUIS A. GOTTSCHALK

Department of Psychiatry and Human Behavior, University of California, Irvine Medical Center,
Orange, CA 92668, U.S.A.

INTRODUCTION

The successful management of a patient's complaint of anxiety depends largely on a thorough diagnostic evaluation. Among other things, one needs to decide whether the anxiety is part of an anxiety disorder per se, part of another psychopathological entity such as schizophrenia, depression, or organic brain syndrome, or whether the anxiety is secondary to an underlying medical illness. One needs to also decide whether the anxiety is part of the stresses of everyday life, in which case antianxiety medication has no role. Once one has decided that antianxiety medication is warranted one has several agents from which to choose.

Rational drug therapy dictates that one should choose agents which are as specific as possible in the successful treatment of the target symptom while minimizing toxicity. At this time, benzodiazepines and beta-adrenoceptor blocking agents most successfully fill this role. Antipsychotics can be effective antianxiety agents but they are not specific to anxiety and have other dangers. For a long time, barbiturates were a mainstay in the treatment of chronic anxiety, but these have an increased risk of addiction, as well as having greater toxicity in overdosage

178

(Wesson and Smith, 1977). Another agent which has a long history of use in these situations is meprobamate and other drugs in that class. Drugs such as these also have a potential for dependence and addiction, as well as an increased toxicity when taken in excessive dosages (Davis, 1981).

While these drugs continue to be used for anxiety (where there is no other major psychopathology), it is generally believed that benzodiazepines and beta-adrenoceptor blocking agents come closest to attaining the ideal of specific antianxiety action and low toxicity (Greenblatt and Shader, 1974; Davis, 1981; Edwards, 1981).

This chapter will describe adverse reactions, cardiotoxicity, and management of overdosage as it applies to the use of benzodiazepines and beta-adrenoceptor blocking agents.

BENZODIAZEPINES

A great deal of clinical and research experience continues to substantiate the belief that benzodiazepines are not only effective as high anxiety agents, but also are quite safe when used in therapeutic dosages (Greenblatt and Shader, 1974; Siassi, 1975; Porter and Lancee, 1978; Richards, 1978; Bellantuono et al., 1980; Korczyn, 1980; Allen and Greenblatt, 1981; Ameer and Greenblatt, 1981; Davis, 1981; Heel et al., 1981; Jerram, 1981). Adverse reactions and cardiotoxicity, as will be described below, tend to be, for the most part, relatively mild and not life-threatening.

Adverse cardiovascular effects

Reviews of the literature (Stimmel, 1979; Edwards, 1981; Risch et al., 1981) suggested that benzodiazepines have virtually no significant effects on the cardiovascular system. It is well known that benzodiazepines have been used with success as antianxiety agents, with concomitant severe acute cardiac illness, such as myocardial infarction. They have been used as adjunctive forms of therapy in cardiac illness, such as arrhythmia requiring cardioversion. They have also been used in angiography and cardiac catheterisation. They do not have a role in the treatment of hypertension.

There are some reports of hypotension as a result of benzodiazepine use (Harrison et al., 1976). This most commonly occurs following intravenous injection of such medications. In most cases, the decrease in blood pressure has no clinical significance.

There have been reports of thrombophlebitis in patients who received intravenous diazepam as a pre-medication for endoscopy (Langdon, 1973). There are some suggestions that the occurrence of thrombophlebitis is not as high in the use of lorazepam and flunitrazepam (Hegarty and Dundee, 1976). In a study of diazepam, mentioned above, the incidence of thrombophlebitis was 3.5 %. One should not inject such medications into an artery for a thrombosis and necrosis can occur (Reed and Normandy, 1980).

There has been an association of ectopic ventricular beats and use of benzodiazepines, though a cause-and-effect relationship has not been documented (Barrett and Hey, 1970).

Respiratory effects

Most of the literature suggests that significant respiratory depression is not a common effect with benzodiazepine use, even in overdosage (Lakshminarayan et al., 1976). This conclusion can only be made, however, for patients who are in good physical health, especially those without significant central nervous system, respiratory, or cardiovascular dysfunction. There are a few reports of respiratory failure induced by benzodiazepines in patients with chronic obstructive pulmonary disease (Clark et al., 1971). Nitrazepam has particularly been shown to aggravate respiratory malfunction in patients with chronic pulmonary disease (Gaddie et al., 1972).

Rapid intravenous injection of benzodiazepines can, however, cause respiratory depression, as well as hypotension and should be avoided even in healthy patients (Korczyn, 1980).

Central nervous system adverse effects

Not surprisingly, the widest variety and severest kind of adverse effects occur in this system.

Probably the commonest mild adverse reaction to benzodiazepines is the degree of excess daytime sedation, particularly with the benzodiazepines with a longer half-life, such as diazepam and chlordiazepoxide (Greenblatt and Shader, 1974; Richards, 1978; Edwards, 1981). Many of these drugs are used as hypnotics while flurazepam has been shown to induce more rapid eye movement (REM) sleep than other hypnotics. Other benzodiazepines do not do this as consistently. One of the results of this appears to be that some patients reported the feeling of 'hangover' (Bond and Lader, 1972). This may partly be the result of REM sleep deprivation or from some other drug effects which are not understood (Harry and Latham, 1980). As a corollary to this, reports of rebound insomnia have been noted when the medication is withdrawn, after even short-term use (Bixler et al., 1978; Kales et al., 1978, 1979). In such cases, reinstitution of the benzodiazepine will diminish the symptom; however, both the physician and the patient may be caught in a vicious cycle with numerous repeated long-term prescriptions of these drugs (see also Chapter 9).

Benzodiazepines have been known to cause anterograde amnesia (Wilson,

1973). This occurs most commonly when benzodiazepines are used intravenously and is sometimes a desired effect, especially before certain diagnostic and therapeutic procedures.

Probably as a direct result of their sedating properties, these drugs can impair psychomotor and mental performance. Reaction time may be increased and vigilance may be decreased. In addition, these drugs have been noted to be able to impair short-term memory. Some patients report difficulty, both subjectively and on objective testing, in consolidating new memory data (Kleinknecht and Donaldson, 1975; Wittenborn, 1979). It may be that some anxious patients perform better when taking these medications as a result of being made less anxious by the drug itself in a specific situation. Nevertheless, frank confusion and disorientation can result, and as is the case with many other kinds of adverse effects, elderly people are more sensitive.

The effect of benzodiazepines on mood has generally been minimal. There have been some reports of depression following use of benzodiazepines, but this is rare (Hall and Jaffe, 1972). Perceptual dysfunctions can occur especially in confused patients and hallucinations may sometimes be reported. These are usually visual.

Syndromes of paradoxical central nervous system effects have been reported (Korczyn, 1980; Jerram, 1981). This can be interpreted as either further central nervous system depression or as a disinhibition, which may take the form of talkativeness, inappropriate social behaviour, and psychomotor agitation. These are most commonly found in young children and in the elderly, especially in situations where other physiological illnesses coexist (Greenblatt et al., 1977b; Korczyn, 1980). In a similar manner there are a few reports of benzodiazepines being implicated in seizure activity (Korczyn, 1980). These have been reported in cases of patients with seizure disorders. Seizure activity was apparently increased while taking benzodiazepines. This was not related to benzodiazepine withdrawal syndrome which will be discussed below. Whereas these drugs usually have anticonvulsant properties this would appear to be a paradoxic effect as well. The reasons are not clear at this time. One particular benzodiazepine, triazolam, has been particularly implicated as a drug in which there is a relatively higher percentage of paradoxic effects than the other benzodiazepines. This medication has a somewhat different structure from the other benzodiazepines, but it is not clear what the mechanism is for triazolam's increased incidence of paradoxic effects. One writer in particular (Van der Kroef, 1979), has recorded a series of patients in which reports of malaise, depression, anxiety, and mood changes have been noted. There has been some concern in the literature that benzodiazepines may increase aggressive behaviour, but the current consensus is that, if anything, these medications decrease aggressive behaviours (Rickels and Downing, 1974; Bond and Lader, 1979).

There are a few reports of benzodiazepines as a possible cause of tardive dyskinesia (Kaplan and Murkofsky, 1978). This would add to a lengthy list of medications which have been implicated in the aetiology of this syndrome, in addition to neuroleptics. While there is a working hypothesis for the development of tardive dyskinesia in neuroleptic drugs, the explanation for such development with the use of benzodiazepines is not forthcoming. While benzodiazepines do appear to have some effects on the gamma-aminobutyric acid (GABA) system, the relationship between that system and the dopaminergic system is yet to be elucidated (Braestrup and Squires, 1978; Haefely, 1978). Some recent research strongly suggests that the benzodiazepine brain receptor is a GABA receptor (Snyder, 1981). These receptors have particularly high concentration in the hippocampus, as well as in areas of the cerebral cortex. Little is understood at this time as to how this system may relate to the dopaminergically mediated tracts, but it has been speculated that in the case of anticonvulsant effects, and perhaps other effects relating to motor activity, that benzodiazepine receptors and, therefore, GABA can modulate neuronal excitability (Snyder, 1981).

Other side effects which appear to be directly the extension of the benzodiazepines' sedating properties in this system include ataxia, vertigo, dizziness, and fatigue (Greenblatt and Shader, 1974; Bellantuono et al., 1980; Korczyn, 1980). A few patients have also reported paraesthesias and nystagmus (Korczyn, 1980). Incidence of such symptoms is always low, considerably below 1%.

It is well known that benzodiazepines exhibit some cross tolerance with alcohol and like alcohol can produce addiction. Within the first 10 days after discontinuation of benzodiazepine therapy it is not uncommon to have withdrawal symptoms which are indistinguishable from those of an alcohol withdrawal syndrome (Preskorn and Denner, 1977; Debard, 1979). One may see headache, seizures, disorientation, abrupt mood change, confusion, hallucinations, paranoia, muscle irritability, tremors, and even coma. It is even possible to see this syndrome in neonates of mothers who habitually use benzodiazepines.

Management of benzodiazepine withdrawal involves reinstitution of benzodiazepines with gradual tapering over a long period of time. Phenobarbital can also be used. It is not uncommon for tolerance to benzodiazepines to occur. And one occasionally hears of remarkably high dosages being used without significant sedation. There is no clear evidence at this time that any one benzodiazepine is more or less prone to induce tolerance or dependence (see also Chapters 8 and 9).

There will be further discussion on central nervous system depression following overdosage with benzodiazepines in the section below on overdoses.

Endocrine and metabolic effects

There are few significant findings in this area. Most of the data are on a case report basis, although one study of 10 patients receiving diazepam revealed a decrease in protein-bound iodine, thyroxine, and free thyroxine (Saldanha et al., 1971). It was suggested that diazepam somehow suppresses thyroid-stimulating hormone. There is no known effect of benzodiazepines on the plasma levels of corticosteroids (Collins et al., 1971).

There is one report of gynaecomastia in a 55-year-old man who had been taking over 80 mg/day of diazepam; the gynaecomastia disappeared when diazepam was withdrawn (Moerck and Magelund, 1979).

Gastrointestinal system

A mild degree of gastrointestinal upset is reported by some patients taking benzodiazepines. Occasionally patients will report constipation, dry mouth, and sometimes hypersalivation (Shader and DiMascio, 1970). One patient who had been receiving clorazepate, 30 mg/day, developed jaundice which resolved completely 5 months after discontinuation of the medication (Parker, 1979). There is some evidence that benzodiazepines can occasionally cause a cholestatic jaundice on a hypersensitivity basis (Shader and DiMascio, 1970). This is a nonspecific, allergic type of reaction that is seen with many other medications.

Dermatological system

Occasionally one will discover a patient with a diffuse rash or urticaria associated with benzodiazepine use in therapeutic dosages (Wintraub and Shiffman, 1979). These are usually time-limited reactions which often respond to discontinuation of the drug or diminution of the dose.

Haematologic system

There are very rare reports of haematological abnormalities attributed to benzodiazepines. Some scattered cases of thrombocytopenia or agranulocytosis have been reported (Cimo et al., 1977).

Effects on pregnancy and lactation

There are now a number of studies and case reports which suggest a teratogenic effect of benzodiazepines (Safra and Oakley, 1975; Korczyn, 1980). There are some significant methodological problems with these studies; nevertheless, one would recommend caution in using such medications, especially during the first trimester of pregnancy. Cleft palate has been the most common abnormality studies in this area (Hartz et al., 1975). This is of course, a relatively common defect in general and this has made it difficult to clarify the cause-and-effect relationship between the drug and the defect.

Use of diazepam during labour usually has a depressant effect upon the infant and hypotonia, decreased sucking, hypothermia, and lower Apgar scores are common (McBride et al., 1979). Since diazepam is a longer-acting drug and metabolic functioning may be immature in the newborn, the effects of diazepam can be felt up to a week or even longer (Greenblatt and Shader, 1974). This clearly has implications for the use of such medications during labour.

Diazepam and other benzodiazepines pass freely in mothers' milk (Cole and Hailey, 1975). As is true in elderly patients, neonates and infants are particularly susceptible to not only toxic but paradoxic effects of these medications and mothers need to be advised accordingly.

Overdosage

It has been said that one of the main advantages of benzodiazepines is their relative safety (Greenblatt et al., 1977). It has been suggested that these drugs are virtually 'suicide-proof'. It is true that it has been difficult to document cases of death directly attributable to benzodiazepines alone in a healthy individual (Finkle et al., 1979). Such deaths have, however, been reported and documented for individuals using chlordiazepoxide, diazepam, and oxazepam (Gottschalk and Cravey, 1980).

Overdosage with benzodiazepines does produce severe central nervous system depression, often leading to coma. There is evidence that the medications do not have the significant respiratory depressive effects of barbiturates and other such medications, and the danger is not as severe. There are no specific features of benzodiazepine-induced coma, which can otherwise aid in its recognition. Cheyne-Stokes breathing is unusual. There is no specific EEG pattern seen in benzodiazepine coma (Greenblatt et al., 1977a; Korczyn, 1980).

There are some suggestions that physostigmine can reverse some of the central nervous system depressant effects (Blitt and Petty, 1975; Larson et al., 1977). Similar claims have been made for naloxone (Bell, 1975). To date, there has been little systematic study of these agents.

Most life-threatening or severe overdosages which involve benzodiazepines also include other agents. Drugs such as tricyclic antidepressants, barbiturates, and other hypnotics present a more imminent danger to life itself, and it is usually necessary to attend to the untoward effects of these medications first. Management of the 'pure' benzodiazepine overdose is largely supportive. There is no specific antidote and a generally supportive approach monitoring respiratory and cardiac functioning will usually suffice. It may also be useful to obtain serial EEGs as a further means of monitoring the return of normal brain functioning. It is important to remember that many of these medications have very long half-lives and the recovery course will be quite slow as a result. The use of stimulant drugs has no place in the management of overdosage, and the body will effectively excrete the toxic substances, albeit slowly.

184

Carcinogenicity

There is no evidence in humans that benzodiazepines have any tumour producing effects. There are a few reports that diazepam facilitated tumour growth in rats in a daily dose of 1 mg/kg of body weight (Guaitani et al., 1979). They also report a similar association of oxazepam in male rats. At this time, consensus is that on the basis of such scanty evidence one need not be concerned about the use of benzodiazepines as it relates to induction of tumour growth or carcinogenicity itself.

BETA-ADRENOCEPTOR BLOCKING DRUGS

Most of the clinical experience with the use of beta-adrenoceptor blocking drugs for the treatment of anxiety has been with propranolol and to a lesser degree, alprenolol. Since the sympathetic nervous system has such a wide variety of roles in the control of physiologic and metabolic function, it should not be surprising that the adverse effects of these medications is also quite varied (Frishman and Silverman, 1979; Carruthers, 1980; Steiner, 1981). It may be useful to consider, as others (Frishman et al., 1980b) have done, the adverse effects of these drugs in two categories: 1) those which appear to be the result of beta-adrenoceptor blockade; and 2) those that do not.

One of the largest major clinical trials that investigated the nature and frequency of side effects was the Boston Collaborative Drug Surveillance Program (Greenblatt and Koch-Weser, 1973). In this program, 319 patients received propranolol primarily for cardiac indications, such as angina and arrhythmias. The average age of the patients was 54 years, half were male and half female. Adverse reactions were noted in 9.4% of these patients. Of these adverse reactions, eight were severe enough to be considered life-threatening and all appeared to be the result of impaired cardiac function. The reactions included pulmonary oedema, bradycardia and shock, complete heart block, and bradycardia and angina. The remainder of the reported reactions were not considered life-threatening, although some did involve impairment of cardiac function, such as, hypotension, bradycardia, and milder forms of heart block. It should be recalled again that these patients were receiving propranolol for cardiac illness, in most cases, and not for anxiety.

In looking at dosage and duration of therapy among these patients, seven of the eight patients who had life-threatening reactions were receiving a daily dose of less than 40 mg/day; there was no direct relationship between dosage and the non-life-threatening reactions. Four of the eight life-threatening reactions occurred within 24 hours of initiation of therapy.

Adverse reactions seemed to be more common among older patients and in patients with azotemia. Other factors, such as sex, specific hospital location, diagnosis, indication for propranolol and other cardioactive drugs did not appear to affect the frequencies of these reactions.

There are some other large studies (Collins and King, 1972; Forrest, 1972; Lubbe, 1978) which investigate the frequency and severity of adverse reactions in other beta-blocking agents, and there appears to be a similar distribution in terms of frequency and severity. The Boston report, for example, reviews 199 patients who received practolol and finds a similar ratio of life-threatening to non-life-threatening adverse reactions, approximately 10%.

Cardiac adverse effects

Adverse cardiac side effects are most common in patients with compromised cardiac functioning, and patients with untreated congestive heart failure should not be given beta-blockers under any circumstances (Frishman et al., 1980b). Also, in any patient with an enlarged heart and impaired myocardial functioning, in which excessive sympathetic stimulation is necessary to maintain compensation, the risk of inducing heart failure is markedly increased. There have been reports of major complications in the use of beta-blockers for the treatment of hypertensive heart failure and heart failure secondary to hyperthyroidism (Laake, 1981). One would withhold beta-blockers in this circumstance as well. If such an agent were deemed clinically indicated, digitalis and diuretics should be used first, before the beta-blocker is added.

To restate the main point, then, congestive heart failure can be precipitated with administration of beta-adrenergic blockers, particularly in patients with already compromised cardiac functioning.

The bradycardia that often occurs with treatment with beta-blockers usually is not symptomatic; however, progressive degrees of atrioventricular dissociation may occur. Again, if there is already a partial or complete conduction defect, then use of such drugs may lead to a serious bradycardia. Propranolol has been implicated in such effects. Other beta-blockers, however, such as pindolol or practolol, do not appear to impair atrioventricular conduction (Laake, 1981).

In a few instances severe hypotension and shock have occurred; again these have been reported in patients with already severely compromised cardiac functioning. Should these occur, the beta-blocking drug should be immediately discontinued and beta-agonist therapy would be indicated, such as isoproterenol.

There has also been some recent concern as to whether acute chest pain can be caused by a beta-blockade. In a series of 296 elderly patients hospitalized with suspected myocardial infarction (Pathy, 1979), 35 patients thoroughly investigated for causes of chest pain remained undiagnosed. It appeared that their chest pain was associated with long-term treatment with beta-blockers. The pain was described as intense and indistinguishable from that of a myocardial infarction. In none of these patients was there significant hypotension or electrocardiographic changes. One hypothesis here may be that coronary artery spasm may have caused the pain; another is that beta-blockers induced a lower cardiac output causing pain. A third alternative has been suggested. Some beta-blockers, particularly alprenolol, can induce an oesophagitis by adhering to the mucosa of the oesophagus, causing inflammation and spasm (Laake, 1981).

It has become well known that a syndrome of beta-adrenoceptor blocker withdrawal exists (Miller et al., 1975; Frishman et al., 1978). Abrupt cessation of beta-blocker therapy after chronic use has led to exacerbation of angina and occasionally acute myocardial infarction. Malignant tachycardias and sudden deaths have been reported as well. Less severe forms of beta-blocker withdrawal include symptoms such as palpitations, tremor, and diaphoresis. It happens most commonly in patients with coronary artery disease and does not appear to be related to the kind of beta-blocker used. Most of the information, however, is based on experience with propranolol.

These findings suggest that there is a form of catecholamine hyperactivity when beta-blockers are discontinued. It has been noted that serum triiodothyronine (T_3) concentrations increase when beta-blockers are discontinued, and some of these symptoms do also appear to be those of hyperthyroidism (Shenkman et al., 1977; Verhoeven et al., 1977). It has also been demonstrated that abrupt withdrawal of beta-blocking agents can cause a hyperaggregability of platelets (Frishman, 1979); this causes an increased production of prostaglandin and, therefore, constriction of coronary arteries resulting in further symptoms of angina. Clinical work-to-date suggests that hypersensitivity of the catecholamine receptors can be blocked by continuing to give beta-blockers in small dosages, such as 10–20 mg of propranolol per day. However, the surest way to avoid this syndrome is to taper beta-blockers gradually and cautiously, especially in patients with ischaemic heart disease.

Adverse respiratory effects

It has been shown that the beta$_2$-adrenoceptors have a bronchodilating effect, and that nonselective beta-blocking agents such as propranolol can block such bronchodilation and, hence, lead to bronchospasm in certain types of patients. However, beta-blockers which are more selectively active on the myocardium are less likely to induce this effect (Frishman et al., 1980b).

Patients with pre-existing pulmonary disease are at an increased risk to develop pulmonary complications from beta-blocker use. Life-threatening bronchospasm has been reported in many patients with asthma or chronic obstructive pulmonary disease and, therefore, all beta-adrenoceptor blocking agents should be used with utmost caution, if at all, in such patients (Richardson and Sterling, 1979).

Some attention has been paid to the interaction of smoking and the use of such drugs. Tobacco smoking causes an increase in adrenaline secretion. This stimulates adrenergic alpha and beta receptors. With beta receptors being blocked the unopposed alpha-adrenergic stimulation may lead to hypertension. It has also been shown that smoking can reduce the effect of treatment of angina with propranolol by this mechanism (Fox et al., 1980). It has been suggested that beta$_1$ selective agents are preferable to the nonselective beta agents. However, this must be weighed against the initial clinical indication for the beta-blocker.

Other findings have been noted but their clinical significance is not yet clear. Healthy subjects given propranolol were found to have a decreased ventilatory response to increasing concentrations of carbon dioxide (Fraley et al., 1980). There is another report of laryngospasm which was attributed to ingestion of propranolol (Laake, 1981); it was however, suggested that the tartrazine dye that is used in the preparation of the propranolol may have been the aetiologic agent.

Peripheral vascular effects

Symptoms of cold hands and feet and diminished or absent pulses have been observed in patients receiving beta-blockers (Greenblatt and Koch-Weser, 1973; Frishman et al., 1980b). Propranolol seems to have the highest incidence of this particular finding. In most cases it is relatively mild and of little concern, and warm clothing will suffice. In a few cases the decreased blood flow has been severe enough to induce cyanosis and even gangrene (Vale et al., 1977). Once again, it should be recalled that patients with impaired cardiac functioning will be more sensitive to such an effect. The combination of reduced cardiac output and decreased peripheral vascular resistence will result in unopposed alpha-adrenoceptor stimulation.

A recent review of the literature (Eliasson et al., 1978) suggests that between 1% and 6% of patients treated with beta-blockers will develop Raynaud's syndrome. In these patients there was no suggestion of a collagen vascular disease.

Some patients with peripheral vascular disease have reported aggravation of symptoms of intermittent claudication (Frolich et al., 1969; Rodger et al., 1976). It is very difficult in such cases to be sure that the beta-blocker is the aggravating agent, since many of these patients have both ischaemic heart disease and peripheral vascular disease. It is not yet known whether cardio-selective beta-blocking agents will protect against this syndrome more than propranolol.

Effects on glucose metabolism

There have been several reports of severe hypoglycaemic reactions during propranolol therapy. Some of these patients were diabetics dependent on insulin; others were non-diabetic (Abramson et al., 1966; Helgeland et al., 1978).

It is known that beta$_2$ stimulation causes mobilisation of glycogen from muscle; mobilisation of glycogen from liver is alpha-mediated. Therefore, the hypoglycaemia caused by insulin can be more severe and of longer duration in persons who are receiving beta-blocking drugs. There would be delayed return of blood sugar to normal in such hypoglycaemia (Allison et al., 1969; Lloyd-Mostyn and Oram, 1975; Deacon et al., 1977). In patients whose glycogen stores are somewhat depleted by fasting or illness, co-administration of beta-blocking agents may retard such recovery (Lager et al., 1979).

Since many of the symptoms of hypoglycaemia are mediated through adrenergic stimulation, the subjective awareness of hypoglycaemia may be decreased. Palpitations, tachycardia, tremor, and diaphoresis are common symptoms of hypoglycaemia and they may not be recognized by the patient receiving beta-adrenoceptor blocking agents. Such people would, in a sense, have to relearn how to recognize hypoglycaemic reactions and symptoms in themselves.

Central nervous system effects

The most common kinds of central nervous system adverse effects are: fatigue, weakness, light headedness, and dizziness (Greenblatt and Koch-Weser, 1973; Carruthers, 1980; Steiner, 1981). In some of these cases these symptoms may be directly the result of decreased cardiac output. In some other cases, however, they may be the effect of direct action of the beta-adrenoceptor antagonists on the central nervous system (Gottschalk, 1981). A variety of other symptoms have been reported, though less frequently (Bengsston et al., 1980). These include: sleep disturbances, hallucinations, extremely vivid dreams, illusions, and depression (Fitzgerald, 1977; Fleminger, 1978). It is very difficult to prove cause-and-effect relationships between such drugs and the more mild psychological symptoms. When such medications are used to treat a psychological symptom such as anxiety, the picture becomes even more obscure. One large study (Bengsston et al., 1980) of 1,302 women investigated such reactions. No significance was noted in the percentage of women reporting sleep disturbances on or off beta-blockers, nor was a significant difference found when nightmares, tiredness, and depression were studied. It may be tentatively concluded from this study that the relationship between beta-blockers and such symptoms is relatively weak.

Some more severe central nervous system reactions have been reported, including psychosis (Kuhr, 1979; Kurland, 1979; Remick et al., 1981). There has been a report of psychosis induced in a 21-year-old healthy woman with no prior psychiatric history (Gershon et al., 1979). There is some suggestion that a 'typical' propranolol psychosis may exist in which a visual hallucination is a very common symptom, as are disorientation and confusion. It does appear, however, that such a presentation has the characteristics of other organic psychoses as well, and a careful mental status examination should be able to differentiate organic from nonorganic psychosis. Not all such psychoses appear to be observed in the first few days of treatment; some have been observed in more long-term treatment, and there is some suggestion that the complication may be related to the rate of increase in dose rather than to the daily dose itself. So far, discontinuation of the beta-adre-noceptor blocking agent that is suspected has always been followed by a marked improvement in the clinical mental status.

Five cases have been reported in which patients receiving pindolol have develop-ed tremor (Hod et al., 1979). This is surprising in view of beta-blockers having been used for the treatment of tremor (Kirk et al., 1973).

There is some association of propranolol and sexual dysfunction in males (Knarr, 1976). It has been difficult to differentiate whether the effects reported are related to peripheral vascular difficulties or centrally acting effects. Neverthe-less, a study of 46 males (Burnett and Chahine, 1979) receiving propranolol for a cardiovascular disease, with no prior history of sexual difficulties, reported the following: complete absence of erections in 7 cases, decreased potency in 13, and decreased libido with normal erections in 2. This was an uncontrolled study; the percentages, however, are quite remarkable. Further studies with careful sexual histories may shed more light on this area.

Gastrointestinal adverse reactions

Overall, between 5 and 10% of patients receiving beta-adrenoceptor blocking agents report mild gastrointestinal symptoms. Diarrhoea, nausea, indigestion, and constipation are most commonly seen (Carruthers, 1980; Frishman et al., 1980b; Steiner, 1981). Usually a change to a different agent or a reduction in dose will relieve these symptoms satisfactorily. A few patients have noted an increase in weight (Laake, 1981). This has been reported with several different beta-blocker agents and the mechanism is not clear. Nevertheless, diuretics have been useful in relieving it.

Allergic and fibrosing disorders

Use of the agent practolol has been implicated in an autoimmune reaction, which has been associated with positive antinuclear antibodies. This syndrome has been referred to as the oculomucocutaneous syndrome (Waal-Manning, 1975; Behan et al., 1976). This syndrome is comprised of a set of eye, skin, ear, and gastrointes-tinal changes which may occur in varying combinations.

The eye symptoms are manifested by a 'gritty' feeling in the eye that can lead to conjunctivitis and keratitis (Wright, 1975). In some cases, the eye changes can be quite severe with corneal damage. A pruritic rash may occur involving the palms and soles of the feet with psoriatic-like plaques appearing. Hearing loss or occa-sional deafness have been noted.

The gastrointestinal syndrome takes the form of sclerosing peritonitis (Windsor et al., 1975; Marshall et al., 1977; Harty, 1978). This disorder usually presents with signs and symptoms suggestive of bowel obstruction. The peritoneum becomes covered with a layer of plaques, but this is usually not discovered until a laparotomy or an autopsy. There is usually massive fibrosis of the small intestine. Ileus is occasionally seen.

An associated finding has been a high incidence of antimitochondrial antibodies in patients receiving beta-blocking agents (Behan et al., 1976). To date, this does not appear to be a clinically significant finding. Anti-mitochondrial antibodies are associated, however, with primary biliary cirrhosis, which has also been associated with autoimmune diseases, such as systemic lupus erythematosus (Harrison et al., 1976; Brown et al., 1978).

The oculomucocutaneous syndrome with or without sclerosing peritonitis appears to be a consequence of long-term treatment with beta-adrenoceptor blocking agents. There is some evidence that there is a causal relationship between the use of acebutolol and increasing titres of anti-nuclear antibody (Booth et al., 1980), and this agent should probably not be given to patients with a history of autoimmune disease.

To date, management of the syndrome has been possible with topical and systemic corticosteroids with antibiotic eye drops and artificial tear solutions as needed. While the syndrome has been well documented for patients receiving practolol, it appears to be exceedingly rare in patients receiving propranolol. Nevertheless, it will be necessary to be watchful for such symptoms, even in patients receiving propranolol.

Other endocrine and metabolic effects

There is an association of hyperkalaemia and usage of beta-adrenoceptor blocking agents. Investigators have studied timolol and found a mild potassium increase (Pedersen and Mikkelsen, 1978). They also found a mild increase in serum uric acid. The significance of this is not yet clear, but it may be that the beta-blocking agents can counteract the hypokalaemic effects of diuretics and aggravate the hyperuricaemic effects.

There is also a suggestion that propranolol and other such agents may increase serum triglycerides (Beinart et al., 1979). This has been noted with atenolol, pindolol, and propranolol. Other miscellaneous endocrine and metabolic changes have included increased plasma phosphate concentrations with propranolol and enhanced release of melanocyte-stimulating hormone (Harrower and Strong, 1977). One patient developed hypermelanosis but did not have increased ACTH or MSH.

Carcinogenicity

Pronethalol was the first beta-adrenoceptor blocking drug in widespread use. It was later withdrawn by its makers because it was found to cause lymphosarcomas and thymic tumours in mice though not in larger animals (Paget, 1963). Later two other beta-adrenoceptor blocking drugs were withdrawn for similar reasons. Alprenolol and practolol have also been implicated in causing tumours in rats (Steiner, 1981). There has been no suggestion yet of malignant tumour development in man related to use of such medications, and in fact, many beta-blocking agents have been rigorously tested for carcinogenicity and found to have none.

Miscellaneous other reactions

The use of such agents in patients with renal disease is a matter of some concern. As these agents may decrease cardiac output and, therefore, renal perfusion, it may be necessary to carefully monitor creatinine clearance in such patients and discontinue the medication if creatinine clearance falls (Swainson and Winney, 1976).

There has been at least one report of alopecia of the scalp. This was associated with propranolol (Martin et al., 1973). Muscle cramps and muscular weakness have been reported as has myopathy (Blessing and Walsh, 1977). Thrombocytopenia has been reported and so has purpura (Laake, 1981). There has also been a case of agranulocytosis with propranolol (Laake, 1981).

Hypertension has been seen in patients with pheochromocytoma who received labetalol (Laake, 1981). There has also been a case of drug fever reported with oxprenolol (Steiner, 1981).

Use in pregnancy and lactation

Propranolol and other beta-blockers cross the placenta (Carruthers, 1980), but so far there has been little to suggest a teratogenic effect. While there has been some concern that such agents would reduce placental blood flow the evidence for the clinical significance of this is small. One study (Pruyn et al., 1979) followed 12 pregnancies in 10 women who were receiving propranolol on a long-term basis for arrhythmia. While one of the babies was born with a significant bradycardia, and three of the babies had mild hypoglycaemia, there was nothing else to suggest a role for propranolol in any untoward effects in these babies. They did, however, tend to be smaller than normal, though not to a marked degree. As is the case with most medications, it is generally best to avoid such agents if possible during pregnancy. If these agents are deemed necessary, then these women should probably be thought of as high risk pregnancies.

Propranolol and other beta-adrenoceptor blocking agents transfer readily to milk (Sandstrom, 1980). The actual amount of available propranolol is limited by its extensive protein binding and, to date, there have been no reports of adverse effects on children of lactating mothers. One would, however, expect that children with moderately compromised cardiovascular status or extremely poor liver functioning may be more sensitive even to minute amounts of propranolol.

Management of overdosage

The major clinical problems in management of overdosage with beta-adrenoceptor blocking drugs are directly the result of the pharmacologic action of the medications (Frishman, 1979). Therefore, hypotension, bradycardia, prolonged atrioventricular conduction times, and symptoms of decreased cardiac functioning are of prime concern (Frishman et al., 1980a). Cardiac failure and cardiogenic shock may be seen, as may bronchospasm and even respiratory depression as a result of decreased cerebral perfusion or a more centrally acting effect (Richards and Prichard, 1978; Buiumsohn et al., 1979).

Since all beta-blocking compounds are rapidly absorbed from the gastrointestinal tract, symptoms will appear relatively rapidly, within 1 to 2 hours. While the half-life of these drugs is between 12 and 24 hours, a decreased cardiac output can increase the plasma half-life to a marked degree.

There is usually a disturbance in consciousness, as well, which can range from delirium to coma. While seizures may be seen, they are not typical.

Electrocardiographic monitoring usually reveals the disturbance in conduction. First degree heart block and bradycardia are most common, and sometimes intraventricular conduction deficits can be seen. There can be a widening of the QRS complex, and occasionally, acute pulmonary oedema (Buiumsohn et al., 1979).

Use of plasma drug levels of beta-adrenoceptor blockers has not been well correlated with the degree of intoxication (Frishman et al., 1980a). The degree of variability of the patient's underlying medical status and resting level of sympathetic tone and metabolism have not made monitoring of plasma levels sufficiently useful. One should also be reminded that most serious overdoses are combinations of medications, and while it is not common clinical experience for beta-adrenoceptor blocking drug overdoses to be fatal by themselves, polydrug overdoses are much more dangerous.

Usually when the patient has been brought to medical attention, recovery has been successful. Most lethal overdoses have been in cases where the individual never received medical treatment.

To summarize the main clinical features again, they are: bradycardia, hypotension, shock, some respiratory depression, disturbances of consciousness, and sometimes convulsions. When death does occur, it is usually due to asystole. For most significant overdosages with these drugs, intensive care unit-type monitoring is necessary; several days are often required.

Gastric lavage and induced vomiting may allow recovery of some uningested tablets; however, since these drugs are absorbed rapidly by the gastrointestinal tract, one cannot expect to recover significant amounts of drug. Propranolol is over 95% protein-bound and, therefore, haemodialysis as a means of decreasing the circulating drug is of little use.

Cardiac monitoring is necessary for discovery of atrioventricular conduction defects and bradycardia (Frishman et al., 1980a). If these occur atropine is the drug of choice and can be given intravenously in dosages of 0.5–3.0 mg in adults or 50 μg/kg in children. If this is not successful, isoproterenol may be given intravenously, at a rate of 4 μg/min. Large doses of this medication have been used at times, and in one report, 115 mg was used. Pulse and blood pressure will have to be monitored for this antidote has vasodilating properties. If hypotension is severe, alpha-adrenergic agents may be necessary, such as noradrenaline or dopamine. In those patients who are not more responsive to isoproterenol, glucagon may be necessary and can be given in an initial bolus of 50 μg/kg followed by continuous infusion of 1–5 mg/hr. If heart block or severe bradycardia cannot be controlled, a pacemaker may be indicated.

Usually the amount of respiratory depression is not significant; however, isoproterenol inhalation or aminophylline may be necessary if tidal volume is not adequate.

Hypoglycaemia as a complication of overdosage is rare, but can, of course, be treated with glucose or glucagon.

Grand mal seizures are usually the result of hypotension, hypoxia, or hypoglycaemia, and if underlying conditions such as these are adequately treated, the seizures will be controlled. However, some of these agents may be central nervous system depressants and can cause seizures on that basis. Intravenous diazepam is usually effective in controlling seizure activity.

As noted earlier, patients with compromised cardiac functioning are more susceptible to withdrawal symptoms from abrupt cessation of beta-adrenoceptor blockers. It should be noted that in such patients who do overdose, the risk for such withdrawal effects may be increased.

REFERENCES

Abramson, E. A., Arky, R. A. and Woeber, K. A. (1966) Effect of propranolol on the hormonal and metabolic responses to insulin-induced hypoglycaemia. Lancet 2, 1386–1389.

Allen, M. D. and Greenblatt, D. J. (1981) Hypnotics and sedatives. In: M. N. G. Dukes (Ed.), Side Effects of Drugs. Excerpta Medica, Amsterdam.

Allen, M. D., Greenblatt, D. J., LaCasse, Y. and Shaden, R. I. (1980) Pharmacokinetic study of lorazepam overdosage. Am. J. Psychiatry 137, 1414–1415.

Allison, S. P., Chamberlain, M. J., Miller, J. E., Ferguson, R., Gillett, A. P., Bemand, B. V. and Saunders, R. A. (1969) Effects of propranolol on blood sugar, insulin and free fatty acids. Diaketologia 5, 339–372.

Ameer, B. and Greenblatt, D. J. (1981) Lorazepam: a review of its clinical pharmaological properties and therapeutic uses. Drugs 21, 161–200.

Barrett, J. S. and Hey, F. B. (1970) Ventricular arrhythmias associated with the use of diazepam for cardioversion. J. Am. Med. Assoc. 214, 1323–1324.

Behan, P. O., Behan, W. M. H., Zacharias, F. J. and Nicholls, J. T. (1976) Immunological abnormalities in patients who had the oculomucocutaneous syndrome associated with practolol therapy. Lancet 2, 984–989.

Beinart, I. W., Cramp, D. G., Pearson, R. M. and Havard, C. W. H. (1979) The effect of metoprolol or plasma lipids. Postgrad. Med. J. 55, 709–714.

Bell, E. F. (1975) The use of naloxone in the treatment of diazepam poisoning. J. Pediatr. 87, 803–806.

Bellantuono, C., Reggi, V., Tognoni, G. and Garattini, S. (1980) Benzodiazepines: clinical pharmacology and therapeutic use. Drugs 19, 195–219.

Bengsston, C., Lennartsson, J., Lindquist, O., Noppa, H. and Biurdsson, J. (1980) Sleep disturbances, nightmares and other possible central nervous disturbances in a population sample of women. Eur. J. Clin. Pharmacol.

Bixler, E. D., Kales, A., Soldatos, C. R., Scharf, M. B., and Kales, J. D. (1978) Effectiveness of temazepam with short, intermediate, and long-term use: sleep laboratory evaluation. J. Clin. Pharmacol. 18, 110–118.

Blessing, W. and Walsh, J. C. (1977) Myotonia precipitated by propranolol therapy. Lancet 1, 73.

Blitt, C. D. and Petty, W. C. (1975) Reversal of lorazepam delirium by physostigmine. Anesth. Analg. Curr. Res. 54, 607–611.

Bond, A. J. and Lader, M. H. (1972) Residual effects of hypnotics. Psychopharmacology. 25, 117–132.

Bond, A. J. and Lader, M. H. (1979) Benzodiazepines and aggression. In: M. Sandler (Ed.), Psychopharmacology of Aggression. Raven Press, New York.

Booth, R. F., Bullock, J. Y. and Wilson, J. D. (1980) Antinuclear antibodies in patients on acebutolol. Br. J. Clin. Pharmacol. 9, 515–522.

Braestrup, C. and Squires, R. F. (1978) Brain-specific benzodiazepine receptors. Br. J. Psychiatry 133, 249–260.

Brown, P. J. E., Lesna, M., Hamlyn, A. N. and Record, C. Q. (1978) Primary biliary cirrhosis after long-term practolol administration. Br. Med J. 1, 1591–1594.

Buiumsohn, A., Evenberg, E., Jacos, H. and Frishman, D. H. (1979) Seizures and intraventricular conduction defect in propranolol poisoning. Ann. Int. Med. 91, 860–862.

Burnett, W. E. and Chahine, R. A. (1979) Sexual dysfunction as a complication of propranolol therapy in men. Cardiovasc. Med. 4, 811–814.

Carruthers, S. G. (1980) Anti-anginal and beta-adrenoceptor blocking agents. In: M.N.G. Dukes (Ed.), Meyler's Side Effects of Drugs. Excerpta Medica, Amsterdam.

Cimo, P. L., Pisciotta, A. V., Desai, R. G., Pino, J. L. and Aster, R. H. (1977) Detection of drug-dependent antibodies by the ^{51}Cr platelet lysis test. Am. J. Hematol. 2, 65–76.

Clark, T. J. H., Collins, J. U. and Tong, D. (1971) Respiratory depression caused by nitrazepam in patients with respiratory failure. Lancet 2, 737–741.

Cole, A. P. and Hailey, D. M. (1975) Diazepam and active metabolite in breast milk and their transfer to the neonate. Arch. Dis. Child 50, 741–742.

Collins, I. S. and King, I. W. (1972) Pindolol, a new treatment for hypertension. Curr. Ther. Res. 14, 185–194.

Collins, J. V., Harris P. W. R., Townsend, J., Clark, T. J. H. and Goulding, R. (1971) Plasma 11-hydroxycorticosteroid levels in drug-induced coma. Lancet 2, 184–187.

Conolly, M. E., Kersting, F. and Dollery, C. T. (1976) The clinical pharmacology of beta-adrenoceptor blocking drugs. Prog. Cardiovasc. Dis. 19, 203–234.

Davis, J. M. (1981) Minor tranquilizers, sedatives and hypnotics. In: H. I. Kaplan, A. M. Freedman and B. J. Sadock (Eds), Comprehensive Textbook of Psychiatry, 3rd edn. Williams and Wilkins, Baltimore.

Deacon, S. P., Karunanayake, A. and Barnett, D. (1977) Acebutolol, atenolol, and propranolol and metabolic responses to acute hypoglycemia in diabetics. Br. Med. J. 2, 1255–1261.

Debard, M. L. (1979) Diazepam withdrawal syndrome. Am. J. Psychiatry 136, 104–105.

Edwards, J. G. (1981) Adverse effects of antianxiety drugs. Drugs 22, 495–514.

Eliasson, K., Lins, L. E. and Sundquist, K.   (1978)   Vasospastic phenomena in patients treated with beta-adrenoceptor blocking agents. Acta Med. Scand. Suppl. 628, 39–49.

Finkle, S. S., McCloskey, V. L. and Goodman, L. S.   (1979)   Diazepam and drug-associated deaths. J. Am. Med. Assoc. 242, 429–434.

Fitzgerald, J. D.   (1967)   Propranolol-induced depression. Br. Med. J. 2, 372–373.

Fleminger, R.   (1978)   Visual hallucinations and illusions with propranolol. Br. Med. J. 1, 1182.

Forrest, W. A.   (1972)   A monitored release study: a clinical trial of exprenolol in general practice. Practitioner 208, 412–416.

Fox, K., Jonathan, A., Williams, H. and Selwyn, A.   (1980)   Interaction between cigarettes and propranolol in treatment of angina pectoris. Br. Med. J. 2, 191–198.

Fraley, D. S., Bruns, F. J., Siegel, D. P. and Adler, S.   (1980)   Propranolol-related bronchospasm in patients without history of asthma. South. Med. J. 73, 238–241.

Frishman, W. H.   (1979)   Clinical pharmacology of the new beta-adrenergic blocking drugs, part I; pharmacodynamics and pharmacokinetic properties. Am. Heart J. 97, 663–671.

Frishman, W. H. and Silverman, R.   (1979)   Clinical pharmacology of the new beta-adrenergic blocking drugs, part II; physiologic and metabolic effects. Am. Heart J. 97, 797–811.

Frishman, W. H., Christodoulou, J., Weksler, B., Smithen, C., Killip, T. and Scheidt, S.   (1978)   Abrupt propranolol withdrawal in angina pectoris: effects on platelet aggregation and exercise tolerance. Am. Heart J. 95, 169–181.

Frishman, W. H., Jacob, H., Eisenberg, E. and Ribner, H.   (1980a)   Self-poisoning with beta-adrenoceptor blocking drugs. In: W.H. Frishman (Ed.), The Clinical Pharmacology of Beta-adrenoceptor Blocking Drugs. Appleton Century Crofts, New York.

Frishman, W. H., Silverman, R., Strom, J. and Elkayam, U.   (1980b)   Adverse effects. In: W.H. Frishman (Ed.), The Clinical Pharmacology of Beta-adrenoceptor Blocking Drugs. Appleton Century Crofts, New York.

Frolich, E. D., Tarazi, R. C. and Dustan, H. P.   (1969)   Peripheral arterial insufficiency: a complication of beta-adrenergic blocking therapy. J. Am. Med. Assoc. 208, 2471–2472.

Gaddie, J., Legge, J. S., Palmer, K. N. U., Petrie, J. C. and Wood, R. A.   (1972)   Effect of nitrazepam in chronic obstructive bronchitis. Br. Med. J. 2, 688–693.

Gershon, E. S., Goldstein, R. E., Moss, A. J. and Van Kammen, D. P.   (1979)   Psychoses with ordinary doses of propranolol. Ann. Int. Med. 90, 938–941.

Gottschalk, L. A.   (1981)   Central and peripheral nervous system mechanisms accounting for psychological and behavioral effects of beta-adrenergic receptor antagonists. Presented at the Second International Bayer Beta-Blocker Symposium, Venice, Italy, October 16–17, 1981.

Gottschalk, L. A. and Cravey, R. H.   (1980)   Toxicological and Pathological Studies on Psychoactive Drug-Involved Deaths. Biomedical Publications, Davis, CA.

Granville-Grossman, K. L. and Turner, P.   (1966)   The effect of propranolol on anxiety. Lancet 1, 788-790.

Greenblatt, D. J. and Koch-Weser, J.   (1973)   Adverse reactions to propranolol in hospitalized medical patients: a report from the Boston Collaborative Drug Surveillance Program. Am. Heart J. 86, 478–488.

Greenblatt, D. J. and Shader, R. I.   (1974)   Benzodiazepines in Clinical Practice. Raven Press, New York.

Greenblatt, D. J., Allen, M. D., Noel, B. J. and Shader, R. I.   (1977a)   Acute overdosage with benzodiazepine derivatives. Clin. Pharmacol. Ther. 21, 497–514.

Greenblatt, D. J., Allen, M. D. and Shader, R. I.   (1977b)   Toxicity of high-dose flurazepam in the elderly. Clin. Pharmacol. Ther. 21, 355-361.

Guaitani, A., Carli, M., Rochetti, M. and Garattini, S.   (1979)   Diazepam and experimental tumour growth. Lancet 1, 1147.

Haefely, W. E.   (1978)   Central actions of benzodiazepines, Br. J. Psychiatry 133, 231–238.

Hall, R. and Jaffe, J. (1972) Aberrant response to diazepam: a new syndrome. Am. J. Psychiatry 129, 738–741.

Harrison, D. C., Markiewicz, W., Hunt, S. and Alderman, E. L. (1976) Circulatory effects of diazepam. J. Clin. Pharmacol. 16, 637–644.

Harrison, T., Sisca, T. S. and Wood, W. W. (1976) Propranolol-induced lupus syndrome. Postgrad. Med. 59, 241–243.

Harrower, A. D. B. and Strong, J. A. (1977) Hyperpigmentation associated with oxprenolol administration. Br. Med. J. 2, 296–297.

Harry, T. V. A. and Latham, A. N. (1980) Hypnotic and residual effects of temazepam in volunteers. Br. J. Clin. Pharmacol. 9, 618–620.

Harty, R. F. (1978) Sclerosing peritonitis and propranolol. Arch. Int. Med. 138, 1424–1427.

Hartz, S. C., Heinonen, O. P., Shapiro, S., Siskind, V. and Slone, D. (1975) Antenatal exposure to meprobamate and chlordiazepoxide in relation to malformations, mental development, and childhood mortality. N. Engl. J. Med. 292, 726–728.

Heel, R. C., Brogden, R. N., Speight, T. M. and Every, G. S. (1981) Temazepam: a review of its pharmacological properties and therapeutic efficacy as a hypnotic. Drugs 21, 321–340.

Hegarty, J. E. and Dundee, J. U. (1977) Sequelae after the intravenous injection of three benzodiazepines-diazepam, lorazepam, and flunitrazepam. Br. Med. J. 2, 1384–1391.

Helgeland, A., Hjermann, I., Leren, P. and Holme, I. (1978) Possible metabolic side effects of beta-adrenergic blocking drugs. Br. Med. J. 1, 828–831.

Hod, H., Har-Zahav, J., Kaplinsky, N. and Frankl, O. (1980) Pindolol-induced tremor. Postgrad. Med. J. 156, 346–348.

Jefferson, J. W. (1974) Beta-adrenergic receptor blocking drugs in psychiatry. Arch. Gen. Psychiatry 31, 681–691.

Jerram, T. C. (1981) Hypnotics and sedatives. In: M.N.G. Dukes (Ed.), Side Effects of Drugs Annual 5. Excerpta Medica, Amsterdam.

Kales, A., Scharf, M. B. and Kales, J. D. (1978) Rebound insomnia: a new clinical syndrome. Science 201, 1039–1041.

Kales, A., Scharf, M. B., Kales, J. D. and Soldatos, C. R. (1979) Rebound insomnia: a potential hazard following withdrawal of certain benzodiazepines. J. Am. Med. Assoc. 241, 1692–1697.

Kaplan, S. R. and Murkofsky, C. (1978) Oral-buccal dyskinesia symptoms associated with low-dose benzodiazepine treatment. Am. J. Psychiatry 135, 1558–1559.

Khatzian, E. J. and McKenna, C. J. (1979) Acute toxic and withdrawal reactions associated with drug use and abuse. Ann. Int. Med. 90, 361–368.

Kirk, L., Baastrup, P. C. and Schou, M. (1973) Propranolol treatment of lithium-induced tremor. Lancet 2, 1086–1087.

Kleinknecht, R. A. and Donaldson, D. (1975) A review of the effects of diazepam on cognitive and psychomotor performance. J. Nerv. Ment. Dis. 161, 399–411.

Knarr, J. W. (1976) Impotence from propranolol. Ann. Int. Med. 75, 259.

Korczyn, A. D. (1980) Hypnotics and sedatives. In: M. N. G. Dukes (Ed.), Meyler's Side Effects of Drugs. Excerpta Medica, Amsterdam.

Kuhr, B. (1979) Prolonged delirium with propranolol. J. Clin. Psychol. 40, 74.

Kurland, M. L. (1979) Organic brain syndrome with propranolol. N. Engl. J. Med. 300, 366.

Laake, K. (1981) Antianginal and beta-adrenoceptor blocking drugs. In: M. N. G. Dukes (Ed.), Side Effects of Drugs Annual 5. Excerpta Medica, Amsterdam.

Lager, I., Blohme, G. and Smith, U. (1979) Effect of cardioselective and non-cardioselective beta-blockade on the hypoglycaemic response in insulin-dependent diabetics. Lancet 1, 458–462.

Lakshminarayan, S., Sahn, S. A., Hudson, L. D. and Weil, J. V. (1976) Effect of diazepam on ventilatory responses. Clin. Pharmacol. Ther. 20, 178–181.

Langdon, D. E., Harlan, J. R. and Bailey, R. L. (1973) Thrombophlebitis with diazepam used intravenously. J. Am. Med. Assoc. 223, 184–185.

Larson, G. F., Hulbert, B. J. and Wingard, D. W. (1977) Physostigmine reversal of diazepam-induced depression. Anesth. Analg. 56, 348–353.

Ledersalle-Pedersen, O., Mikkelsen, E., LanngNielsen, J. and Christensen, N. J. (1979) Abrupt withdrawal of beta-blocking agents in patients with arterial hypertension. Europ. J. Clin. Pharmacol. 15, 215–222.

Liljequist, R. and Mattila, M. J. (1979) Acute effects of temazepam and nitrazepam on psychomotor skills and memory. Acta Pharmacol. Toxicol. 44, 364–369.

Lloyd-Mostyn, R. H. and Oram, S. (1975) Modification by propranolol of cardiovascular effects of induced hypoglycaemia. Lancet 1, 1213–1215.

Lubbe, W. F. (1978) Clinical usefulness of the beta-adrenergic antagonists. S. Afr. Med. J. 54, 139–148.

Marshall, A. J., Baddeley, H., Barritt, D. W., Davies, J. D., Lee, R. E. J., Low-Beer, T. S. and Read, A. E. (1977) Practolol peritonitis: a study of 16 cases and a survey of small bowel function in patients taking beta-adrenergic blockers. Q. J. Med. 46, 135–146.

Martin, C. M., Southwick, E. F. and Maibach, H. I. (1973) Propranolol-induced alopecia. Am. Heart J. 86, 236.

Matthew, H. and Lawson, A. (1979) Treatment of Common Acute Poisonings, 4th edn. Churchill Livingstone, Edinburgh.

McBride, R. J., Dundee, J. W., Moore, J., Toner, W. and Howard, P. J. (1979) A study of the plasma concentration of lorazepam in mother and neonate. Br. J. Anaesth. 51, 971–978.

Miller, R. R., Olsen, H. G., Amsterdam, F. A. and Mason, D. T. (1975) Propranolol withdrawal rebound phenomenon. N. Engl. J. Med. 293, 416–419.

Moerck, H. J. and Magelund, G. (1979) Gynaecomastia and diazepam abuse. Lancet 2, 1344.

Paget, G. E. (1963) Carcinogenic actions of pronethalol. Br. Med. J. 2, 1266–1277.

Parker, J. L. W. (1979) Potassium clorazepate induced jaundice. Postgrad. Med. J. 55, 908–911.

Pathy, S. (1979) Acute central chest pain in the elderly. Am. Heart J. 98, 168–180.

Pedersen, O. L. and Mikkelsen, E. (1978) Beta blockers and uric acid excretion. Lancet 2, 1160.

Porter, W. R. and Lancee, W. J. (1978) A multicenter evaluation of lorazepam. Clin. Ther. 2, 31–43.

Preskorn, S. H. and Denner, L. J. (1977) Benzodiazepines and withdrawal psychosis. J. Am. Med. Assoc. 237, 36–38.

Pruyn, S. C., Phelan, U. P. and Buchonan, G. C. (1979) Long-term propranolol therapy in pregnancy. Am. J. Obstet. Gynecol. 135, 485–500.

Reed, M. and Normandy, J. (1980) Accidental intra-arterial injection of diazepam. Br. Med. J. 2, 289–290.

Remick, R. S., O'Kunie, J. and Sparling, T. G. (1981) A case report of toxic psychosis with low-dose propranolol therapy. Am. J. Psychiatry 138, 850.

Richards, D. A. and Prichard, B. N. (1978) Self-poisoning with beta-blockers. Br. Med. J. 1, 1623.

Richards, D. J. (1978) Clinical profile of lorazepam, a new benzodiazepine tranquilizer. J. Clin. Psychiatry 39, 56–61.

Richardson, P. S. and Sterling, G. M. (1969) Effects of beta-adrenergic receptor blockade on airway conductance and lung volume in normal and asthmatic subjects. Br. Med. J. 3, 143–145.

Rickels, K. and Downing, R. W. (1974) Chlordiazepoxide and hostility in anxious outpatients. Am. J. Psychiatry 131, 442–444.

Rickels, K., Gordon, P., Jenkin, W., Perloff, M., Sacks, T. and Stepansky, W. (1970) Drug treatment in depressive illness. Dis. Nerv. Syst. 31, 30–41.

Risch, S. C., Groom, G. P. and Janowsky, D. S. (1981) Interfaces of psychopharmacology and cardiology, part two. J. Clin. Psychiatry 42, 47–56.

Rodger, V. C., Sheldon, C. D., Lerski, R. A. and Livingstone, W. R.   (1976)   Intermittent claudication complicating beta-blockade. Br. Med. J. 1, 1125–1127.

Safra, M. J. and Oakley, Jr., G. P.   (1975)   Association between cleft lip with or without cleft palate and prenatal exposure to diazepam. Lancet 1, 478–480.

Saldanha, V. F., Bird, R. and Havard, C. W. H.   (1971)   Effect of diazepam on dialysable thyroxine. Postgrad. Med. J. 47, 326–331.

Sandstrom, B.   (1980)   Metoprolol excretion into breast milk. Br. J. Clin. Pharmacol. 9, 518–525.

Shader, R. I. and DiMascio, A.   (1970)   Psychotropic Drug Side Effects. Williams and Wilkins, Baltimore.

Shenkman, L., Podrid, P. and Lowenstein, J.   (1977)   Hyperthyroidism after propranolol withdrawal. J. Am. Med. Assoc. 238, 237–241.

Siassi, I., Thomas, M. and Vanov, S. K.   (1975)   Evaluation of the safety and therapeutic effects of lorazepam on long-term use. Curr. Ther. Res. 18, 163–171.

Simpson, F. O.   (1974)   Beta-adrenergic receptor blocking drugs in hypertension. Drugs 7, 85–105.

Snyder, S. H.   (1981)   Benzodiazepine receptors. Psych. Ann. 11 (Suppl.), 19–23.

Steiner, J. A.   (1981)   Anti-anginal and beta-adrenoceptor blocking drugs. In: M.N.G. Dukes (Ed.), Side Effects of Drugs Annual, No. 4. Excerpta Medica, Amsterdam.

Stimmel, B.   (1979)   Cardiovascular Effects of Mood-Altering Drugs. Raven Press, New York.

Swainson, C. P. and Winney, R. J.   (1976)   Effect of beta-blockade in chronic renal failure. Br. Med. J. 1, 459.

Tyrer, P. J. and Lader, M. H.   (1974)   Physiological and psychological effects of propranolol and diazepam in induced anxiety. Br. J. Clin. Pharmacol. 1, 379–385.

Vale, J. A., Van de Pette, S. J. and Price, T. M.   (1977)   Peripheral gangrene complicating beta-blockade. Lancet 2, 412–414.

Van der Kroef, C.   (1979)   Letter. Lancet 2, 526.

Verhoeven, R. P., Visser, T. J., Docter, R., Nennemann, G. and Schalekamp, M. D.   (1977)   Plasma thyroxine 3, 3′ 5-triiodothyronine and 3,3′ 5′-triiodothyronine during beta-adrenergic blockade in hyperthyroidism. J. Clin. Endocrinol. Metab. 44, 1002–1005.

Waal-Manning, H.   (1975)   Problems with practolol. Drugs 10, 336–341.

Wesson, D. and Smith, D. E.   (1977)   Barbiturates: Their Use, Misuse, and Abuse. Human Sciences Press, New York.

Wilson, J.   (1973)   Lorazepam as a premedicant for general anesthesia. Curr. Med. Res. 1, 308–316.

Windsor, W. O., Kurrein, F. and Dyer, N. H.   (1975)   Fibrinous peritonitis: a complication of practolol therapy. Br. Med. J. 2, 468–471.

Wintraub, B. U. and Shiffman, N. J.   (1979)   Adverse cutaneous reactions to drugs. In: T. B. Fitzpatrick et al., (Eds), Dermatology in General Medicine. McGraw-Hill, New York.

Wittenborn, J. R.   (1979)   Effects of benzodiazepines on psychomotor performance. Br. J. Clin. Pharmacol. 7 (Suppl.), 61–67.

Wright, P.   (1975)   Ocular reactions to beta-blocking drugs. Br. Med. J. 2, 577.

Editorial   (1978) Self-poisoning with beta-blockers. Br. Med. J. 1, 1010.

Editorial   (1980) Beta-blocker poisoning. Lancet 1, 803–804.

Burrows/Norman/Davies (eds) Antianxiety agents
© *Elsevier Science Publishers B.V., 1984*

Chapter 13

Newer antianxiety agents

GERTRUDE RUBINSTEIN

and

TREVOR R. NORMAN

Department of Psychiatry, University of Melbourne, Austin Hospital, Heidelberg, 3084 Victoria,
Australia.

INTRODUCTION

Although several classes of drugs have been used for the treatment of anxiety states (see Chapter 8, this volume), the benzodiazepines are usually the drugs of first choice. They have assumed pre-eminence, mainly because of their demonstrated efficacy, safety on overdosage and comparative lack of interaction with other commonly prescribed drugs. Since chlordiazepoxide was first introduced 20 years ago, the number of benzodiazepines has proliferated. Many of the drugs are metabolised to or undergo chemical conversion to desmethyldiazepam. Others are metabolites of desmethyldiazepam. Even though clear pharmacokinetic differences exist between the drugs, clinical differences are not readily established.

Several new antianxiety agents representing different classes of drugs are discussed. Variations on the 1,4-benzodiazepine structure as well as a new class of anxiolytic represented by buspirone, provide a number of examples of potential new anxiolytics. The emphasis is placed on clinical evaluations and the potential advantages of new drugs over those already available.

HALAZEPAM

Recently introduced into the United States as an anxiolytic the pharmacokinetic profile of halazepam has been studied by Greenblatt and Shader (1982). After single oral doses, halazepam is transformed into desmethyldiazepam with only low levels of the parent drugs being detected in the blood. This suggests that during multiple oral dosing only minimal accumulation of halazepam will occur, while desmethyldiazepam will accumulate extensively. Halazepam's pharmacokinetic profile would indicate that it is unlikely to be any different clinically from other benzodiazepines such as diazepam, chlorazepate or prazepam. Controlled clinical trials support the pharmacokinetic observations – halazepam has been shown to be as effective as other standard benzodiazepines (Rickels et al., 1977, 1978, Fann et al., 1982). It is unlikely that halazepam offers any advantages over other long-acting benzodiazepines and in one study it was suggested that the high doses of halazepam necessary for an antianxiety effect caused excessive sedation (Rickels et al., 1978).

CLOBAZAM

Clobazam, a 1,5-benzodiazepine (see Fig. 1) is biotransformed by N-demethylation to yield the pharmacologically active metabolite, N-desmethyl clobazam (Tedeschi et al., 1981). The metabolite persists for longer in plasma than the parent drug during both single and multiple oral dosing. Clinical research on this drug is extensive and has been reviewed elsewhere (Clobazam Workshop, 1979; Brogden et al., 1980).

Controlled trials of clobazam in anxiety or in anxiety associated with organic or functional disorders have shown it to be an effective drug in doses of 30–80 mg/day (Brogden et al., 1980). Open evaluations in hospitalised patients or outpatients over varying lengths of drug administration have confirmed the antianxiety effects. More importantly, double-blind controlled comparisons with placebo, diazepam or chlorazepate have shown clobazam to be more efficacious than placebo and at least as effective as either 1,4-benzodiazepine. Some of these trials are summarized in Table 1.

In patients with mild or moderate anxiety accompanying gastrointestinal disorders, Laudano et al. (1977) found similar effects of clobazam 30 mg and diazepam 15 mg. Coste-Simonin and Krantz (1975) found a reduction in anxiety in patients with cardiovascular disease who received clobazam. In patients with cardiac symptoms but no organic heart disease, clobazam appeared to be superior to diazepam (Coste-Simonin and Krantz, 1975). Koeppen (1979) summarized 45 double-blind studies comparing clobazam with diazepam and placebo (3,824 patients) in anxiety disorders. The trials lasted from 3 months to 3.5 years. Doses ranged from 5 mg in children to 120 mg in adult psychiatric inpatients. The usual

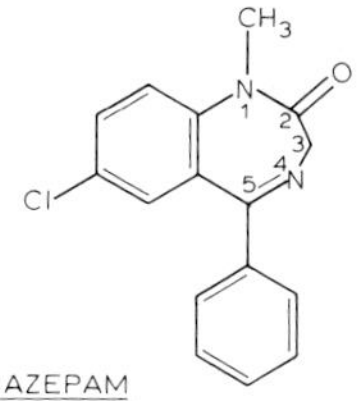

Fig. 1.

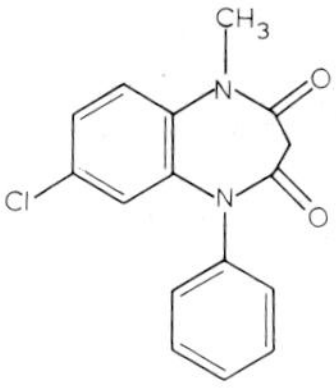

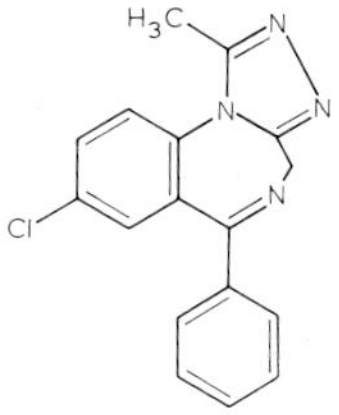

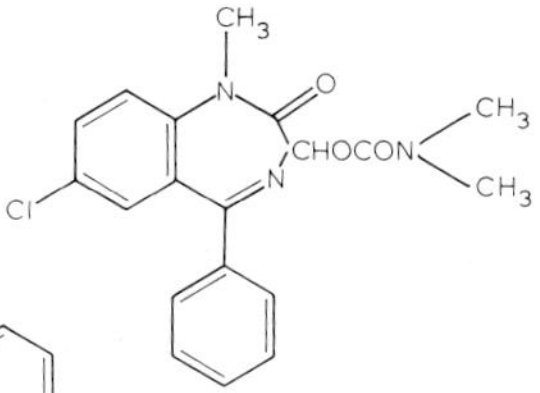

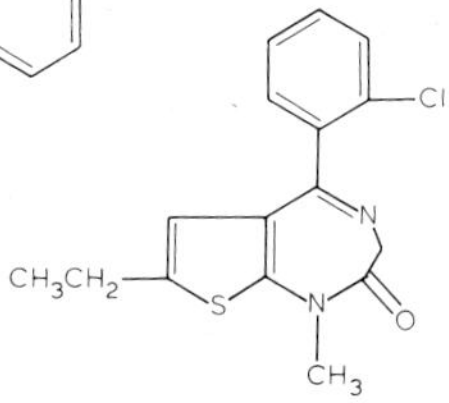

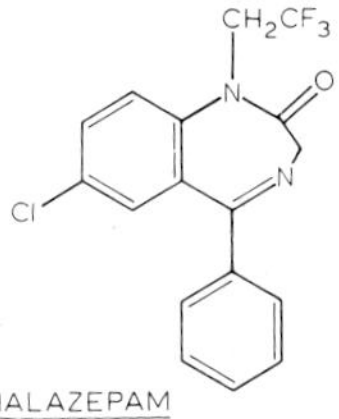

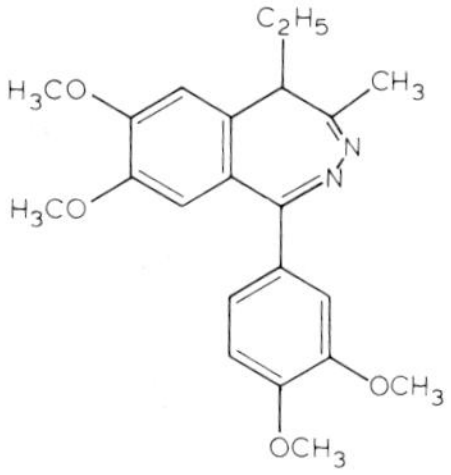

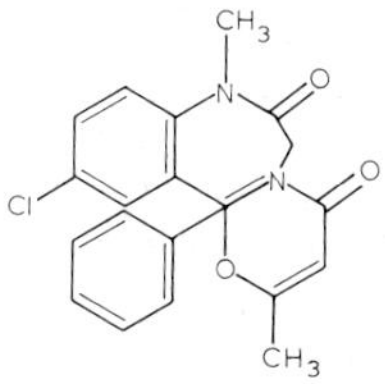

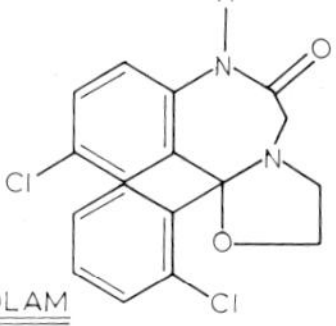

TABLE 1

Some clinical trails of clobazam in anxiety states.

Study population	Dose (mg/day)	Duration of treatment (wks)	Assessment methods	Results	Authors
18 inpatients anxiety symptoms	up to 30	8	Hamilton, CGI	C, anxiolytic	Nielsen et al. (1981)
45 anxious patients	20 C 15 D	4	Hamilton	C>D*	Botter (1980)
159 outpatients anxiety	57 C 30 D	4	Hamilton, CGI, HSCL	C=D>P	Rickels (1981)
30 elderly inpatients anxiety	30 C 3 L	4	Hamilton, CGI, VAS	C=L	Paes de Sousa et al. (1981)
41 outpatients anxiety	30 C 9 B	4	Hamilton, CGI, Zung	C=B	Ponciano et al. (1981)
30 outpatients anxiety neurosis	80 C 40 D	3	Hamilton, CGI, Zung	D>C	Ananth and Van den Steen (1979)
36 outpatients anxiety or depressive neurosis	30–60 C 15–30 D	4	Hamilton, CGI, BPRS	C=D	Ban and Amin (1979)
42 outpatients anxiety neurosis	80 C 40 D	5	Hamilton, CGI, self-rating, ASI	C=D	Mendels et al. (1978)

* On the item anxious mood of Hamilton.
C = clobazam; D = diazepam; B = bromazepam; L = lorazepam; P = placebo.

outpatient dosage was 20–30 mg daily, the most common duration of trial 2–4 weeks. Clobazam was concluded to be an efficacious anxiolytic, well-tolerated in neurotic and psychosomatic disorders.

Psychomotor effects. Brogden et al. (1980) have reviewed a large number of studies on the changes in psychomotor performance after administration of clobazam. The subjective conclusion was that general alertness was reduced the morning after a night-time dose, but this was not confirmed by objective measurement of arousal and psychomotor performance.

In a comparative study of clobazam, lorazepam and placebo, lorazepam was consistently rated intermediate between clobazam and placebo (Hindmarch and Gudgeon, 1980). This was an actual driving test with experienced volunteer female drivers. Sittig et al. (1981) compared performance tests after administration of 1,4- and 1,5-benzodiazepines, using pharmaco-EEG, and tests related to psychomotor performance. Clobazam was superior in the psychomotor performance tests. This may be an area of specific advantage for clobazam over the 1,4-benzodiazepines.

Arnau et al. (1982) concluded that single or divided daily doses produced similar effects, therefore where compliance is a problem, a single daily dose can be used with safety. Divoll et al., (1982) found that concomitant food intake slows but does not reduce absorption of the drug, therefore it is of no consequence whether medication is taken with or without meals.

Withdrawal. Two cases of typical withdrawal symptoms on discontinuation of clobazam have been reported. Both had been transferred to clobazam from other benzodiazepines, withdrawal from clobazam alone has not yet been reported, but the authors expect it eventually (Petursson and Lader, 1981).

Side effects and overdosage. Clobazam is generally well tolerated, side effects being drowsiness, sedation and hangover. Generally similar effects occur between clobazam and half the dosage of diazepam. On overdosage of 300 mg of clobazam, there was no loss of consciousness or changes in vital signs (Donlon et al., 1977). There is no marked effect on the cardiovascular system or respiration at normal therapeutic dosages (Fielding and Hoffman, 1979).

Drug interactions. There is no evidence of interaction with anticoagulants, diuretics, digitalis derivatives and clofibrate (see Coste-Simonin and Krantz, 1975). A study by Rupp et al. (1977) on clobazam and nomifensine in healthy volunteers showed no evidence of interaction, while Wieck (1979) commented that no adverse interactions with antidepressants had been reported.

Interaction of clobazam and alcohol appears to be quantitatively similar to that of alcohol and diazepam. The combination of drugs is more hazardous for driving than alcohol alone (Berry et al., 1974).

No hypersensitivity reactions to clobazam have been observed in patients receiving the drug, but in patients with known sensitivity to the 1,4-benzodiazepines, cross-sensitivity to the 1,5-benzodiazepines should be assumed. Clobazam is contraindicated in myasthenia gravis and should be avoided in the first trimester of pregnancy. The use of the drug in children under 3 years of age is not recommended.

ALPRAZOLAM

Alprazolam is a triazolo benzodiazepine closely related in structure to the hypnotic agent triazolam (see Fig. 1). The drug is metabolised by hydroxylation to produce pharmacologically active compounds (Eberts et al., 1980). Little if any of these metabolites reach the systemic circulation and so are of little clinical importance (Greenblatt et al., 1983). The plasma half-life of elimination is short to intermediate, i.e. in the range 10–15 hours.

Open evaluations of alprazolam with anxious outpatients and inpatients found it to be an effective antianxiety agent (Itil et al., 1973; Fabre and Harris, 1974). In both studies it was suggested that the drug was without significant side effects. Later double-blind studies comparing alprazolam with placebo, diazepam or chlordiazepoxide were conducted. In a 4-week study, alprazolam was superior to placebo and equivalent to diazepam in patients with psychoneurotic anxiety (Fabre and McLendon, 1979). The optimum dose of alprazolam was 2 mg/day given as a divided dose. Alprazolam produced fewer side effects than diazepam or placebo with nausea, vomiting, diarrhoea, constipation and confusion being the commonly noted effects. Greiss and Fogari (1980) also showed alprazolam to be superior to placebo in anxious patients treated for 4 weeks. Drowsiness was the major side effect of alprazolam and the mean effective dose was 1.35 mg/day. Similar results were reported by Aden and Thein (1980) as well as by Itoh et al. (1980) and Cohn (1981).

Alprazolam was as effective as chlordiazepoxide in treating the symptoms of alcohol withdrawal in alcoholic inpatients (McLendon and Fabre, 1980). The mean dose of alprazolam was 2.7 mg/day. Drowsiness was most often reported with a higher incidence in alprazolam-treated patients. Kolin and Linet (1981) demonstrated equivalent efficacy for alprazolam and diazepam in alcohol withdrawal.

In addition to its usefulness in the treatment of generalised anxiety disorders, alprazolam may be efficacious in the treatment of panic disorders and depressive illness. Chouinard et al. (1982) found that alprazolam in dosages of 0.25–3 mg/day given for 8 weeks to 14 panic-disorder patients was significantly better than placebo given to six similar patients. Additional controlled studies in panic disorders are indicated.

Rickels et al. (1982) compared alprazolam with imipramine in 199 unipolar depressed outpatients who fulfilled the DSM III criteria for a major depressive disorder, most belonging to the anxious-agitated type. In the last weeks of the trial, mean daily dose was 3.0 mg alprazolam, or 150 mg imipramine. Side effects were more apparent with imipramine, mainly drowsiness or dry mouth. Anticholinergic effects were imipramine 72 %, placebo 52 %, alprazolam 28 %. Both active compounds were superior to placebo in alleviating the symptoms of depression, whether the diagnosis was for the reactive or endogenous category. Alprazolam may have special significance for the treatment of elderly depressed patients in view of its relative lack of sedative and anticholinergic effects compared with imipramine. A pilot study by Weissman et al. (1983) compared alprazolam with imipramine and placebo in a group of ambulatory elderly patients (age 60–85 years). Side effects were significantly fewer with alprazolam, but at the end of treatment all patients were doing well. The authors cite a multicentre trial by Fawcett and Kravitz (1982) which like their trial showed more rapid onset of improvement with alprazolam, but no such effect was noted by Rickels et al. (1982). Individual psychotherapy was used throughout the Weissman et al. trial. They consider as a result of this trial that alprazolam is particularly promising for treatment of the depressed elderly.

Information on drug interactions with alprazolam is lacking, however, it seems likely, in view of the reported incidence of drowsiness, that CNS depressant effects of alcohol, barbiturates and hypnotics will be potentiated when coadministered with alprazolam. The drug is contraindicated in myasthenia gravis and known hypersensitivity to other benzodiazepines. Although information on the use of alprazolam in pregnancy is lacking, it is generally not recommended, nor is its use in children.

KETAZOLAM

Ketazolam has pharmacological properties similar to the better known benzodiazepines. It is metabolised mainly to desmethyldiazepam and can be categorised as a long elimination half-life benzodiazepine (Greenblatt et al., 1983). Ketazolam is suitable for once-daily dosage and if administered at night may help with problems of insomnia and improve compliance.

The anxiolytic properties of ketazolam have been studied in a number of clinical evaluations. Gallant et al. (1973) studied the drug in 15 alcoholic inpatients with prominent symptoms of anxiety and tension for 4 weeks. Improvement in symptomatology was noted in 13 patients receiving average daily doses of 250 mg. Amelioration of anxiety symptoms was noted in 25 inpatients treated for 4 weeks with ketazolam (Fabre and Harris, 1974). A wide range of doses from 25 to 230 mg/day (median 70 mg/day) were used. Side effects were generally mild with dizziness or drowsiness being most often reported. In a double-blind comparison, Fabre and colleagues (1976) showed ketazolam (mean dose 47 mg/day) to be more effective than placebo in psychoneurotic anxiety. The drug was administered as a single nocte dose and side effects were fewer in ketazolam- than placebo-treated patients. Similar results have been observed in other trials. Ketazolam has been shown to be as effective as diazepam (Fabre et al., 1978; Feighner, 1980; Rickels et al., 1980; Fabre et al., 1981), lorazepam (Perez-Rincon et al., 1981) clorazepate (Fabre and McLendon, 1979; Nair et al., 1982) and more effective than placebo (Bowden, 1978; Cohn and Gottschalk, 1980). The dosage of ketazolam for symptomatic treatment of anxiety is 50–70 mg/day from most studies. Side effects are generally reported as less than those with comparative substances. Drowsiness and light headedness are most commonly reported for the drug usually on initiation of therapy or on increasing the dose.

Fabre et al. (1981) carried out an extended (6 months) trial comparing diazepam and ketazolam. Therapeutic effect did not diminish over the period, but a rebound effect of acute anxiety was manifest after stopping medication. The authors considered both drugs to be safe over this period, without development of tolerance, but advocated gradual reduction of dose leading up to cessation.

Information on the use of ketazolam in pregnancy, nursing mothers and children, is not available. Drug interactions with ketazolam have not been studied, but interactions with alcohol and other CNS depressants similar to those with other 1,4-benzodiazepines should be assumed.

CAMAZEPAM

Camazepam is a carbamyloxy derivative of temazepam. The drug has not been well characterised pharmacokinetically, but, studies in animals suggest that it has an intermediate plasma elimination half-life (Legheand et al., 1982) and that there is considerable penetrance of unchanged drug into the brain (Marcucci et al., 1978). In animals, camazepam is converted to temazepam and oxazepam but metabolic data in humans is not available (Garattini et al., 1981).

Relatively few clinical studies have been carried out with the drug. Two double-blind studies have compared camazepam (30 mg/day) with diazepam (15 mg/day) or temazepam (30 mg/day) in psychoneurotic patients with symptoms of anxiety (Cesa-Bianchi et al., 1974; Deberdt, 1975). In both of these small outpatient trials, camazepam demonstrated anxiolytic properties, was well tolerated with few side effects and was as efficacious as the reference compound. Placebo controlled studies in anxiety are lacking.

Camazepam (20 mg) has been compared with diazepam (10 mg) as a premedicant before endoscopy (Celli and Santagostino, 1974; Galli, 1976). In both studies camazepam was reported as more useful than diazepam particularly as it did not cause drowsiness or interfere with secretion and peristalsis.

Nicholson and Stone (1982) have compared performance effects of camazepam and lormetazepam, another analogue of temazepam, in healthy volunteers. Temazepam, which has a short half-life and no long-acting metabolite, is a useful hypnotic for persons carrying out skilled work because of its relative lack of hangover effects. With camazepam 10–20 mg changes in sleep were minimal, non-anxious subjects reported being more relaxed the day after a night-time dose, and there was improved performance on the digit symbol substitution test. With 40 mg camazepam there was distortion of the normal sleep EEG, and impairment of performance in the morning.

The lack of recent information on this drug suggests that camazepam has failed to find acceptance as an anxiolytic despite promising comparisons with diazepam. Information on drug interactions, use in children, pregnancy and nursing mothers is lacking and the routine use of the drug in these patients should be avoided until more is known.

TOFISOPAM

Tofisopam is a benzodiazepine anxiolytic chemically similar to diazepam but as seen in Fig. 1 different from it in the position of the nitrogen atoms in the heterocyclic ring. In 29 European clinical trials involving about 1,200 patients, tofisopam demonstrated anxiolytic effects but also had a mild stimulatory property. A daily dose of tofisopam of 200–300 mg produced anxiolysis with a concomitant reduction in psychosomatic complaints. In a double-blind study tofisopam was compared with placebo in 57 outpatients with symptoms of anxiety and depression (Goldberg and Finnerty, 1979). After 4 weeks of treatment tofisopam was considered to be an effective anxiolytic with the best results in patients with somatic difficulties. Tofisopam was effective in an open evaluation in 30 patients with a mixed anxiety-depressive syndrome (Molcan et al., 1981). The average daily dose was 158 mg. Side effects were minimal. Filip et al. (1981) showed that tofisopam was more effective than placebo in 50 outpatients with anxiety treated for 4 weeks. Side effects were mimimal but drowsiness and fatigue were noted. Analysis of the items of the Hamilton anxiety scale showed tofisopam to have a marked effect on the item 'fears' suggesting antiphobic properties. This has not been further explored. Clearly, further studies are needed to assess the place of tofisopam as a treatment for anxiety symptoms.

Both subjective and objective evaluation of psychomotor function performed by Lammintausta et al. (1980) indicated that tofisopam, in contrast to diazepam and lorazepam, produced no significant impairment. It is of interest but of unknown significance that Lammintausta et al. (1980) found that tofisopam unlike diazepam, caused no change in serum growth hormone. Kangas et al. (1980) compared tofisopam as a preoperative medication with nitrazepam and placebo. Tofisopam was found to have an anxiolytic effect but no sleep-inducing properties consistent with the mild stimulant effects noted in some clinical studies.

Bond and Lader (1982) compared tofisopam with diazepam and placebo on a series of measures in healthy normal subjects. The psychotropic profile of diazepam included EEG changes, pronounced sedation, and psychomotor impairment. Tofisopam produced no EEG changes, no impairment on the psychological tests but a mild stimulation. Since the stimulant effect occurred only 3–5 hours after drug administration, Bond and Lader (1982) suspected that tofisopam may be a prodrug for an active metabolite or that it penetrates the brain slowly.

Seppala et al. (1980) cited a trial on young lorry drivers in which Gerevich et al.

(1975) found improvement rather than impairment after treatment with tofiso-pam. From the results of a wide range of psychomotor tests, Seppala et al. con-cluded that unlike diazepam, tofisopam did not impair performance either as a single dose or as repeated doses. However, either of these benzodiazepines in con-junction with alcohol impaired performance.

Data on drug interactions and the use of tofisopam in pregnancy, children, lac-tating women or myasthenia gravis is not available.

CLOXAZOLAM

This novel benzodiazepine was found in the process of screening derivatives of oxazolam, and showed promise in animal experiments as an effective minor tran-quillizer (Kamioka et al., 1972).

A number of multicentre trials in Europe and Japan and complementary trials in other countries were recently collated by Fischer-Cornelssen (1981). There were in all nearly 3,000 patients, with a diagnosis of chronic anxiety of medium to severe intensity. Improvement rates were considered to be higher with cloxazolam than either lorazepam or diazepam. The tolerance of cloxazolam was good com-pared with the active agents or placebo, unless cloxazolam exceeded 3 mg twice daily.

No interaction was reported with concomitant non-psychotropic drugs, which included antihypertensive agents and anticoagulants, and no effect was observed on either glucose tolerance or insulin-secretion activity.

Over a 6-week period, patients suffering from endogenous or psychogenic depression were treated with cloxazolam and dibenzepin comcomitantly. Onset of action was claimed to be quicker than with single agents, side effects of similar occurrence to single agents.

Vollmer et al. (1981) compared cloxazolam and dibenzepin administered oral-ly, individually and simultaneously, by pharmaco-EEG. The sedative effect was considered to indicate a potentiating effect of cloxazolam on the antidepressant drug.

CLOTIAZEPAM

Clotiazepam is a thienodiazepine derivative (Fig. 1) which is metabolised by demethylation and hydroxylation to yield pharmacologically active metabolites (Arendt et al., 1982). The drug has a short to intermediate plasma half-life, but only preliminary data are available at present (Arendt et al., 1982). Nakanishi and Setoguchi (1972) have summarized the pharmacology of clotiazepam and in animal-screening tests it has properties similar to the benzodiazepines. Three studies cited by these authors claimed effectiveness of clotiazepam in psychoneu-rotic and psychosomatic disorders, and in preoperative sleep disturbance. Clearly

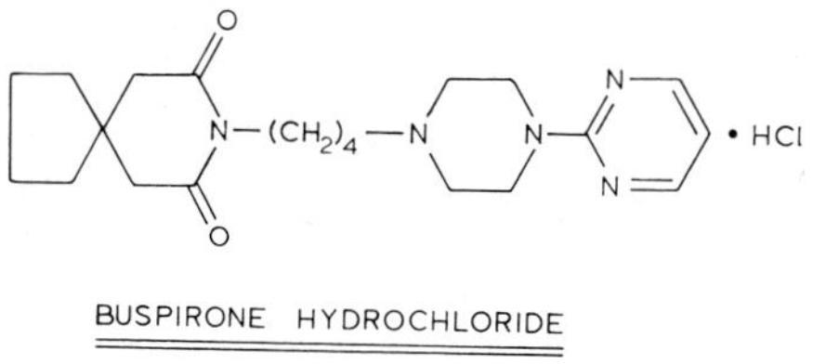

BUSPIRONE HYDROCHLORIDE

Fig. 2.

further clinical evaluations are required.

BUSPIRONE

Buspirone is a potential antianxiety agent chemically and pharmacologically distinct from the benzodiazepines. In animal studies buspirone lacks anticonvulsant, sedative-hypnotic or muscle-relaxant properties. It also appears to lack the potential for physical dependence or abuse in animal models (Riblet et al., 1982). Buspirone has no effect on ^{3}H-benzodiazepine binding but possesses properties of a dopamine agonist and antagonist (Temple et al., 1982).

A number of clinical trials of buspirone has been conducted and are summarized in Table 2. The results of these studies suggest that buspirone has anxiolytic properties equivalent to the benzodiazepines and more effective than a placebo. The abuse liability of buspirone compared to diazepam, methaqualone and placebo in recreational sedative users was considerably less (Cole et al., 1982). Newton et al. (1982) reviewed the incidence of side effects in buspirone-treated patients compared with benzodiazepine- or placebo-treated patients from a number of clinical trials. They concluded that sedation, lethargy and depression were less with buspirone and that other side effects occurred with a similar frequency in buspirone- and benzodiazepine-treated patients. Using the same data base, Gershon (1982) reached the same conclusion, but added that the use of a variety of medications did not affect the side effect profile of buspirone.

Bond and Lader (1981) compared the psychological and physiological effects of single doses of diazepam (10 mg), buspirone (10 or 20 mg) and a placebo in 12 normal healthy volunteers. Subjects felt sedated on both active compounds but cognitive performance was not impaired by buspirone and psychomotor performance was impaired only at high dose. Diazepam affected both functions. The psychotropic effects of repeated oral dosing of buspirone was studied in normal volunteers and compared with diazepam and placebo (Lader, 1982). Drowsiness and dizziness increased following buspirone, but irritability and physical tiredness decreased. Psychological measures were impaired primarily by diazepam, but no effects were seen with buspirone.

TABLE 2

Some clinical studies with buspirone

Study population	Dose (mg/day)	Duration of treatment (wks)	Assessment methods	Results	Authors
100 outpatients with generalized anxiety disorder	16.5 B 15.0 D		Hamilton, Covi, Raskin SCL-56	B=D	Feighner et al. (1982)
54 anxious outpatients	20 B 20 D		Hamilton, Covi, Raskin SCL-56	B=D>P	Goldberg and Finnerty (1982)
56 anxious outpatients	16.0 B 20.4 CL		Hamilton, Covi, Raskin SCL-56	B=CL	Goldberg and Finnerty (1982)
56 psychoneurotic outpatients	19.6 B 18.7 D 21.3 P	4		B=D>P	Goldberg and Finnerty (1979)
131 anxious patients	30 B 30 D 30 P	3	Hamilton	B=D>P	Wheatley (1982)
240 anxious patients	20 B 20 D 20 P	4	Hamilton, Covi	B=D>P	Rickels et al. (1982)

B = buspirone; D = diazepam; P = placebo; CL = chlordiazepoxide.

Little if any interaction between alcohol and acutely administered buspirone (Mattila et el., 1982; Seppala et al., 1982) or chronically administered drug (Moskowitz and Smiley, 1982) has been observed. The latter study showed little or no impairment on skills related to driving tasks.

Buspirone may prove to be a useful alternative to the benzodiazepines if its anxiolytic action can be substantiated in further clinical trials.

SUMMARY AND CONCLUSIONS

A number of new drugs has been investigated for their clinical anxiolytic potential. Most are related to the well known and clinically proven 1,4-benzodiazepines and some (e.g. halazepam, ketazolam, camazepam) function as prodrugs for these better known compounds. Clearly these agents would appear to offer little or no advantage over their better known counterparts. Some of the new drugs may prove to have specific advantages over compounds presently in use. For example, if confirmed in placebo-controlled comparisons, the specific antipanic effect claimed for alprazolam and tofisopam will no doubt add a new dimension to the treatment of phobic disorders. The apparent lack of abuse liability of buspirone is of particular clinical interest given the recent concern over dependence problems with the benzodiazepines. Buspirone is enigmatic, since unlike other drugs used for anxiolysis it does not have sedative, muscle-relaxant or anticonvulsant effects (Taylor et al., 1982). It provides a challenge to current views of the neurochemical basis of anxiety, since buspirone does not interact directly with the benzodiazepine/GABA system, yet has agonist and antagonist effects at dopamine receptors. Perhaps there is a role for dopamine in the aetiology of anxiety? An understanding of the neurochemistry of anxiety will no doubt lead to drugs with more specific actions. Already the identification of multiple benzodiazepine binding sites in the brain has led to the hypothesis of separate physiological endpoints for the receptor subtypes, e.g. sedation for one; anxiolytic and anticonvulsant effects for the other (Martin, 1982). The clinical evaluation of compounds like CL-218872, which is specific for one type of benzodiazepine receptor is awaited with interest. The development of specific benzodiazepine antagonists, such as ROIS-1788 and CGS 8216, is also at potential clinical value. Future developments may see the production of an antianxiety agent without muscle-relaxant or anticonvulsant effects. The clinical desirability of the separation of such effects may be questionable. For the present some of the new drugs discussed here appear to have some specific advantage over the established agents, while others, even at this early stage of development, offer none.

REFERENCES

Aden, G. C. and Thein, S. G. (1980) Alprazolam compared to diazepam and placebo in the treatment of anxiety. J. Clin. Psychiatry 41, 245–248.

Ananth, J. and Van den Steen, N. (1979) Clobazam in the treatment of anxiety neurosis; a double-blind study. Curr. Ther. Res. 26, 119–126.

Arendt, R., Ochs, R. and Greenblatt, D. J. (1982) Electron capture GLC analysis of the thienodiazepine clotiazepam. Arzneim. Forsch. 32, 453–455.

Arnau, C., Costa Molinari, J. M., Pina, C. and Vallve, C. (1982) Clobazam: single or divided doses? Eur. J. Clin. Pharmacol. 22, 235–238.

Ban, T. A. and Amin, M. M. (1979) Clobazam: uncontrolled and standard controlled clinical trials. Br. J. Clin. Pharmacol. 7, 135S–138S.

Berry, P. A., Burtles, R., Grubb, D. J. and Hoare, M. V. An evaluation of the effects of clobazam on human motor co-ordination, mental acuity and mood. Br. J. Clin. Pharmacol. 1, 346P.

Bond, A. J. and Lader, M. H. (1981) Comparative effects of diazepam and buspirone on subjective feelings, psychological tests and the EEG. Int. Pharmacopsychiatry 16, 212–220.

Bond, A. J. and Lader, M. H. (1982) A comparison of the psychotropic profiles of tofisopam and diazepam. Eur. J. Clin. Pharmacol. 22, 137–142.

Botter, P. A. (1980) Single daily dose treatment of anxiety with clobazam: a double-blind study

212

versus normal multiple-dose treatment with diazepam. Curr. Med. Res. Opin. 6, 593–597.

Bowden, C. L. (1978) Double-blind placebo-controlled trial of ketazolam in anxiety. Curr. Ther. Res. 24, 170–178.

Brogden, R. N., Heel, R. C., Speight, T. M. and Avery, G. S. (1980) Clobazam: a review of its pharmacological properties and therapeutic use in anxiety. Drugs 20, 161-178.

Celli, L. and Santagostino, C. (1974) Camazepam versus diazepam: a double-blind study during endoscopy inspection. Curr. Ther. Res. 16, 457–460.

Cesa-Bianchi, M., Ghirardi, P. and Ravaccia, F. (1974) A preliminary double-blind study with SB5833 (Camazepam), a new benzodiazepine derivative. Arzneim. Forsch. 24, 2032–2035.

Chouinard, G., Annable, L., Fontaine, R. and Solyom, L. (1982) Alprazolam in the treatment of generalized anxiety and panic disorders: a double-blind placebo-controlled study. Psychopharmacol 77, 229–233.

Clobazam Workshop (1979) Br. J. Clin. Pharmacol. 7, Suppl. 1, 7S–151S.

Cohn, J. (1981) Multicenter double-blind efficacy and safety study comparing alprazolam, diazepam and placebo in clinically anxious patients. J. Clin. Psychiatry 42, 347–351.

Cohn, J. and Gottschalk, L. A. (1980) Double-blind comparison of ketazolam and placebo using once-a-day dosing. J. Clin. Pharmacol. 20, 676–680.

Cole, J. O., Orzack, M. H., Beake, B., Bird, M. and Bar-Tab, Y. (1982) Assessment of the abuse liability of buspirone in recreational sedative users. J. Clin. Psychiatry 43, 69–75.

Coste–Simonin, A. and Krantz, D, (1975) Étude clinique d'un nouvel anxiolytique en cardiologie: le clobazam. Gaz. Med. Fr. 82, 4460–4464. Abstracted in Clobazam Workshop, 131S, see above.

Deberdt, R. (1975) Camazepam versus diazepam: a double-blind trial on psychoneurotic patients. Curr. Ther. Res. 17, 32–39.

Divoll, M., Greenblatt, D. J., Ciraulo, D. A., Surendra, K. P., Irwin, H. O. and Shader, R. I. (1982) Clobazam kinetics: intrasubject variability and effect of food on absorption. J. Clin. Pharmacol. 22, 69–73.

Donlon, P. R., Green, W. and Johnson, M. (1977) Clobazam vs. placebo for neurotic anxiety and tension. Curr. Ther. Res. 22, 894–899.

Eberts, F. S., Philopoulos, Y., Reineke, L. M. and Vliek, R. W. (1980) Disposition of 14-C-alprazolam, a new anxiolytic-antidepressant, in man. Pharmacologist 22, 279.

Eberts, F. S., Philopoulos, Y., Reineke, L. M. and Vliek, R. W. (1981) Triazolam disposition. Clin. Pharmacol. Ther. 29, 81–93.

Fabre, L. F. and Harris, R. T. (1974a) Pilot open study on U31,889 in anxious inpatients. Curr. Ther. Res. 16, 1010–1013.

Fabre, L.F. and Harris, R.T. (1974b) Pilot open-label study on U-28,774, in anxious inpatients. Curr. Ther. Res. 16, 848–852.

Fabre, L. F. and McLendon, D. M. (1979a) A double-blind study comparing the efficacy and safety of alprazolam with diazepam and placebo in anxious out-patients. Curr. Ther. Res. 25, 519–526.

Fabre, L. F. and McLendon, D. M. (1979b) Ketazolam administered once a day compared to clorazepate T.I.D. and placebo in a double-blind study of anxious out-patients. Curr. Ther. Res. 25, 710–720.

Fabre, L. F., Harris, R. T. and Stubbs, D. F. (1976) Double-blind placebo-controlled efficacy study of ketazolam (U-28,774). J. Int. Med. Res. 4, 50–54.

Fabre, L. F., McLendon, D. M. and Gainey, A. (1978) Double-blind comparison of ketazolam administered once a day with diazepam and placebo in anxious outpatients. Curr. Ther. Res. 24, 875–883.

Fabre, L. F., McLendon, D. M. and Stephens, A. G. (1981) Comparison of the therapeutic effect, tolerance and safety of ketazolam and diazepam administered for six months to out-patients with chronic anxiety neurosis. J. Int. Med. Res. 9, 191–198.

Fann, W. E., Pitts, W. M. and Wheless, J. C. (1982) Pharmacology, efficacy and adverse effects of halazepam, a new benzodiazepine. Pharmacotherapy 2, 72–79.

Fawcett, J. and Kravitz, H. M. (1982) Alprazolam: pharmacokinetics, clinical efficacy and mechanism of action. Pharmacotherapy 2 (5) 243–254.

Feighner, J. P. (1980) Ketazolam once-a-day in the treatment of anxiety: a double-blind comparison with placebo. Curr. Ther. Res. 28, 425–431.

Feighner, J. P., Merideth, C. H. and Hedricksen, G. A. (1982) A double-blind comparison of buspirone and diazepam in outpatients with generalized anxiety disorder. J. Clin. Psychiatry 43, 103–108.

Fielding, S. and Hoffman. I. (1979) Pharmacology of anti-anxiety drugs with special reference to clobazam. Br. J. Clin. Pharmacol. 7, Suppl. 1, 7S-15S.

Filip, V., Sladka, R., Dostalova, J., Haskovcova, V., Jarosova, M., Faltus, F. and Slanska, J. (1981) A double-blind, placebo-controlled study with tofizopam in anxiety neurosis. Aggressologie 22, 27–30.

Fischer-Cornelssen, K. A. (1981) Multicenter trials and complementary studies of cloxazolam, a new anxiolytic drug. Arzneim. Forsch. 31, 1757–1765.

Gallant, D. M., Guerrero-Figueroa, R. and Swanson, C. (1973) U-28,774 (Ketazolam): an early evaluation of a new antianxiety agent. Curr. Ther. Res. 15, 123–126.

Galli, G. (1976) Camazepam (SB/5833) in preparation for endoscopy inspection: open and double-blind study versus diazepam. Curr. Ther. Res. 19, 316–319.

Garattini, S., Caccia, S., Carli, M. and Mennini, T. (1981) Notes on kinetics and metabolism of benzodiazepines. In: B. Angrist, G.D. Burrows, M.H. Lader, O. Lingjaerde, G. Sedvall and D. Wheatley (Eds), Recent Advances in Neuropsychopharmacology. Pergamon Press, Oxford, pp. 351–364.

Gerevich, J., Bolla, K., Toth, K. and Sebo, J. (1975) The effect of Grandaxin on lorry drivers. Ther. Hung. 23, 143–146.

Gershon, S. (1982) Drug interactions in controlled clinical trials. J. Clin. Psychiatry 43, 95–98.

Goldberg, H. L. and Finnerty, R. J. (1979a) Comparative efficacy of tofisopam and placebo. Am. J. Psychiatry 136, 196–199.

Goldberg, H. L. and Finnerty, R. J. (1979b) The comparative efficacy of buspirone and diazepam in the treatment of anxiety. Am. J. Psychiatry 136, 1184–1187.

Goldberg, H. L. and Finnerty, R. J. (1982) Comparison of buspirone in two separate studies. J. Clin. Psychiatry 43, 87–91.

Greenblatt, D. J. and Shader, R. I. (1982) New anxiolytics: are they really new? Psychopharmacol. Bull. 18, 58–61.

Greenblatt, D. J., Divoll, M., Abernethy, D. R., Ochs, H. R. and Shader, R. I. (1983) Clinical pharmacokinetics of the newer benzodiazepines. Clin. Pharmacol. 8, 233-252.

Greiss, K. C. and Fogari, R. (1980) Double-blind clinical assessment of alprazolam, a new benzodiazepine derivative, in the treatment of moderate to severe anxiety. J. Clin. Pharmacol. 20, 693–699.

Hindmarch, I. and Gudgeon, A. C. (1980) The effect of clobazam and lorazepam on aspects of psychomotor performance and car handling ability. Br. J. Clin. Pharmacol. 10, 145–150.

Itil, T. M., Polvan, N., Egilmez, S., Saletu, B. and Marasa, J. (1973) Anxiolytic effects of a new triazolo-benzodiazepine, U-31,889. Curr. Ther. Res. 15, 603–615.

Itoh, H., Takahashi, R. and Miura, S. (1980) Alprazolam, a new type anxiolytic in neurotic patients: a pilot study. Int. Pharmacopsychiatry 15, 344-349.

Kamioka, T., Tagaki, H., Kobayashi, S. and Suzuki, Y. (1972) Pharmacological studies on 10-chloro-11b-2-(2-chlorophenyl)-2,3,4,5,6,7,11,6 hexahydrobenzo 6,7-1,4-diazepino 5,4-6 oxazol-6-one (CS-370), a new psychosedative agent. Arzneim. Forsch. 22, 884–891.

Kangas, L., Kanto, J., Pakkanen, A. and Mansikka, M. (1980) Comparison of sedatory and anx-

214

iolytic properties of placebo, tofisopam and nitrazepam as oral premedicants. Abstracts of the 12th CINP Congress, Göteborg, Sweden p. 197.

Koeppen, D. (1979) Review of clinical studies on clobazam. Br. J. Clin. Pharmacol. 7, Suppl. 1, 139S–150S.

Kolin, I. and Linet, O. I. (1981) Double-blind comparison of alprazolam and diazepam for subchronic withdrawal of alcohol. J. Clin. Psychiatry 42, 169–173.

Lader, M. H. (1982) Psychological effects of buspirone. J. Clin. Psychiatry 43, 62–67.

Lammintausta, R., Kangas, L., Lammintausta, O. and Nieminen, A. (1980) Pharmacological profile of tofizopam – a different benzodiazepine. Abstracts of the 12th CINP Congress, Göteborg, Sweden, p. 216.

Laudano, O., Peralta, M., Lujan, L., Aparicio, N. and Moizeszowicz, J. (1977) Effect of a new benzodiazepine derivative, clobazam, in anxious patients with a gastrointestinal disorder. J. Clin. Pharmacol. 17, 441–446.

Legheand, J., Cuisinaud, G., Bernard, N., Riotte, M. and Sassard, J. (1982) Pharmacokinetics of intravenous camazepam in dogs. Arzneim. Forsch. 32, 752–756.

Marcucci, F., Mussini, E., Cotelessa, L., Ghirardi, P., Parenti, M., Riva, R. and Salva, P. (1978) Distribution of Camazepam in rats and mice. J. Pharm. Sci. 67, 1470–1471.

Martin, I. L. (1982) The benzodiazepines: recent trends. Psychol. Med. 12, 689–693.

Mattila, M. J., Aranko, K. and Seppala, T. (1982) Acute effects of buspirone and alcohol on psychomotor skills. J. Clin. Psychiatry 43, 56–61.

McLendon, D. M. and Fabre, L. F. (1980) A double–blind comparison of the efficacy of alprazolam, chlordiazepoxide hydrochloride and placebo in the chronic withdrawal period from alcohol. Curr. Ther. Res. 28, 447–455.

Mendels, J., Secunda, S., Schless, A., Sandler, K. and Singer, J. (1978) A double-blind comparison of clobazam and diazepam in the treatment of anxiety neurosis. J. Clin. Pharmacol. 18, 353–357.

Molcan, J., Novotny, V., Korinkova, V. and Konikova, M. (1980) Tofisopam in the therapy of anxious-depressive syndroms. Aggressologie 22D, 23-24.

Moskowitz, H. and Smiley, A. (1982) Effects of chronically administered buspirone and diazepam on driving-related skills performance. J. Clin. Psychiatry 43, 45–55.

Nair, N. P. V., Singh, A. N., Lapierre, Y., Saxena, B. M., Nestoros, J. N. and Schwartz, G. (1982) Ketazolam in the treatment of anxiety: a standard- and placebo-controlled study. Curr. Ther. Res. 31, 679–691.

Nakanishi, M., Tsumagari, T., Takigawa, Y., Shuto, S., Kenjo, T. and Fukuda, T. (1972) Studies on psychotropic drugs XIX: Psychopharmacological studies of 1-methyl-5-O-chlorophenyl-7-ethyl-1,2-dihydro-3H-thieno 2,3-e 1,4 diazepin-2-one (Y-6047) Arzneim. Forsch. 22, 1905–1914.

Newton, R. E., Casten, G. P., Alms, D. R. Benes, C. O. and Marunycz, J. D. (1982) The side effect profile of buspirone in comparison to active controls and placebo. J. Clin. Psychiatry 43, 100-102.

Nicholson, A. N. and Stone, B. (1982) Hypnotic activity and effects on performance of lorazepam and camazepam – analogues of temazepam. Br. J. Clin. Pharmacol. 13, 433-439.

Nielsen, N. P., Zizolfi, S., Sesso, M., Koeppen, D., Taeuber, K. and Uihlein, M. (1981) Multiple dose kinetics of clobazam and N-desmethyl clobazam in anxious psychiatric in-patients. In: I. Hindmarch and P. Stonier (Eds), Royal Society of Medicine International Congress and Symposium Series, No 43. Clobazam. Academic Press, London. pp. 97–102.

Paes de Sousa, M., Figuiera, M. L., Loureiro, F. and Hindmarch, I. (1981) Lorazepam and clobazam in anxious elderly patients. In: I. Hindmarch and P. Stonier (Eds), Royal Society of Medicine International Congress and Symposium Series, No 43. Clobazam. Academic Press, London. pp. 119–123.

Perez-Rincon, H., Alvarez-Rueda, J. M. and Trujillo, A. (1981) A comparative double-blind study between ketazolam and lorazepam in the treatment of anxiety. Curr. Ther. Res. 29, 936–942.

Petursson, H. and Lader, M. H. (1981) Withdrawal action from clobazam. Br. Med. J. 282, 1931–1932.

Ponciano, E., Relvas, J., Mendes, F., Lameiras, A., Vaz Serra, A. and Hindmarch, I. (1981) Clinical effects and sedative activity of bromazepam and clobazam in the treatment of anxious outpatients. In: I. Hindmarch and P. Stonier (Eds), Royal Society of Medicine International Congress and Symposium Series, No 43. Clobazam. Academic Press, London. pp. 125–131.

Riblet, L. A., Taylor, D. P., Eison, M. S., and Stanton, H. C. (1982) Pharmacology and neurochemistry of buspirone. J. Clin. Psychiatry 43, 11–17.

Rickels, K., Pereira-Ogan, J., Csanalosi, I., Morris, R.J., Rosenfeld, H., Sablowsky, L., Schless, A. and Werblowsky, J. H. (1977) Halazepam and diazepam in neurotic anxiety: a double-blind study. Psychopharmacology 52, 129–136.

Rickels, K., Case, W. G., Chung, H., Downing, R. W. and Vlahovich, J. (1978) Diazepam and halazepam in anxiety: some prognostic indicators. Int. Pharmacopsychiatry 13, 118–125.

Rickels, K., Csanalosi, I., Greisman, P., Mirman, M. J., Morris, R. J., Weiss, C. C. and Weiss, G. (1980) Ketazolam and diazepam in anxiety. A controlled study. J. Clin. Pharmacol. 20, 281–289.

Rickels, K., Cohen, D., Csanalosi, I., Harris, H., Koepke, H. and Werblowsky, J. (1982a) Alprazolam and imipramine in depressed outpatients: a controlled study. Curr. Ther. Res. 32, 157–164.

Rickels, K., Weisman, K., Norstad, N., Singer, M., Stoltz, D., Brown, A. and Danton, J. (1982b) Buspirone and diazepam in anxiety: a controlled study. J. Clin. Psychiatry 43, 81–86.

Rupp, W., Heptner, W., Uihlein, M., Bender, R. and Taeuber, K. (1977) Kinetic interaction of nomifensine with a 1,5 benzodiazepine (clobazam). Br. J. Clin. Pharmacol. 4, 143S–146S.

Seppälä, T., Palva, E., Mattila, M. J. Korttila, K. and Shrotriya, R. (1980) Tofisopam, a novel 3,4-benzodiazepine: multiple-dose effects on psychomotor skills and memory. Comparison with diazepam and interactions with alcohol. Psychopharmacology 69, 209–218.

Seppälä, T., Aranko, K., Mattila, M. J. and Shrotriya, R. (1982) Effects of alcohol on buspirone and lorazepam actions. Clin. Pharm. Ther. 32, 201–207.

Sittig, W., Badian, M., Rupp, W. and Taeuber, K. (1981) The effect of clobazam and diazepam on computer EEG vigilance and psychomotor performance. In: I. Hindmarch and P. Stonier (Eds), Royal Society of Medicine International Congress and Symposium Series, No 43, Clobazam. Academic Press, London. pp. 39–40.

Taylor, D. P., Riblet, L. A., Stanton, H. C., Eison, A. S., Eison, M. S. and Temple, D. L. (1982) Dopamine and antianxiety activity. Pharmacol. Biochem. Behav. 17, Suppl. 1, 25–35.

Tedeschi, G., Riva, R. and Baruzzi, A. (1981) Clobazam plasma concentrations: pharmacokinetic studies in healthy volunteers and data in epileptic patients. Br. J. Clin. Pharmacol. 11, 619–622.

Temple, D. L., Yevich, J. P. and New, J. S. (1982) Buspirone: chemical profile of a new class of anxioselective agents. J. Clin. Psychiatry 43, 4–9.

Vollmer, R., Matejcek, M., Knor, K. and Jellinger, K. (1981) Evidence for potentiating effect of two different psychotropic compounds (cloxazolam and noveril) by means of pharmaco-encephalography and polarity profiles. Psychopharmacol. Bull. 17, 95.

Weissman, M. M., Prusoff, B. A., Sholomskas, A. J. and Berry, C. (1983) The pharmacologic treatment of the depressed elderly: a pilot study of alprazolam (Xanax[tm]), imipramine (Tofranil) or placebo. In: G. D. Burrows, T. R. Norman and K. P. Maguire (Eds), Selected papers from the 13th CINP Conference, Jerusalem 1982. John Libbey and Co, London. pp. 167–174.

Wheatley, D. (1982) Buspirone: multicenter efficacy study. J. Clin. Psychiatry 43, 92–94.

Wieck, H. H. (1979) Mode of action of modern tranquillizers from the benzodiazepine group; a clinical view. Br. J. Clin. Pharmacol. 7, Suppl. 1, 107S–108S.

Burrows/Norman/Davies (eds) Antianxiety agents
© *Elsevier Science Publishers B.V., 1984*

Chapter 14

Benzodiazepines and sleep

IAN HINDMARCH

Human Psychopharmacology Research Unit, University of Leeds, Leeds LS 16 SNT, U.K.

Traditional hypnotic drugs; chlormethiazole, chloral hydrate, barbiturates, glute-thimide and methyprylon; induce unconsciousness and so promote and maintain sleep. They are clinically efficacious although being exceptionally toxic and liable, in overdose, to produce respiratory depression, coma and death. Their effects are potentiated by many other psychotropic agents – especially alcohol – and pro-longed use of the drugs leads to dependency and the potential for abuse. Some of these older hypnotics produce gastric irritation and are unpleasant to taste, factors which pose problems for elderly patients and those with concurrent gastro-intestinal illness.

Compared to these early hypnotics the benzodiazepine derivatives are much safer in clinical use being relatively free from toxic effects and having a lower potential for interaction with other drugs. The benzodiazepines possess a 5-fold clinical activity being efficacious in reducing anxiety, producing muscle relaxation, possessing anti-convulsant activity, producing amnesia and inducing and maintaining sleep. Their widespread clinical utility in treating anxious, epileptic and sleep-disturbed patients and their use as premedications, e.g. endoscopies, reflect their broad spectrum of clinical pharmacological action. Individual derivatives can be classed as primarily anti-anxiety or anti-convulsant or sedative-hypnotic dependent upon the profile of action shown on the five clinical aspects.

However, it is not only sedative-hypnotic benzodiazepines which have some usefulness as treatments for sleep disturbance and before considering the various available benzodiazepines it is worthwhile reviewing the manifestations of 'sleep disturbance' found in general practice situations.

SLEEP DISORDERS

There are six major groups of patients who seek treatment for sleep-related disorders:

1) *Physical illness.* Patients with nocturnal pain and rheumatic/muscular discomfort may not need a specific hypnotic medication as their problem might be alleviated following analgesic and anti-inflammatory medications. Sleep apnoea, due to obesity, can readily be treated via diet and exercise regimens without recourse to a benzodiazepine and likewise problems of painful and frequent nocturnal micturition and nocturnal myoclonus might be susceptible to psycho- as opposed to pharmacotherapy. Indeed the respiratory depressant effect of many benzodiazepine hypnotics might augment rather than reduce some problems of sleeplessness, produced by apnoeic episodes and respiratory distress.

2) *Physiological disorders.* Many patients create their own sleep problem by drinking strong coffee immediately prior to bedtime, or by overindulging in alcohol and/or nicotine. Excessively hot or cold bedrooms and noisy, humid or strange environments can induce sleeplessness. Elderly patients need less sleep than their younger counterparts. These physiological disturbers of sleep are best counteracted, not by a prescribed medicine but by changing the patient's life style and discouraging the use of late night caffeine-containing beverages. There is little cause, in the first instance, to advocate the use of an hypnotic. Ear plugs, double glazing, heated blankets etc., could be regarded as first line therapy.

3) *Psychological disturbance.* The commonest cause of sleep disturbance is a psychological one. Patients are unable to get to sleep because of anxieties about the future or worries about their past experiences. Nightmares and disturbing dreams might cause intra-sleep restlessness and waking. Early morning waking seems to be particularly associated with depressive illness, but not in the absence of other, more characteristic, symptoms. Depressed patients need not be given a nocturnal hypnotic in conjunction with their antidepressant medication as the effects of the latter are usually sufficient to reduce the sleep disturbance along with the other depressive symptoms. Anxiety states are amenable to treatment with benzodiazepines which can be given nocturnally or on a conventional daily treatment regimen.

4) *Idiosyncratic life styles.* Shift workers and international travellers often have sleep problems associated only with the peculiar sleep wakefulness cycles they need, from time to time, to adopt. The short-term treatment of such chronicity problems is viable using benzodiazepines, but long-term manipulation of sleep/wake cycles is best done via other methods. The bizarre sleep/wake cycles of students working for exams and late night party-goers gives rise to problems with sleeping at conventional times. Such problems disappear, usually, with a return of normality. Hypnotic agents are not recommended for such patients. Some elderly

patients suffer excessive daytime drowsiness and respond by taking 'catnaps' during the day. Many patients underestimate the time they are asleep during the day. Sleep during the day will make it more difficult for patients to fall asleep and remain asleep at night. Patients should be encouraged to adopt a different life style where daytime activities are intended to maintain wakefulness.

5) *Iatrogenic disturbance.* Many prescriptions for antihistamines and medicines for the treatment of respiratory disorders contain somnorific substances which act as 'hypnotics'. If taken on their usual daily treatment regimens excessive daytime somnolence and drowsiness will occur, thus creating difficulties in falling asleep later in the day. In such cases the physician is unwittingly producing the sleep disturbance. The most effective treatment would not involve nocturnal hypnotics but a cessation of the use of the sedative giving rise to the problem, or a change of dose regimen to a nocturnal treatment schedule.

6) *Idiopathic sleep disorder.* Patients who complain of sleep-related disorder without any of the other five factors being present can be labelled as idiopathic as there is no obvious physical or psychological cause for their complaint. Although relatively rare these patients are an important group in general practice.

If none of the alternative therapies are suitable then there exists a bewildering range of benzodiazepines with potential utility for sleep-disturbed patients. There are two basic ways in which benzodiazepines function as sleep improvers. Some derivatives are primarily sedative/hypnotics which promote and maintain sleep via sedation and the induction of 'unconsciousness'. Such compounds are clinically equivalent to the barbiturates, although they do not have the toxicity or so widespread a depression of CNS functions. The alternative approach is to use a benzodiazepine with anxiolytic properties and so reduce or remove the anxiety or stress state which is causing the sleep disturbance.

An ideal drug would be one that allowed a patient to fall asleep quickly, and/or maintain sleep, without any residual sequelae which might interfere with subsequent daytime behaviour. Residual sedation, or anti-anxiety activity, can be useful in certain clinical conditions where daytime tranquillisation is needed. However, 'hangover' of a subjective or objective nature is not required in ambulant patients who could well be placed at risk of accident should their daytime performance be affected by nocturnal doses of benzodiazepines.

In differentiating between the benzodiazepines to find the most appropriate derivative for a particular patient there are three factors to be borne in mind: pharmacokinetic, pharmacodynamic and clinical.

Pharmacokinetic factors

The rate of a drug's absorption, distribution and elimination are important factors to consider in separating one derivative from another. In drugs which exert an

TABLE 1

Elimination half-lives (hrs) of benzodiazepine hypnotics (+active metabolites) in young healthy volunteers.

Midazolam	1.5–3
Triazolam	2–4
Loprazolam	6–8
Temazepam	6–10
Lormetazepam	10–12
Flunitrazepam	15–30
Nitrazepam	18–33
Flurazepam	24–48

hypnotic effect by promoting 'unconsciousness' a rapid absorption is required and the elimination half-life should be such that there is not a sufficient concentration of active compound, or metabolites, remaining to produce sedation the next day. If the elimination half-life of the drug is in excess of 24 hours then an accumulation of active substance could occur with repeated dosing as residual blood levels of the drug will be present when the next and subsequent doses are taken.

Table 1 lists a variety of currently available hypnotic benzodiazepines and illustrates the range of elimination half-lives found with these drugs.

Most of the pharmacokinetic data used to arrive at the data in Table 1 were taken from healthy young volunteers. It is worthwhile remembering that patients, especially the elderly, might exhibit different elimination characteristics, most usually manifest as an increase in the time taken to metabolise and excrete the drug.

The half-lives shown in Table 1 suggest a three-way classification of these drugs into 'short' (midazolam, triazolam, temazepam and loprazolam), 'medium' (lormetazepam, flunitrazepam) and 'long' (nitrazepam, flurazepam) elimination times. The implications of this classification will be discussed later.

Most of the compounds listed are sufficiently readily absorbed to quickly induce drowsiness although the rate of absorption can be facilitated by presenting the compound, e.g. temazepam, in a more bio-available form such as a soft gelatin capsule (Fucella, 1979). The use of different galenic formulations, e.g. elixirs and suppositories might be of clinical importance in increasing the rate of absorption and, therefore, speed of sleep induction.

Table 2 lists a selection of drugs, and their elimination half-lives, primarily for the treatment of anxiety, but which could well be used to treat sleep disturbance. Other compounds: clorazepate, ketazolam, prazepam can be regarded as pro-drugs or precursors of N-desmethyldiazepam and as having pharmacokinetic elimination times of similar magnitude.

TABLE 2

Elimination half-lives (hrs) of some benzodiazepines, which can be used for sleep disturbance.

Diazepam	20–70
Desmethyldiazepam	40–120
Lorazepam	10–20
Oxazepam	5–12
Clobazam	40–60

Drugs of this group will be expected to reduce the anxiety state of the patient and so assist sleep and need not necessarily act as hypnotics.

Lorazepam and diazepam have noticeable direct sedative action, but desmethyldiazepam (and related compounds) are less sedative and clobazam is, relative to the other compounds, not sedative. Oxazepam has sedative activity, although it is somewhat slowly absorbed, and has the shortest elimination half-life of this group of drugs.

Pharmacodynamic considerations

The relevance of pharmacodynamics rests in the extent to which residual drug levels produce a 'sedative hangover' which is measurable the morning following treatment and the extent to which this 'hangover' has clinical pertinence to the everyday behaviour of patients taking nocturnal doses of benzodiazepines.

The residual effects of psychoactive drugs can be measured with accuracy using a variety of objective techniques (Hindmarch, 1981). One of the most consistent measures of sedation is the choice reaction time task (CRT). This task measures the speed of motor response to the presentation of a visual stimulus. The coordination of the stimulus recognition and the motor response components of the task is via the brain and the CNS. The administration of a substance with a sedative action will reduce the capacity of the brain and CNS to coordinate sensori-motor behaviour. The extent of sedation will be reflected in the increased time taken to react and respond to the critical stimulus. The CRT task also has a high degree of 'face validity' in that speed of reaction forms an important basic component of the performance of many daily activities, for example, car driving. High correlations have been demonstrated between the scores on CRT tests and those obtained in 'on-the-road' assessments of car driving (Gudgeon and Hindmarch, 1980; Parrott et al., 1982). It could, therefore, be argued that drugs with residual sedation, as measured on the CRT, could also impair the vehicle handling and machine operating skills of patients taking them.

As well as producing objectively determined sedation, benzodiazepine hypnotics affect the sleep of patients taking them in a subjective manner. There does not

222

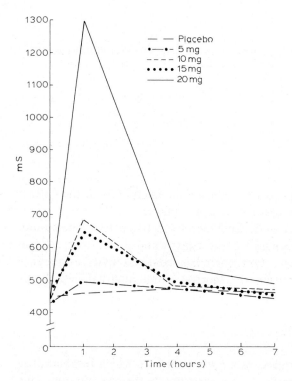

Fig. 1. Total reaction time for midazolam.

seem to be an agreed definition of 'normal' sleep and, as there are great differences between individuals in the duration and quality of non-medicated sleep, it is not appropriate to measure the perceived action of a drug using 'normalised' data. Instead a scale is needed which is sensitive to the change in state produced by the administration of an hypnotic. Using the 10 cm line visual analogue rating scale technique the Leeds Sleep Evaluation Questionnaire (LSEQ) was constructed to observe the subjective response to psychoactive drugs on sleep and early morning behaviour (Hindmarch, 1975; Parrott and Hindmarch, 1978, 1980). The LSEQ measures four sleep factors viz. the ease of getting to sleep, the quality of sleep, the ease of waking and the integrity of behaviour following waking.

The CRT measure is used as an index of sedation and, as illustrated in Fig. 1, the time course of action of a particular drug and its dose-response characteristics can be readily seen. Normal subjects can be selected and the experimental assessments and treatment regimens controlled to a far greater extent than could be obtained with even compliant patients. Dose range and time-based studies of this type are very necessary if the clinical activity of a compound is to be monitored. The CRT data in Fig. 1 show that 6 hours after acute doses of 5–20 mg midazolam there will be no objectively assessed sedative activity. If a patient then claims residual tiredness and sedation following the use of this drug it is reasonable to assume that the tiredness is a psychological, and not a residual pharmacological effect. Without information of this nature from normal volunteers it is impossible to determine the nature or origins of any residual sedative activity in the clinical situation. These dose ranging studies also indicate the level at which sedation is objectively discernable (increased reaction time) and so indicate the clinically effective dosage schedules.

We have already indicated that residual sedation the morning following medication might have important consequences for ambulant patients performing the tasks of everyday living. Table 3 presents data obtained on the CRT task the morning following nocturnal treatment with a variety of benzodiazepine hypnotics.

Although the CRT measures provide objective evidence of sedation it is also necessary to investigate the subjective response to drug administration overnight. All the LSEQ studies summarised in Table 4 are placebo-controlled, double-blind crossovers with subjects in each study acting as their own controls. All the studies had a similar experimental protocol but the significant placebo and drug differences found on the LSEQ are appropriate only within each particular study.

The results in Table 4 show a clear and significant sleep-inducing effect to be perceived following both acute and repeated doses of a variety of benzodiazepines. The hypnotic effect is clearly dose-related. Not all derivatives are effective in maintaining sleep and improving its perceived quality. Some benzodiazepines are primarily sleep inducers, some maintain sleep, others have a residual sedative effect which might have clinical application in the management of agitated patients or those on surgical wards where daytime sedation is needed, but could lead to impaired performance of everyday tasks in ambulant out-patients.

It is apparent that the benzodiazepines differ significantly from one another in the extent to which there are 'objective' and 'subjective' sequelae the morning following nocturnal treatment. The presence or absence of a measurable hangover is not wholly dependent upon pharmacokinetic considerations. Nitrazepam and clorazepate both have long elimination half-lives yet clorazepate is without any residual effects on CRT whereas nitrazepam produces significant impairments (Table 3). The elimination characteristics of benzodiazepines should be relatively independent of the dose administered yet low doses of temazepam are without hangover and high doses (30 mg or more) are associated with significant residual sedation (Table 3).

Subjective appreciation of hypnotic and residual activity as measured on the LSEQ (Table 4) shows no clear correlation between elimination half-life and psychological response to the administration of a benzodiazepine.

Clobazam, ketazolam and clorazepate are of similar elimination characteristics yet have totally different effects on ratings of the ease of waking and early morning behaviour. Significant hangovers are perceived following lorazepam, loprazo-

224

TABLE 3

The effects of nocturnal doses of benzodiazepines on choice reaction time (CRT) measures of sedation the morning following treatment (with respect to placebo controls) (from Hindmarch, 1982).

	Dose (mg)	CRT (ms)
Nitrazepam	2.5 × 1	=
	5.0 × 1	−
	10.0 × 1	−*
	5.0 × 4	−*
	10.0 × 4	−*
Flunitrazepam	1.0 × 1	=
	1.0 × 4	−
Lormetazepam	0.5 × 1	=
	0.5 × 7	=
	1.0 × 1	=
	1.0 × 7	=
	2.0 × 1	=
	2.0 × 7	−
Loprazolam	1.0 × 1	=
	1.0 × 4	=
	2.0 × 1	−
	2.0 × 4	−
Temazepam	10.0 × 1	=
	10.0 × 4	=
	20.0 × 1	=
	20.0 × 4	=
	30.0 × 1	−*
	30.0 × 4	−*
	40.0 × 1	−***
	40.0 × 4	−***
	60.0 × 1	−*
	60.0 × 4	−**
Triazolam	0.5 × 1	=
	0.5 × 4	+
Ketazolam	30.0 × 3	=
Oxazolam	30.0 × 3	=

Midazolam	5.0 × 1	=
	10.0 × 1	=
	15.0 × 1	=
	20.0 × 1	−
Clorazepate	15.0 × 3	=

= No change between placebo and drug conditions
+ A trend for an improvement of CRT scores.
− A trend for an impairment of CRT scores.
Significant changes (* = $p<0.05$; ** = $p<0.01$; *** = $p<0.001$ – all two-tailed values).

TABLE 4

Leeds Sleep Evaluation Questionnaire ratings (drug/placebo differences) following doses of benzodiazepines in healthy volunteers (from Hindmarch, 1982).

	Dose (mg)	Getting to sleep	Quality of sleep	Ease of awaking from sleep	Behaviour following waking
Nitrazepam	2.5 [a]	=	=	=	=
	5.0 [a]	+*	+**	−	=
	10.0 [b]	+*	+*	−*	−*
Flurazepam	15.0 [c]	+**	+**	−*	=
Flunitrazepam	1.0 [d]	+***	=	−	−
Midazolam	10.0 [e]	+**	+*	−	−
	15.0 [e]	+**	+*	+	+
Clorazepate	15.0 [c]	=	+*	−	=
Lorazepam	1.0 [g]	+*	+*	−*	−*
Clobazam	10.0 [g]	+*	+	−	=
	20.0 [d]	+*	+*	=	=
	30.0 [d]	+*	+*	−	−
	40.0 [d]	+*	+*	−	−*
Temazepam	10.0 [d]	=	+	=	=
	20.0 [d]	+*	+	−	=
	30.0 [d]	+*	=	−*	−*
	40.0 [d]	+***	+***	−***	−***
	60.0 [d]	+***	+***	−*	−**
Triazolam	0.5 [d]	+**	+*	−*	=

226

	Dose (mg)	Getting to sleep	Quality of sleep	Ease of awaking from sleep	Behaviour following waking
Loprazolam	0.5 b	+	+***	−	−***
	1.0 d	+**	+*	−**	−**
	2.0 b	+***	+***	−	−
Lormetazepam	0.5 f	=	+	=	−
	1.0 f	+*	+*	−	−
	2.0 f	+*	+*	=	−
Ketazolam	30.0 c	+*	+**	−**	−**
Oxazolam	30.0 c	+	+	+	+

a After an acute dose.
b After two consecutive nocturnal doses
c After three consecutive nocturnal doses
d After four consecutive nocturnal doses
e After six consecutive nocturnal doses
f After seven consecutive nocturnal doses
g After t.d.s. for 3 days.
= No change between placebo and drug conditions.
+ A trend for improvement.
− A trend for impairment.
Significant changes. (* = $p<0.05$; ** = $p<0.01$; *** = $p<0.001$ – all two-tailed values).

lam, nitrazepam and high doses of temazepam – yet all the drugs have dissimilar elimination half-lives.

The relationship between 'short', 'medium' and 'long' elimination half-lives and duration of pharmacodynamic activity is neither simple nor obvious from the results presented here. The duration of action of a drug is determined by more than its pharmacokinetic profile.

Clinical considerations

The previous results have been obtained from healthy volunteers and it could be argued that patients with poor sleep might behave differently and experience less 'hangover' as they have some complex 'need' for the drug treatment. It is, however, worth considering the number of 'non-patients' who use benzodiazepines to assist sleep during international travel, shift work and acute stress situations. The use of volunteers is, therefore, not without clinical relevance.

There is a dearth of objective data on the residual sequelae of benzodiazepines

TABLE 5

The effects of benzodiazepines on patients' psychomotor function the morning following nocturnal treatment. Mean changes from pre-drug or placebo baselines on choice reaction time and card sorting tests (from Hindmarch, 1982).

	Dose (mg)	CRT (ms)	Card sorting (s)
Temazepam	20.0 × 7	30 −	
	40.0 × 7	42 −	
	60.0 × 7	42 −	
Triazolam	0.125 × 1		5 −
	0.125 × 5		14 −
Nitrazepam	2.5 × 1		18 −
	2.5 × 5		34 − *
Flunitrazepam	0.5 × 1	14 −	
	0.5 × 4	28 +	
	0.5 × 7	29 − *	
Clobazam	20.0 × 7	29 +	
	20.0 × 14	13 +	
	40.0 × 7	36 −	
	40.0 × 14	25 −	

+ A trend for improvement.
− A trend for impairment.
Significant changes (* = $p<0.05$).

in patients due mainly to the experimental and ethical constraints governing work in the clinical field. The patient who complains simply of sleep disturbance, without pain or physical or mental disorder, and is not anxious, is a very rare phenomenon. The majority of patients using hypnotic medications on a chronic basis are usually in receipt of other medications. The interaction of drug treatments, the lack of a homogeneous patient group of 'sleep-disturbed' individuals and the logistics of experimental control in out-patients make for difficulties in psychopharmacological studies.

A limited number of controlled studies have been performed (see Tables 5 and 6) using the objective and subjective measures described earlier.

Table 5 shows that in patient populations significant 'hangovers', as an impairment of CRT performance, can be demonstrated following some compounds. Again the lack of objectively determined hangover is not related to elimination half-life. Clobazam, with one of the longest elimination half-lives, is without any significant residual effects especially following 20 mg nocte. At this dose cloba-

TABLE 6

Patients' evaluation of the effectiveness and tolerability of nocturnal treatment with benzodiazepines. The mean changes produced on the Leeds Sleep Evaluation Questionnaire with respect to pre-drug or placebo baselines (from Hindmarch, 1982).

	Dose (mg)	Getting to sleep	Quality of sleep	Ease awaking from sleep	Behaviour following waking
Temazepam	20.0 × 7	25+*	20+*	7+	5+
	40.0 × 7	31+*	25+*	3−	1+
	60.0 × 7	32+*	24+*	1+	2+
Triazolam	0.125 × 1	30+*	29+*	2−	2−
	0.125 × 5	22+*	22+*	1−	1−
Nitrazepam	2.5 × 1	15+	18+*	7−	8−
	2.5 × 5	29+*	19+*	3−	8−
Flunitrazepam	0.5 × 1	25+*	23+	23+	15+
	0.5 × 4	24+*	20+	20+	19+
	0.5 × 7	29+*	13+	11+	5+
Clobazam	20.0 × 7	12+*	13+*	3+	8+
	20.0 × 14	13+*	14+*	14+	12+
	40.0 × 7	24+*	34+*	9−	7+
	40.0 × 14	19+*	31+*	3−	14+*

+ A trend for improvement.
− A trend for impairment.
Significant changes (* = $p < 0.05$).

zam is perceived as significantly better (Table 6) than placebo in promoting and maintaining the quality of sleep (Hill et al., 1981).

The studies performed with patients included chronic insomniacs (temazepam), hospitalised geriatric patients (nitrazepam and triazolam), ambulant general practice patients with idiopathic sleep disturbance (flunitrazepam) and anxious patients in general practice (clobazam).

The importance of the LSEQ ratings in Table 6 is that patients do not feel any significant subjective hangover following a range of hypnotics yet, as the results in Table 5 illustrate, an objectively measured impairment of reaction time is present in some instances.

The reason that the duration of action of a drug cannot be simply explained by pharmacokinetic variables is that such measures do not take account of the psychological response to the administration of a psychoactive substance.

The importance of the psychological response has been illustrated in both volunteer and patient populations.

It is important for prescribing physicians to be aware of the residual effects of benzodiazepines used in the management of sleep disturbance.

The choice of a suitable derivative for a particular patient might be governed by pharmacokinetic considerations but it is felt that pharmacodynamic factors will ultimately prove more useful in deciding which of the numerous available drugs is to be prescribed.

REFERENCES

Fucella, L. M. (1979) Bioavailability of temazepam in soft gelatin capsules. Br. J. Clin. Pharmacol. 8, 31S–35S.

Gudgeon, A. C. and Hindmarch, I. (1980) The effect of 1,4 and 1,5 benzodiazepines on aspects of car driving behaviour. A preliminary investigation. In: D. J. Oborne and J. A. Levis (Eds.), Human Factors in Transport Research, Vol. 2. Academic Press, London, pp. 303–310.

Hill, A. J., Walsh, R. D. and Hindmarch, I. (1981) Tolerability of nocturnal doses of clobazam in anxious patients in general practice. Royal Society of Medicine International Congress and Symposium Series, No. 43, 133–140.

Hindmarch, I. (1975) A 1,4 benzodiazepine, temazepam: its effect on some psychological aspects of sleep and behaviour. Arnzeim. Forsch. (Drug Research) 25, (II), 1836–1839.

Hindmarch, I. (1981) Tests of psychomotor function. In: M. Lader and A. Richens (Eds.), The Central Nervous System. MacMillan, London, pp. 30–49.

Hindmarch, I. (1982) Hypnotics and residual sequelae. In: A.N. Nicholson (Ed.), Hypnotics in Clinical Practice. Medicine Publishing Foundation, Oxford, pp. 7–16.

Parrott, A. C. and Hindmarch, I. (1978) Factor analysis of a sleep evaluation questionnaire. Psychol. Med. 8, 325–329.

Parrott, A. C. and Hindmarch, I. (1980) The Leeds Sleep Evaluation Questionnaire in psychopharmacological investigations – a review. Psychopharmacology 71, 173–179.

Parrott, A. C., Hindmarch, I. and Stonier, P. D. (1982) Clobazam in combination with nomifensine (HOE8476): effects on mood, sleep and psychomotor performance relating to car driving ability. Drug Dev. Res. Suppl. 1, 47-55.

Subject index

A